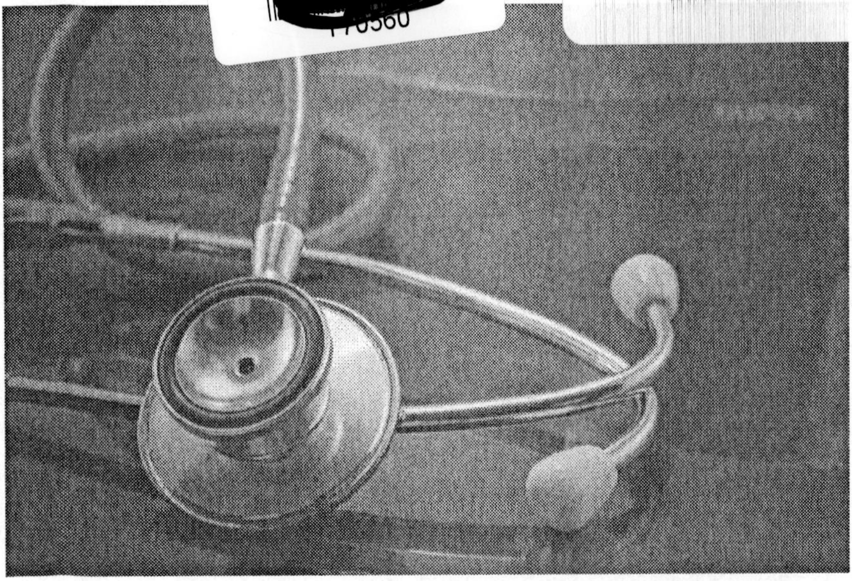

Succeeding in the UKCAT (UK Clinical Aptitude Test)

Comprising over 800 practice questions including detailed explanations, two mock tests and comprehensive guidance on how to maximise your score

Fifth Edition

Matt Green, Graham Blackman, Riaz Gulab and James Rudge

BPP
LEARNING MEDIA

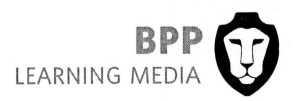

First edition 2008
Fifth edition July 2015

ISBN 9781 4727 2784 8
Previous ISBN 9781 4453 8165 7
e-ISBN 9781 4727 4478 4

British Library Cataloguing-in-Publication Data
A catalogue record for this book is available from the British Library

Published by
BPP Learning Media Ltd
BPP House, Aldine Place
London W12 8AA

www.bpp.com/health

Printed in the United Kingdom
by RICOH UK Limited

Unit 2
Wells Place
Merstham
RH1 3LG

Your learning materials, published by BPP Learning Media Ltd, are printed on paper sourced from sustainable, managed forests.

The views expressed in this book are those of BPP Learning Media and not those of UCAS. BPP Learning Media are in no way associated with or endorsed by the UCAS or the NHS.

The contents of this book are intended as a guide and not professional advice. Although every effort has been made to ensure that the contents of this book are correct at the time of going to press, BPP Learning Media, the Editor and the Author make no warranty that the information in this book is accurate or complete and accept no liability for any loss or damage suffered by any person acting or refraining from acting as a result of the material in this book.

Every effort has been made to contact the copyright holders of any material reproduced within this publication. If any have been inadvertently overlooked, BPP Learning Media will be pleased to make the appropriate credits in any subsequent reprints or editions.

A note about copyright

Dear Customer

What does the little © mean and why does it matter?

Your market-leading BPP books, course materials and e-learning materials do not write and update themselves. People write them on their own behalf or as employees of an organisation that invests in this activity. Copyright law protects their livelihoods. It does so by creating rights over the use of the content.

Breach of copyright is a form of theft – as well as being a criminal offence in some jurisdictions, it is potentially a serious beach of professional ethics.

With current technology, things might seem a bit hazy but, basically, without the express permission of BPP Learning Media:

- Photocopying our materials is a breach of copyright
- Scanning, ripcasting or conversion of our digital materials into different file formats, uploading them to facebook or e-mailing them to your friends is a breach of copyright

You can, of course, sell your books, in the form in which you have bought them – once you have finished with them. (Is this fair to your fellow students? We update for a reason.) But the e-products are sold on a single user license basis: we do not supply 'unlock' codes to people who have bought them secondhand.

And what about outside the UK? BPP Learning Media strives to make our materials available at prices students can afford by local printing arrangements, pricing policies and partnerships which are clearly listed on our website. A tiny minority ignore this and indulge in criminal activity by illegally photocopying our material or supporting organisations that do. If they act illegally and unethically in one area, can you really trust them?

Contents

About the Publisher

BPP Learning Media is dedicated to supporting aspiring professionals with top quality learning material. BPP Learning Media's commitment to success is shown by our record of quality, innovation and market leadership in paper-based and e-learning materials. BPP Learning Media's study materials are written by professionally-qualified specialists who know from personal experience the importance of top quality materials for success.

Reaching your Goal

The process of applying to medical school can be a somewhat long and arduous process but the rewards of a career within Medicine and Dentistry are infinite. BPP Learning Media and BPP University School of Health are committed to supporting aspiring and current doctors and dentists to progress their career through our comprehensive range of books, personal development courses and degree programmes. I often say there is no other vocation that provides such breadth and depth of career options for the individual to follow and specialise in. Whether it is the fast paced nature of the A&E department or the measured environment of Pathology, there is something for everyone.

There is no greater privilege than being responsible for leading the treatment of patients and sharing in their recovery. There are few other careers that provide such diversity on a daily basis. A passion for helping others, clear communication skills especially empathy, excellent team working and leadership qualities as well as the ability to strike a work-life balance are all skills that an accomplished doctor or dentist should possess.

The decision to follow a career in Medicine or Dentistry is something that should not be taken lightly and you should undertake careful research to ensure it really is for you. A career in Medicine or Dentistry is not for everyone and I would urge readers to ensure they have undertaken sufficient work experience to gain a balanced insight into what becoming a doctor or dentist really entails.

I first began mentoring aspiring medical and dental students ten years ago when it was clear that many individuals were not gaining access to the help and support they required to successfully apply to medical and dental school. It was with this in mind that I embarked on publishing our Entry to Medical School Series to provide a clear insight into the various facets of successfully getting into medical and dental school. Whether it is help with choosing the right medical school, how to prepare an outstanding personal statement or how to succeed in your medical and dental school interview, our comprehensive range of books provide the advice that is so often hard to find.

I would like to take this opportunity to wish you the very best of luck with your application and hope that you pass on some of the gems of wisdom that you acquire along the way to other aspiring medics and dentists.

Matt Green
Series Editor – Entry to Medical School
Medical Publishing Director

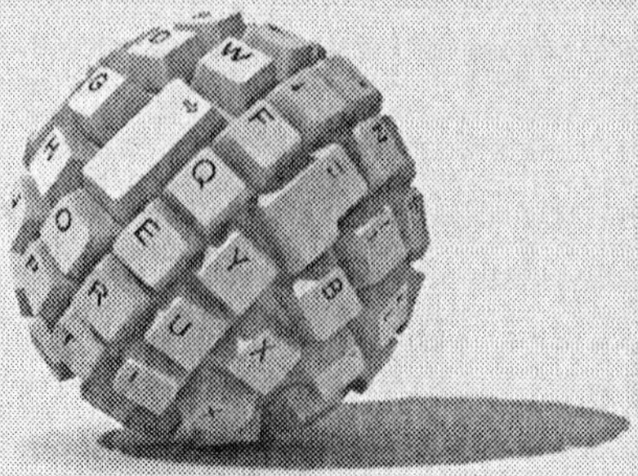

Free Companion Material

Readers can access further practice tests and answer sheets for free online.

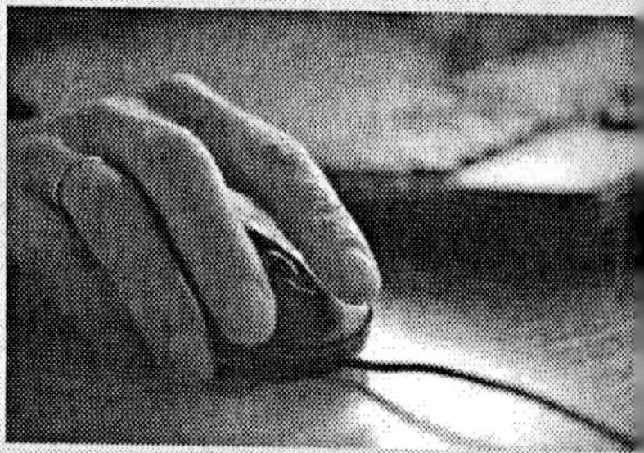

To access the above companion material please visit **www.bpp.com/freehealthresources**

About the Authors

Matt Green, BSc (Hons), MPhil

Matt Green has spent the last ten years directly helping thousands of individuals prepare for and pass their UKCAT. Matt has now used this extensive experience to write this book with the aim of assisting prospective medical and dental students to be successful in the UKCAT as part of their application to university.

Graham Blackman, BSc (Hons)

Graham attained First Class Honours in Psychology at the University of Bath, which included a one-year internship at Harvard University. Since graduating he has held research positions at the MRC Institute of Hearing Research and the University of Nottingham, and is currently a student on the Graduate Entry MBChB course at the University of Birmingham. Graham is an enthusiastic teacher and has helped prospective medical and dentistry school students prepare for the UKCAT since 2008.

Riaz Gulab BSc, (Hons), MSc

Riaz is a medical student on the Graduate Entry Programme at the University of Birmingham, having previously gained First Class Honours in Biology. He plays an active role in university life as a liaison officer. He is a keen advocate of supporting the local community as a young person support worker and has worked with students of all ages. Riaz understands the importance of the UKCAT and with his experience hopes to help more students to follow their dreams and achieve their true potential.

James Rudge, BSc (Hons)

James graduated from the University of Sheffield with first class Honours in Biomedical Science, and is currently studying Medicine at the University of Birmingham on their four-year Graduate Entry course. While studying for his undergraduate degree James acted as a course ambassador, providing academic and welfare support to new students. At Birmingham, James is currently the acting course representative, providing information and guidance to new applicants embarking on a career in medicine.

Acknowledgement

We would like to thank all the students who have contributed such valuable feedback on our UKCAT revision exercises.

Preface

The aim of this revision guide is to help you prepare yourself fully for your approaching UKCAT. With the introduction of this test for the majority of UK medical and dental schools, applicants need to ensure that they are more prepared than ever to succeed in their application.

This guide addresses each of the four sections of the UKCAT, providing the reasoning behind each section of the test, together with example questions. It culminates in two entire mock UKCAT tests that you should complete under timed conditions. To gain the full benefit, we recommend that you visit our website to download a free answer sheet to use when working through the example and mock test questions.

From all at BPP Learning Media we would like to wish you the best of luck with your application to medical or dental school.

Chapter 1

Introduction to the UKCAT

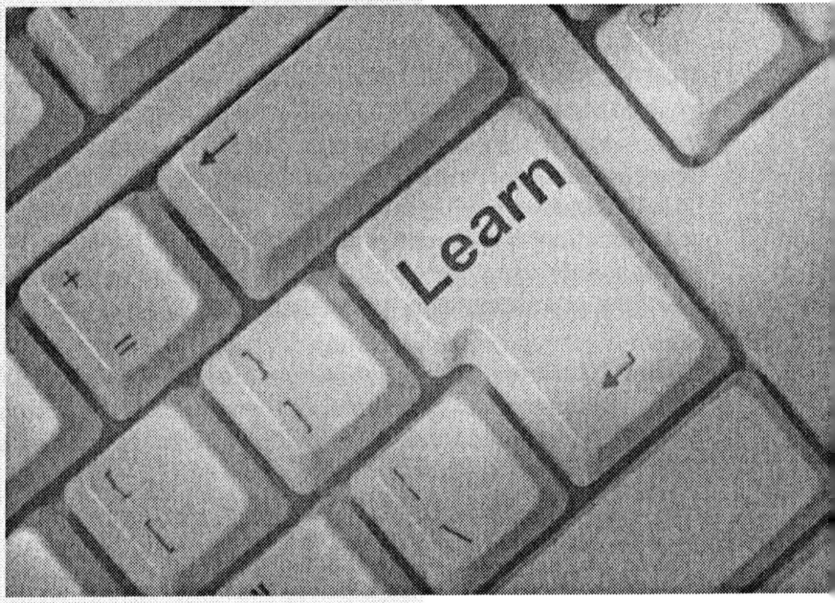

How do I prepare?

It is sometimes said that you cannot prepare for the UKCAT, but this is not the case. It is our opinion that three month's extensive practice will enable you to achieve a higher score than if you had not prepared. Last minute cramming will be counter productive to a good night's sleep before the exam – you need to feel refreshed and alert on the day. By completing practise tests you will have a clearer idea of what to expect and will feel more confident. We would encourage you to read carefully through the UKCAT website so that you have a clear understanding of the test process and the interface that is used in the test centre. To ensure that you are fully prepared for your UKCAT, work through this book and practise what you have learnt by completing the mock tests (see Chapters 8 and 10) under timed conditions.

The first part of this guide explains each subtest of the UKCAT and why it used, and it also provides practice questions for you to work through to ensure that you follow through on what you have learnt. The second part comprises two full mock tests that you can undertake under timed conditions. We would recommend that you visit our website to download our free blank Answer Sheet, on which you can record your answers, which will make it easier to refer your answers back to the guide. There are also further mock tests available to subscribe to at www.bpp.com/freehealthresources.

Chapter 2

Succeeding in the UKCAT

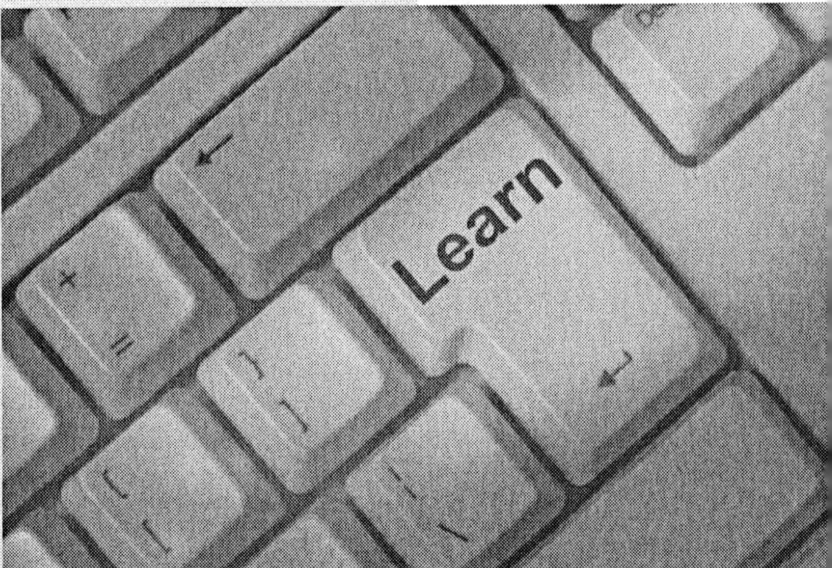

Succeeding in the UKCAT

Practice makes perfect

As with any test it is essential to practise example questions to ensure you are familiar with the structure and type of content you will be tested on. The UKCAT is no exception despite what people may tell you!

The following chapters will enable you to practise each of the different subtests which together form the UKCAT. This will enable you to familiarise yourself with the format and style of the UKCAT and hopefully help you to realise that the questions are not to be feared.

However, this is not to say that the UKCAT test is of an easy nature, otherwise it would not be a useful tool in the selection process. Although the UKCAT may measure general ability you will find that you only have a limited amount of time for each subtest.

Each of the subtests is individually timed, therefore it is not possible for you to make up for lost time in the other remaining subtests. It is vital that you complete each section fully as you progress through the test and do not leave any questions unanswered. By doing so, if you find that you do not have time to go back and check your answers, you will at least stand a chance of scoring a mark.

The aim of this book is to ensure that, on the day of your test, you are faced with something you are already familiar with. This book culminates with two full mock tests for you to complete under timed conditions. This will enable you to enhance your time management skills, increase your confidence and also alleviate any anxiety you may have. To help you record your answers, a blank Answer Sheet can be downloaded free of charge from www.bpp.com/freehealthresources.

What are multiple choice tests?

The UKCAT is set out in a multiple choice format. Multiple choice tests are commonly used within the field of selection and assessment. The test questions are designed to test a candidate's awareness and understanding of a particular subject.

The subtests within the UKCAT are based on an answer format known as *'A-Type questions'*, which is the most commonly used design in multiple choice tests. This specific design helps to make transparent the number of choices which need to be selected. These questions usually consist of a 'Stem' and 'Lead-in question' which are followed by a series of choices. To illustrate this, below is an example of a Quantitative Reasoning question:

Stem

This is generally an introductory statement, question or passage of relevant information which elicits the correct answer. The stem on the whole provides all the information for the question, or questions which will follow, for example:

'There are 100 students who go on a school trip to a science park.'

Lead-in question

This is the question which identifies the exact answer required, for example:

'If 35% of the students were female, how many female students were there?'

Choices

In a multiple choice test, the choices will generally consist of one correct answer. However, depending on the type of question, you may be required to select two or even three correct answers. Wherever there are correct answers there are also incorrect answers, which are known as the *'distracters'*.

For this example, typical choices could be as follows:

A 25
B 67
C 35 – correct answer (35% of 100 students = 35 female students)
D 65

General tips for answering multiple choice tests

- Read and reread the question to ensure you fully understand what is being asked, not what you want to be asked.
- Try to answer the question before looking at the choices available to you.
- Eliminate any incorrect answers you know are wrong.
- Do not spend too much time on one question – remember you only have a set amount of time per section so, as a rule of thumb, you should spend x amount per question (where x = time of section ÷ number of questions).
- Do not keep changing your mind – research has shown that the first answer that appeals to you is often the correct one.
- If you cannot decide between two answers, look carefully and decide whether for one of the options you are making an unnecessary assumption – trust your gut instinct.
- Always select an answer for a given question even if you do not know the answer – never leave any answers blank.
- Pace yourself – you will need to work through the test at the right speed. Too fast and your accuracy may suffer, too slow and you may run out of time. Use this guide to practise your timekeeping and approach to answering each question – you need to do what works for you, not what might work for someone else.
- In the actual test, you will be given the opportunity to mark your questions for review, so do try to remember and go back and check that you have answered all the questions to the best of your ability.
- To familiarise yourself with the way the online test will be conducted, visit the online testing demonstration which is available on the UKCAT web site.
- Remember you will only be awarded marks for correct answers, and marks will not be deducted for incorrect answers. Therefore try to answer every single question, even ones you are unsure of.
- When you take the test, listen carefully to the administrator's instructions.
- If you are unsure about anything, remember to ask the test administrator before the test begins. Once the clock begins ticking, interruptions will not be allowed.
- You may be presented with a question which you simply cannot answer due to difficulty, or if the wording is too vague. If you have only 20 seconds per question, and you find yourself spending five minutes determining the answer for each question, then your time management skills are poor and you are wasting valuable time.

Chapter 3

The Verbal Reasoning subtest

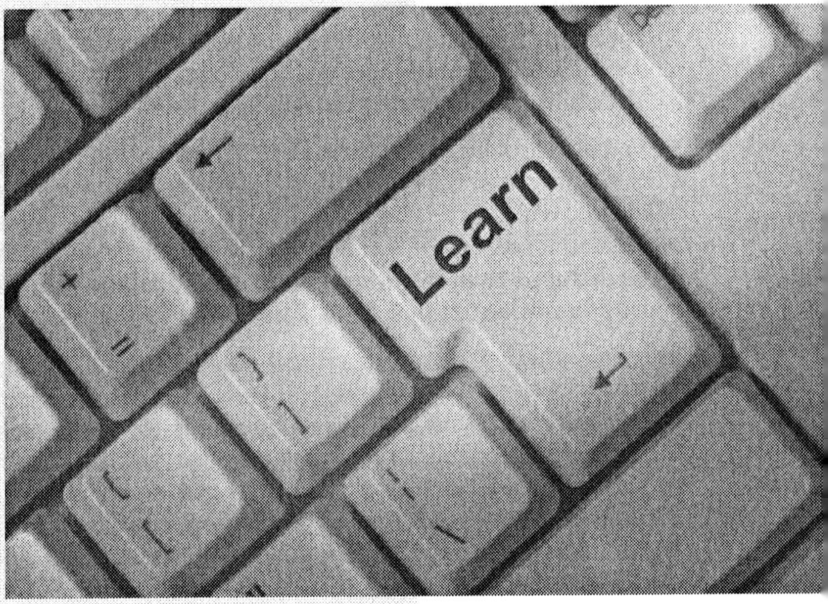

Choices

Your task will be either to decide whether the lead-in question is 'True', 'False' or 'Can't tell' or to select the most appropriate answer to an incomplete sentence or question based purely on the evidence given in the stem. In the UKCAT subtests it can be distracting to monitor exactly how long you spend on answering each question, especially when you have a stem to read through. Therefore a more useful time management approach is to divide each subtest into four quarters. In the case of the Verbal Reasoning subtest, with a time limit of 22 minutes, after approximately six minutes you should be working on the fourth passage, after approximately 11 minutes you should be commencing the seventh passage, and so on. If you find yourself falling behind at these points you know that you need to pick up the pace.

Example of a Verbal Reasoning question

There have been two noteworthy events which make the need for effective time management non-negotiable for doctors. You will be aware of the introduction of the European Working Time Directive (Working Time Relations, 2003). It came into force in August 2004 to protect the health and safety of doctors in training by reducing hours worked per week to a maximum of 58 and imposing minimum rest requirements with a maximum of 13 hours of work in any 24 and at least 11 hours of rest between shifts. The next challenge has arrived with the full implementation of this directive on 1st August 2009, which takes the maximum working hours per week down to 48. In early 2009 it was suggested that up to 50% of trusts in the United Kingdom may not be compliant and in some regions this figure was thought to be as low as 30%. The Workforce Review Team analysed 11 broad specialty groups and found that anaesthetics, medicine, obstetrics & gynaecology and surgery had the most doctors working more than 48 hours each week. These specialties all have a high out-of-hours commitment. It is clear that healthcare provision is faced with a big challenge and that significant changes are required to achieve Working Time Directive compliance. In the light of this new standard the need for effective time management has critical implications which cannot be ignored.

The second significant influence on doctors in relation to time management in the United Kingdom is the introduction and implementation of the Medical Leadership Competency Framework which has been jointly developed by The Academy of Medical Royal Colleges and the NHS Institute for Innovation and Improvement, in conjunction with a wide range of stakeholders. The Medical Leadership Competency Framework applies to all medical students and doctors and is designed to introduce students and doctors at all levels into management and leadership competencies. Although some may not realise it, time management is an important management skill. The ability to be able to organise oneself is the key to eventually being able to organise the activities of whole teams and to understand how to make the best use of the time available.

Inevitably service delivery and patient care will be positively impacted by successful time management, as processes and systems are implemented and maintained by a well organised team. The NHS Institute for Innovation and Improvement (2008) outlines three main career stages that have been identified and used throughout the MLCF. Stage 1 covers up to the end of undergraduate training, Stage 2 up to the end of postgraduate training and the final Stage 3 extends up to five years or equivalent post-specialist certification experience.

From *Effective Time Management Skills for Doctors.*

Q: The effective management of time will impact negatively on service delivery in the NHS.
Answer: True, False or Can't tell

Verbal Reasoning hints and tips

- **Ensure the answer you give is determined solely by the information contained within the passage and not your assumptions or background knowledge on the topic in question.** A common mistake that candidates often make is to allow their previous knowledge on a subject to interfere with and bias the information and facts that are presented in the passages (often these are of a conflicting nature).
- Therefore, it is important that you **read the passages very carefully**.
- Look out for misleading words such as *'all'*, *'everything'* and *'completely'*– these are words which suggest that the whole of a particular object, person, area or group is wholly affected.
- Understand that *'may'*, *'could'*, *'should'* and *'probably'* do not mean that something has definitely occurred.
- Other potentially misleading words include *'virtually'*, *'almost'*, *'particularly'*, *'nearly'* and *'close to'* – these are words which refer to something *close to* happening rather than actually happening.

- Remember that each of the passages is **deliberately manipulated to influence the candidate** to a particular perspective or point of view.
- Often you may find that a passage states information which may subsequently alter, or be contradicted further on in the passage.
- Ensure that you are aware of any changes or contradictions and reflect these when selecting your answers.
- **Do not waste too much time thinking about a difficult question.** All questions are marked equally, therefore a difficult question will not be worth more than an easy question. If you are having difficulty understanding a passage, flag it and move on to the next passage, ensuring that you come back to it later.
- Remember that **time management is key throughout** the test, and in the Verbal Reasoning subtest you have only 30 seconds to consider an answer.
- If you find a question particularly difficult you can flag it, so that you can return to it before you move on to the next subtest. When flagging a question in this way we recommend that you still select an answer in case you do not have time to return to the question.
- **Attempt all questions** as you will not be penalised for getting questions wrong, but you will lose marks if you leave an answer blank.

Seven simple steps to Verbal Reasoning

Step 1

Browse through the passages (answering each question systematically) and try to gain a feel for what the passage is trying to portray. Remember not to let previous knowledge on a subject interfere with what is actually presented in the passage.

Step 2

Note any changes, or contradictions, in terms of information, or valid points.

Step 3

Read through each question and determine exactly what you are being asked.

Step 4

Read through the passage again if necessary and answer each of the questions. Remember to take into account any changes or contradictions from Step 2.

Step 5

Eliminate answers which are obviously incorrect.

Step 6

Try to answer the questions as accurately as possible and do not leave any answers blank, even if you are not sure of the answer.

Step 7

If you are having trouble answering any of the questions, still select an answer and flag it so you can return to it later.
Learn to **manage your time efficiently**. Go through practice mock papers and time yourself as if you were in a real exam. By familiarising yourself with the types of questions you will be faced with, you will be able to analyse where your weaknesses are and remove them. Read through newspapers and other varied sources of literature which use elaborate and detailed language. This will enhance your skills in reading and also enable you to consider in-depth critical arguments and perspectives.

Verbal Reasoning practice examples

The following part of this chapter will enable you to work through various examples of Verbal Reasoning questions together with evaluating your answers against explanations. Remember, you can download a free Answer Sheet from www.bpp.com/freehealthresources to make it easier for you when working through these examples.

Example 1

There have been two noteworthy events which make the need for effective time management non-negotiable for doctors. You will be aware of the introduction of the European Working Time Directive (Working Time Relations, 2003). It came into force in August 2004 to protect the health and safety of doctors in training by reducing hours worked per week to a maximum of 58 and imposing minimum rest requirements with a maximum of 13 hours of work in any 24 and at least 11 hours of rest between shifts. The next challenge has arrived with the full implementation of this directive on 1st August 2009, which takes the maximum working hours per week down to 48. In early 2009 it was suggested that up to 50% of trusts in the United Kingdom may not be compliant and in some regions this figure was thought to be as low as 30%. The Workforce Review Team analysed

11 broad specialty groups and found that anaesthetics, medicine, obstetrics & gynaecology and surgery had the most doctors working more than 48 hours each week. These specialties all have a high out-of-hours commitment. It is clear that healthcare provision is faced with a big challenge and that significant changes are required to achieve Working Time Directive compliance. In the light of this new standard the need for effective time management has critical implications which cannot be ignored.

The second significant influence on doctors in relation to time management in the United Kingdom is the introduction and implementation of the Medical Leadership Competency Framework which has been jointly developed by The Academy of Medical Royal Colleges and the NHS Institute for Innovation and Improvement, in conjunction with a wide range of stakeholders. The Medical Leadership Competency Framework applies to all medical students and doctors and is designed to introduce students and doctors at all levels into management and leadership competencies. Although some may not realise it, time management is an important management skill. The ability to be able to organise oneself is the key to eventually being able to organise the activities of whole teams and to understand how to make the best use of the time available.

Inevitably service delivery and patient care will be positively impacted by successful time management, as processes and systems are implemented and maintained by a well organised team. The NHS Institute for Innovation and Improvement (2008) outlines three main career stages that have been identified and used throughout the MLCF. Stage 1 covers up to the end of undergraduate training, Stage 2 up to the end of postgraduate training and the final Stage 3 extends up to five years or equivalent post-specialist certification experience.

From *Effective Time Management Skills for Doctors.*

1. **The effective management of time will impact negatively on service delivery in the NHS.**
   A. True
   B. False
   C. Can't tell

2. **Those working within Obstetrics & Gynaecology are more likely to work more than 48 hours a week due to high out-of-hours commitment.**
   A. True
   B. False
   C. Can't Tell

3. **The EWTD came into force on the 21st August 2004.**
   A. True
   B. False
   C. Can't Tell

4. **The Academy of Medical Royal Colleges and the NHS Institute for Innovation and Improvement developed the MLCF independently.**
   A. True
   B. False
   C. Can't Tell

Example 2

The concept of clinical governance has been transferred from the commercial sector. In 1992, a number of incidents led the government to recommend standards for financial management to companies in the private sector for adopting new rules on accountability and conduct. These ideas were transferred to healthcare, with clinical governance becoming a requirement for the NHS (Committee on Standards in Public Life 1995). Clinical governance was (and still is) defined as: 'A framework through which NHS organisations are accountable for continuously improving the quality of their services and safeguarding high standards of care by creating an environment in which excellence in clinical care will flourish.' (Scally & Donaldson, 1998).

Initially, six facets of clinical governance were identified, including clinical audit. The other five were education and training, clinical effectiveness, research and development, openness and risk management. These components still make up the core of most clinical governance meetings today. However, categorising and isolating a set number of elements is now considered too simplistic, and probably carries a risk of ignoring other key components. All activities leading to the maintenance and improvement of clinical excellence should be within the remit of clinical governance.

> Partner or Consultant – they may have more experience in this area. As well as safeguarding patients, ensure that your underperforming colleague has sufficient support to help deal with their problems.

From *Succeeding in the GPST Stage 3 Selection Centre.*

1. **A Ward Sister can be considered a senior colleague.**
   A. True
   B. False
   C. Can't Tell

2. **GMC stands for Global Medical Constitution.**
   A. True
   B. False
   C. Can't Tell

3. **If an individual feels a colleague is under performing in their role, they should leave the matter for the HR department to address and not become involved.**
   A. True
   B. False
   C. Can't Tell

4. **If an individual is in a situation where they are unsure of what to do, one of the actions the GMC advise is to contact the Citizens Advice Bureau.**
   A. True
   B. False
   C. Can't Tell

Example 4

> Managing people and their performance takes time, as does planning the correct resources for any service or project. Planning itself is time consuming and it is something often overlooked by busy doctors. When you already feel overwhelmed by a lack of time in which to achieve everything on your list, it may seem too challenging to have to find extra time in which to plan. However, you will find as you progress through this book, that planning will be a key part of organising your working week, and you will reap the benefits of allocating some time to this essential activity.

The sub-groupings of Improving Services are:

- Facilitating transformation
- Encouraging innovation
- Critically evaluating
- Ensuring patient safety

These principles focus heavily on the strategic aspect of a doctor's role and will affect you at some point in your medical career, even if that circumstance has not yet arisen. Strategic thinking requires a considerable amount of uninterrupted time, as does the creation of plans. Many operational responsibilities will have to be delegated in order for you to secure the time you need to focus on improving the services your department or team provides.

The sub-groupings of Setting Direction are:

- Evaluating impact
- Making decisions
- Applying knowledge and evidence
- Identifying the contexts for change

These are capabilities which require experience and practice, as setting direction is a fundamental leadership skill involving the competencies of strategic thinking and decision making. Poor decision making is one of the major causes of failure for time management, as it prevents progress on the commitments which require action. At first glance the MLCF appears to be relevant to management and leadership only, but as this chapter shows, it is a strong driver for the improvement of time management skills. In order for any doctor to achieve proficiency in these framework attributes it will be necessary to possess robust organisational skills.

From *Effective Time Management Skills for Doctors.*

1. **Making poor decisions is one of the key contributors to the failure of managing time effectively.**
   A. True
   B. False
   C. Can't Tell

2. **Planning requires quiet thinking time.**
   A. True
   B. False
   C. Can't Tell

3. **The MLCF is known as the Medical Leadership Competency Framework.**
   A. True
   B. False
   C. Can't Tell

4. **Setting direction involves making decisions, assessing the impact of a given event, identifying the reasons for change and applying knowledge and evidence.**
   A. True
   B. False
   C. Can't Tell

Example 5

Fundamental of traffic signals
Traffic Signals are one of the more familiar types of intersection control. Using either a fixed or adaptive schedule, traffic signals allow certain parts of the intersection to move while forcing other parts to wait, delivering instructions to drivers through a set of colourful lights (generally, of the standard red-yellow (amber)-green format). Some purposes of traffic signals are to (1) improve overall safety, (2) decrease average travel time through an intersection, and (3) equalise the quality of services for all or most traffic streams. Traffic signals provide orderly movement of intersection traffic, have the ability to be flexible for changes in traffic flow, and can assign priority treatment to certain movements or vehicles, such as emergency services. However, they may increase delay during the off-peak period and increase the probability of certain accidents, such as rear-end collisions. Additionally, when improperly configured, driver irritation can become an issue. Traffic signals are generally a well-accepted form of traffic control for busy intersections and continue to be deployed. Other intersection control strategies include signs (stop and yield) and roundabouts. Intersections with high volumes may be grade separated.

http://en.wikibooks.org/wiki/Fundamentals_of_Transportation/Traffic_Signals

1. **Traffic signals may increase accidents involving:**
   A. Pedestrians using the road
   B. Rear end collisions
   C. Head on collisions
   D. Breakdowns

2. **Based on the passage each of these statements are false except:**
   A. The use of traffic signals are being phased out
   B. One of the limitations of traffic signals is their inflexibility as a result of changes to traffic flow
   C. Driver irritation can become an issue when Traffic Signals are not properly configured
   D. Level crossings is another strategy to controlling intersections

3. **Traffic signals provide many benefits. From the passage it can inferred that this is achieved by:**
   A. Improving overall safety and decreasing average travel time
   B. Increase delay times
   C. Reducing the frustrations of drivers
   D. The implementation of roundabouts

4. **Which of the following statements is best supported by the passage?**
   A. Traffic signals are incredibly inflexible
   B. Emergency services are given equal priority to oncoming traffic
   C. Traffic signals communicate via a series of signals that are depicted by colour
   D. Traffic signals only deliver a fixed schedule

Example 6

The doctor-patient relationship is a sacred one, and confidentiality should be maintained at all times. However, there may be some situations where confidentiality must be broken, for example, to safeguard the safety of others. If you feel that this is necessary, then you must inform the patient that you are going to do so. The GMC has guidance about when it is acceptable to breach confidentiality:

- If the patient consents to disclosure of information.
- If disclosure of information is required by law, for example with notifiable diseases. Patients should be informed about the disclosure but their consent is not required.
- If a judge or presiding officer of a court order instructs you to disclose information. However, you must not disclose information to respectable members of the community which include solicitors, police officers or fire officers who are not appointed to act on behalf of the judge in an official capacity. A presiding officer can be any

respectable member of the community appointed by a judge.

- If the disclosure is in the public interest. That is, if the benefits of the disclosure to an individual or society outweigh the public and the patient's interest in keeping the information confidential.

In all cases where you consider disclosing information without consent from the patient, you must weigh the possible harm (both to the patient, and the overall trust between doctors and patients) against the benefits which are likely to arise from the release of information. Wherever possible, it is still advisable to inform the patient that you are planning to disclose the information. An example where it is acceptable to break confidentiality would be when a patient is driving against medical advice, for example after a fit. This is something that can come up in the patient consultation task, where you would be required to advise a patient of the risks of driving when they have had a fit, and the guidance about this. The GMC states that

'The DVLA is legally responsible for deciding if a person is medically unfit to drive. The Agency needs to know when driving licence holders have a condition which may now, or in the future, affect their safety as a driver.'

In the first instance, you should make sure that the patient in question understands that their condition can impair their ability to drive. In situations where they are unable to understand this information, for example in patients with dementia, then you should inform the DVLA immediately. With competent patients you should also explain to them that they have a legal duty to inform the DVLA. If they continue to drive, you must make a reasonable effort to persuade them to stop. This may include discussing with their next of kin if they consent to this. However, if you cannot persuade them to stop, or there is evidence that they are continuing to drive, then you should disclose relevant medical information to the medical adviser at the DVLA. Before you do this, you should advise the patient that you are doing so, and afterwards, write to the patient informing them that disclosure has been made.

From *Succeeding in the GPST Stage 3 Selection Centre*.

1. **The GMC can decide whether or not someone is able to drive a minibus.**
   A. True
   B. False
   C. Can't Tell

2. A doctor must ring the patient in question to inform them that he or she is going to report them to the DVLA as being unfit to drive.
   A. True
   B. False
   C. Can't Tell

3. A police officer with a court order can request a doctor to disclose confidential patient information.
   A. True
   B. False
   C. Can't Tell

4. A doctor cannot break confidentiality.
   A. True
   B. False
   C. Can't Tell

Example 7

The evolution of music
By the 9th century Western music had become standardised into a notational form called nuemes which were shapes that represented notes. One line was used to indicate the middle pitch with nuemes above the line being higher in pitch and the nuemes below the line being lower in pitch. This primitive notational system was more of a memory aid rather than a complete notational system showing exact pitch and duration. To read nuemes you needed to be familiar with the piece of music beforehand. In the 10th century Guido d'Arezzo, a Benedictine monk and Choir Master, extended the one line to four lines and set the exact pitch of each note. This new invention of the stave allowed music to be notated more precisely. Guido d'Arezzo also devised the solfeggio system where a different syllable is sung to each note of an ascending scale:
Do - Re - Mi - Fa - Sol - La - Ti
Today a scholarly approach has been applied to the music of the past in relation to ensuring that the notation is interpreted correctly. An example is baroque music where modern research into the instruments, techniques and approach of this period has led today's musicians to revise their interpretation and performance of Baroque notation.

http://en.wikibooks.org/wiki/Guitar/Scale_Theory

1. **Based on the information it is most likely that modern day musicians perform music, based on Baroque notation, as it was originally intended to be heardv because:**
   A. Modern musical instruments are constructed to a much higher standard
   B. The way modern musicians are educated is much better today
   C. Of a discovery by musicians of a plethora of well-preserved music sheets
   D. Recent research has enabled a more accurate interpretation of the way this particular music is played

2. **Based on the passage each of the following statements are true except:**
   A. The solfeggio system follows that multiple syllables are sung to the same note
   B. Guido d'Arezzo lived in the 10th Century
   C. The introduction of the Stave enabled music to be noted more accurately
   D. The use of Nuemes was not a very accurate system

3. **According to the passage adopting a uniform approach to noting music had formalised:**
   A. In the 10th Century
   B. Towards the middle of the 8th Century
   C. In the 9th Century
   D. By the 9th Century

4. **Which of the following statements is correct based on the passage**
   A. Neumes is an advanced notation system that aids memory
   B. Nuemes is arranged using a 6-point ascending scale
   C. Nuemes is a basic notation system that required prior knowledge of the song
   D. Nuemes was invented in the 10th Century

Example 8

Some of you will already have teaching experience from before you attended medical school. Most of you will not. Again, if you are reading this early in your medical career then there are several actions you can put into motion to gain some teaching experience and skills before the applications. This is where you have an advantage compared to later on in your career. Although it may not seem it now, you have more time on your hands, as trying to gain teaching experience when working full-time is quite a stretch!

At some point after the end of your pre-clinical or second years at medical school, approach the Anatomy department and see if they need a hand with some voluntary anatomy-demonstrating during the free sessions you have in the week. As there are very few paid medical demonstrator jobs these days, it is likely that your offer of help will be very well received! This is also excellent practice for those of you who intend to become surgeons or pathologists, as the best way to consolidate your knowledge about a subject is to teach it. There is usually an Academic Consultant in charge of the medical education of junior medical students; approach them and ask if you can help to facilitate at Integrated Learning Activities or Problem-Based Learning sessions. Lastly, during the summer months when most of the first- and second-year students have gone home, the unfortunate few from each year who have failed their end-of-year exams must remain for extra tuition and revision sessions before the re-sits at the end of summer. Volunteer yourself as a study-buddy via the medical school to see if any of the junior medical students want extra help. This will not only give you some excellent material for your CV, it will introduce you to the possibility of becoming involved in medical education further down the road of your career, which is an area you may wish to involve yourself in. Make sure that you get some feedback for your teaching; this need not be any weighty graphically designed form, just a simple feedback form asking the student to outline the positive aspects of your teaching session and areas for improvement. A simple way to do this is to give each student different coloured post-it notes and ask them to put the positive points on one colour and the suggestions for improvement on another.

From *Preparing the Perfect Medical CV.*

1. **Those wishing to follow a career in Cardiology should gain experience as an anatomy demonstrator.**
   A. True
   B. False
   C. Can't Tell

2. **Gaining teaching experience now rather than later is advisable because you have more time.**
   A. True
   B. False
   C. Can't Tell

3. **To run the Medical Education function of junior medical students at medical school an individual must be an Academic Consultant.**
   A. True
   B. False
   C. Can't Tell

4. **Medical teachers should obtain feedback from students they teach.**
   A. True
   B. False
   C. Can't Tell

Example 9

The precise format of the patient simulated exercise will vary across Deaneries. You will be given a brief; a sheet of paper or card with the background to the case written on it. This will normally be a short paragraph however it may even be a simple sentence such as , 'Mr Smith, aged 46, has come to see you with regard to his chest pain.' For most of the Deaneries you will be given five minutes before the exercise starts to read the brief and information given to you. These five minutes are crucially important and we will explain later how to gain as much information as you can from the brief and use this time to your advantage. You will also have an opportunity during your five minutes to rearrange the furniture in the room if required. The importance of this will be discussed in more detail later. The examiners will ensure that you have understood the information given to you and you will have a chance to ask them any questions if something in the brief is not clear before you start. The patient or simulator at this time is usually outside the room and thus after reading the brief you will be expected to invite the patient into the room. The actual time allocated to the consultation may vary between Deaneries. For most, there will be 20 minutes to complete the consultation but you do not have to use all of the time available.

Some Deaneries use an OSCE-like format where you will have ten minutes to complete the consultation. Thus it is important to find out in advance from your Deanery how much time you will have for the exercise. You will be expected to bring the consultation to a natural close yourself within your allocated time. The examiners may give you a warning when your time is about to run out or they may simply not say anything until your time is up. If you are in the OSCE-type exam a bell may simply ring at the end of the allocated time. To avoid being caught out and having your consultation ended abruptly by the examiners, it is a good idea to keep an eye on the time yourself. Therefore you may want to bring a digital watch or stop clock with you. Failing this you could ask the assessors to give you a warning when you have a certain amount of time remaining.

From *Succeeding in the GPST Stage 3 Selection Centre.*

1. **A Deanery is a regional body responsible for co-ordinating and administering the training of junior doctors in England.**
   A. True
   B. False
   C. Can't Tell

2. **The actual patient simulation exercise itself will last for 20 minutes in all Deaneries.**
   A. True
   B. False
   C. Can't Tell

3. **OSCE stands for Objective Structured Clinical Examination.**
   A. True
   B. False
   C. Can't Tell

4. **Some Deaneries will give individuals ten minutes before the exercise to familiarise themselves with the background of the scenario.**
   A. True
   B. False
   C. Can't Tell

Example 10

Procrastination is a critical enemy of effective time management. It means to put off a task or action until a later time. The word comes from the Latin word procrastinatio: pro- (forward) and crastinus (of tomorrow). Procrastination can be described as a coping mechanism for dealing with the anxiety associated with starting a particular task or project. Although it is normal for people to delay difficult or dreaded tasks to some degree it doesn't actually help. Many people feel stressed at the thought of doing a particular task or activity.

For example, imagine you have been asked by a senior colleague to make a presentation at an important meeting in a month's time. You are expected to prepare a 60-minute talk with slides and to speak confidently about a topic of which you have limited knowledge. It is likely that the prospect of giving this presentation is daunting for you and the necessary preparation will require a lot of effort on your part. You now have a choice about how you wish to handle this assignment. You may perceive it as a great career opportunity and a chance to create a good impression of yourself to your senior colleagues. With that in mind you will probably embark upon the task with energy and excitement. Or you may feel very anxious about the event and decide to put off any work associated with it for as long as possible. You may even believe that in doing so you can relieve your anxieties and put the event out of your mind for at least another three weeks. What you will discover, however, is what effective time managers already know. When you procrastinate you actually increase your feelings of stress, not diminish them. The feeling of fear never leaves you and becomes an added burden for you to carry around during the forthcoming month.

All the time you are putting off the preparation of that future task or project you will also experience feelings of guilt. You know you should be getting on with it but you cannot face it. This is another common reaction to putting things off and, as is the case with stress, feelings of guilt do not go away until the task is complete.

From *Effective Time Management Skills for Doctors.*

1. **All individuals who have been asked to give a presentation will feel better by putting off preparing the event for another three weeks.**
   A. True
   B. False
   C. Can't Tell

2. **Feelings of guilt about putting off a task will not go away until the task is complete.**
   A. True
   B. False
   C. Can't Tell

3. **The meaning of 'procrastination' derives from the Latin language.**
   A. True
   B. False
   C. Can't Tell

4. **If an individual is considered to be procrastinating then they can also be perceived by others to be unproductive.**
   A. True
   B. False
   C. Can't Tell

Example 11

Sensory Memory

This type of memory has the shortest retention time, only milliseconds to five seconds. Roughly, Sensory Memory can be subdivided into two main kinds:

- Iconic Memory (visual input)
- Echoic Memory (auditory input)

While Iconic and Echoic Memory have been well researched, there are other types of Sensory Memory, like haptic, olfactory, etc., for which no sophisticated theories exist so far. It should be noted, though, that according to the Atkinson and Shiffrin (1968) Sensory Memory was considered to be the same thing as Iconic Memory. Echoic Memory was added to the concept of Sensory Memory due to research done by Darwin and others (1972). Let us consider the following intuitive example for Iconic Memory: Probably we all know the phenomenon that it seems possible to draw lines, figures or names with lighted sparklers by moving the sparkler fast enough in a dark environment. Physically, however, there are no such things as lines of light. So why can we nevertheless see such figures? This is due to Iconic Memory. Roughly speaking, we can think of this subtype of memory as a kind of photographic memory, but one which only lasts for a very short time (milliseconds, up to a second). The image of the light of a sparkler remains in our memory (persistence of vision) and thus makes it seem to us like the light leaves lines in the dark. The term "Echoic Memory", as the name already suggests, refers to auditory input. Here the persistence time is a little longer than with Iconic Memory (up to five seconds).

http://en.wikibooks.org/wiki/Cognitive_Psychology_and_Cognitive_Neuroscience/Memory

1. **One conclusion that can be drawn from the passage is:**
   A. Darwin played a key role in Echoic Memory being grouped under the concept of Sensory Memory
   B. There is much research still to be done to understand Sensory Memory
   C. All aspects of Sensory Memory encompass the principles of photographic memory
   D. Echoic Memory is not the only type of memory that falls under Sensory Memory

2. **According to the passage which of the below options best supports the statement 'The key players in establishing the fundamental theory on Sensory Memory' were:**
   A. Atkinson and Shriffin
   B. Darwin, Atkinson and Shriffin
   C. Darwin
   D. Darwin, Atkinson, Shriffin & others

3. **Iconic Memory can be described as:**
   A. Is why it hurts an individual's eyes when they stare at the sun
   B. Is influenced by sounds
   C. A medium term form of memory
   D. A form of photographic memory

4. **Which of the following statements regarding Sensory Memory based on the passage is correct:**
   A. It is not restricted to visual and auditory input
   B. It includes haptic, olfactory and taste
   C. Linden and others have contributed significantly to research in the area of Iconic Memory
   D. It relates to information that is retained for up to 10 seconds

Example 12

Patients in hospital and in the community often give presents to their doctors, such as chocolates to express their gratitude for help with their treatment. But what is the guidance on this? The GMC states that:

'You must not encourage patients to give, lend or bequeath money or gifts that will directly or indirectly benefit you. You must not put pressure on patients or their families to make donations to other people or organisations.'

(Good Medical Practice)

We should not encourage patients to give you gifts, but what if they were to give you a gift, should you accept it? In general, you would need to look at whether the gift is appropriate, for example, a box of chocolates after a ward stay is more reasonable than giving £200 to a particular doctor. Scenarios involving this situation could come up in any part of the assessment. Each situation would need to be analysed individually. It is important to ascertain whether the patient thinks they are obliged to give the present in order to receive good quality healthcare, and you must make sure that they realise that this is not the case. If the concern is a colleague accepting gifts, then the facts would need to be ascertained to find out whether they are coercing the patient to do so. If you decline a gift that seems inappropriate, do so sensitively and explain to the patient your reasons for doing so.

Some parts of the Stage 3 assessment may involve issues of handover and cover, for example, going off duty when there is nobody to hand over to. The main point here is to ensure that patient safety is not put at risk. Therefore if your shift has ended but the next doctor has not arrived then you must wait until you can hand over. If you feel patient safety is at risk for any reason, for example by there not being enough doctors on the ward due to illness, then it would be worth saying that you would inform appropriate people to ensure that this is rectified, such as your Consultant or the department lead so that locum cover can be arranged.

From *Succeeding in the GPST Stage 3 Selection Centre.*

1. **In the event that a doctor feels patient safety is being put at risk due to insufficient staff numbers the doctor should inform the HR Manager that this is the case.**
   A. True
   B. False
   C. Can't Tell

2. **The GMC advises that doctors should not discuss the issue of receiving gifts with the patients involved.**
   A. True
   B. False
   C. Can't Tell

3. **A box of chocolates is considered to be a reasonable gift compared to a significant monetary gift.**
   A. True
   B. False
   C. Can't Tell

4. **Patients always give their doctor a present after receiving treatment for a particular illness.**
   A. True
   B. False
   C. Can't Tell

Example 13

The Council of Heads of Medical Schools, in consultation with the Department of Health and British Medical Association, have produced a statement setting out guiding principles for the selection and admission of students to medical schools. These are:

1. Selection for medical school implies selection for the medical profession.

   A degree in Medicine confirms academic achievement and in normal circumstances entitles the new graduate to be provisionally registered by the General Medical Council.
2. The selection process attempts to identify the core academic and non-academic qualities of a doctor:
   - Honesty, integrity and an ability to recognise one's own limitations and those of others, are central to the practice of medicine.
   - Other key attributes include having good communication and listening skills, an ability to make decisions under pressure, and to remain calm and cope with stress.
   - Doctors must have an understanding of teamwork and respect for the contributions of others. Desirable characteristics include curiosity, creativity, initiative, flexibility and leadership.
3. A high level of academic attainment will be expected. Understanding science is core to the understanding of medicine, but medical schools generally encourage diversity in subjects studied by candidates.
4. The practice of medicine requires the highest standards of professional and personal conduct. Put simply, some students will not be suited to a career in medicine and it is in the interests

of the student and the public that they should not be admitted to medical school.

5. The practice of medicine requires the highest standards of professional competence. However, a history of serious ill health or disability will not jeopardise a career in medicine unless the condition impinges upon professional fitness to practise.
6. Candidates should demonstrate some understanding of what a career in medicine involves and their suitability for a caring profession. Medical schools expect candidates to have had some relevant experience in health or related areas. Indeed, some medical schools stipulate a defined minimum period of relevant work experience.
7. The primary duty of care is to patients. All applicants to medical schools will be expected to understand the importance of this principle.
8. Failure to declare information that has a material influence on a student's fitness to practise may lead to termination of their medical course.

From *Succeeding in your Medical School Application.*

1. **A doctor's primary duty of care is to their colleagues.**
   A. True
   B. False
   C. Can't Tell

2. **Leadership is a valued non-academic quality of a doctor.**
   A. True
   B. False
   C. Can't Tell

3. **An individual who is wheelchair-bound will not be able to follow a career in Medicine.**
   A. True
   B. False
   C. Can't Tell

4. **An individual is unlikely to succeed in their application if they do not undertake any work experience prior to their application.**
   A. True
   B. False
   C. Can't Tell

Example 14

Control Engineering

The study and design of automatic Control Systems, a field known as control engineering, has become important in modern technical society. From devices as simple as a toaster or a toilet, to complex machines like space shuttles and power steering, control engineering is a part of our everyday life. Control engineering is a very large field. Control systems are components that are added to other components, to increase functionality, or to meet a set of design criteria. For example: We have a particular electric motor that is supposed to turn at a rate of 40 RPM. To achieve this speed, we must supply 10 Volts to the motor terminals. However, with 10 volts supplied to the motor at rest, it takes 30 seconds for our motor to get up to speed. This is valuable time lost.

This simple example, however can be complex to both users and designers of the motor system. It may seem obvious that the motor should start at a higher voltage, so that it accelerates faster. Then we can reduce the supply back down to 10 volts once it reaches ideal speed. This is clearly a simplistic example, but it illustrates an important point: we can add special 'Controller units' to preexisting systems, to improve performance and meet new system specifications. Classical and Modern control methodologies are named in a misleading way, because the group of techniques called 'Classical' were actually developed later than the techniques labeled 'Modern'. However, in terms of developing control systems, Modern methods have been used to great effect more recently, while the Classical methods have been gradually falling out of favor. Most recently, it has been shown that Classical and Modern methods can be combined to highlight their respective strengths and weaknesses.

http://en.wikibooks.org/wiki/Control_Systems/Introduction

1. **Which of the following statements is false based on the passage of information?**
   A. At the ideal speed an electric motor will spin at a rate 40 RPM with a 10V supply
   B. Control Engineering can be used in cars
   C. Control systems work in a standalone capacity
   D. Increasing the voltage delivered to a motor upon starting can prevent time being lost

2. **Which of the following statements can be inferred from the passage?**
   A. The principles of Control Engineering could be used in vacuum hoovers
   B. The principles of Control Engineering rely heavily on chemical theories
   C. Control Engineering was discovered in the late 18th Century
   D. The principles of Control Engineering can only be implemented on new systems

3. **One conclusion that can be drawn from the passage is:**
   A. 'Classical' and 'Modern' methods of Control Systems cannot be combined
   B. The use of the 'Classical' and 'Modern' terminology is self-explanatory to someone unfamiliar with Control Systems
   C. Classical methods of Control Systems are becoming more common
   D. Modern methods of Control Systems have had a positive impact in recent times

4. **Which of the following statement can inferred from the passage?**
   A. Supplying a higher voltage to a motor will slow the motor down
   B. Control Engineering has contributed to putting man into space.
   C. The field of Control Engineering is a very niche field
   D. Delivering a higher voltage to an electric motor will decrease its RPM

Justifications of Verbal Reasoning practice examples

Example 1

1 **False.** The statement: *'Inevitably service delivery and patient care will be positively impacted by successful time management, as processes and systems are implemented and maintained by a well organised team'* contradicts this, and this statement is therefore false.

2 **True.** The following supports this statement: *'The Workforce Review Team analysed 11 broad specialty groups and found that anaesthetics, medicine, obstetrics & gynaecology and surgery had the most doctors working more than 48 hours each week. These specialties all have a high out-of-hours commitment.'*

3 **Can't tell.** Although the passage states that the EWTD came into force in August 2004 it is not possible to confirm that the exact date is 21st August: *'It came into force in August 2004 to protect the health and safety of doctors in training'.*

4 **False.** Although the passage states that the MLCF was developed jointly developed by the Academy of Medical Royal Colleges and the NHS Institute for Innovation and Improvement it also states that a wide range of stakeholders were involved: *'the Medical Leadership Competency Framework which has been jointly developed by The Academy of Medical Royal Colleges and the NHS Institute for Innovation and Improvement, in conjunction with a wide range of stakeholders'.*

Example 2

1 **False.** Although the passage appears to confirm this statement, upon closer inspection the actual year stated is 1999: *'From April 1999, acute and community NHS trusts had developed established structures and processes for effective clinical governance'.*

2 **Can't tell.** Although the passage confirms that Chief Executives are indeed accountable it does not confirm whether or not they can be punished with a custodial sentence if found to be infringement of clinical governance principles: *'In the 1990's chief executives of NHS trusts and primary care trusts for the first time became directly accountable for the quality of service provided by their organisations'.*

3 **False.** Financial reporting is not mentioned as one of the six original facets of clinical governance in the passage: *'Initially, six facets of clinical governance were identified, including clinical audit. The other five were education and training, clinical effectiveness, research and development, openness and risk management'.*

3 **True.** This is confirmed by the definition provided: *'A framework through which NHS organisations are accountable for continuously improving the quality of their services'.*

Example 3

1 **Can't tell.** Although the passage mentions a number of roles that constitute a senior colleague, whether a ward sister is considered to be a senior colleague is not mentioned: *'As detailed above, if you cannot deal with the matter yourself you should involve an appropriate senior colleague, such as a Registrar, Partner or Consultant – they may have more experience in this area'.*

2 **Can't tell.** Although most readers will know that GMC stands for 'General Medical Council' the passage neither confirms nor contradicts this statement.

3 **False.** The passage clearly states that you should take action if you suspect a colleague is underperforming: *'You must protect patients from risk of harm posed by another colleague's conduct, performance or health. The safety of patients must come first at all times. If you have concerns that a colleague may not be fit to practise, you must take appropriate steps without delay, so that the concerns are investigated and patients are protected where necessary.'*

4 **False.** Although this could be a reasonable course of action to take, the passage makes no mention of contacting the Citizens Advice Bureau and is therefore not an option advised by the GMC: *'If you are not sure what to do, discuss your concerns with an impartial colleague or contact your defence body, a professional organisation, or the GMC for advice.'*

Example 4

1 **True.** The passage confirms that making poor decisions is indeed a key contributor to the failure of managing time effectively: *'Poor decision making is one of the major causes of failure for time management, as it prevents progress on the commitments which require action'.*

2 **True.** This statement is confirmed by the following in the passage: *'Strategic thinking requires a considerable amount of uninterrupted time, as does the creation of plans'.*

3 **Can't tell.** Although the MLCF is indeed known as the Medical Leadership Competency Framework the passage does not state this, therefore it is not possible to confirm this from the passage.

4 **True.** The statement is confirmed by the following bullet-pointed information:

'The sub-groupings of Setting Direction are:

- *Evaluating impact*
- *Making decisions*
- *Applying knowledge and evidence*
- *Identifying the contexts for change'.*

Example 5

1. **The correct answer is B.** The passage states: 'However, they may increase delay during the off-peak period and increase the probability of certain accidents, such as rear-end collisions'.
2. **The correct answer is C.** The passage states 'Additionally, when improperly configured, driver irritation can become an issue'.
3. **The correct answer is A.** Some purposes of traffic signals are to (1) improve overall safety, (2) decrease average travel time through an intersection, and (3) equalise the quality of services for all or most traffic streams.
4. **The correct answer is C.** Delivering instructions to drivers through a set of colourful lights (generally, of the standard red-yellow (amber)-green format).

Example 6

1 **False.** The DVLA is the body responsible for determining whether an individual is medically fit to drive: *'The DVLA is legally responsible for deciding if a person is medically unfit to drive. The Agency needs to know when driving licence holders have a condition which may now, or in the future, affect their safety as a driver'.*

2 **Can't tell.** Although the passage states a doctor must inform a patient they are going to report them to the DVLA the passage does not stipulate how: *'Before you do this, you should advise the patient that you are doing so, and afterwards, write to the patient informing them that disclosure has been made'.*

3 **True.** The passage states that a presiding officer of the court can be any responsible member of the community, which includes a policeman, appointed by a judge. This is confirmed by the following bullet point: *'If a judge or presiding officer of a court order instructs you to disclose information. However, you must not disclose information to respectable members of the community, which include solicitors, police officers or fire officers, who are not appointed to act on behalf of the judge in an official capacity. A presiding officer can be any respectable member of the community appointed by a judge'.*

4 **False.** This statement is false based on the following in the passage: *'However, there may be some situations where confidentiality must be broken, for example, to safeguard the safety of others'.*

Example 7

1. **The correct answer is D.** Today a scholarly approach has been applied to the music of the past in relation to ensuring that the notation is interpreted correctly. An example is baroque music where modern research into the instruments, techniques and approach of this period has led today's musicians to revise their interpretation and performance of Baroque notation.
2. **The correct answer is A.** Guido d'Arezzo also devised the solfeggio system where a different syllable is sung to each note of an ascending scale.
3. **The correct answer is D.** By the 9th century Western music had become standardised into a notational form called nuemes which were shapes that represented notes.
4. **The correct answer is C.** This primitive notational system was more of a memory aid rather than a complete notational system showing exact pitch and duration. To read nuemes you needed to be familiar with the piece of music beforehand.

Example 8

1 **Can't tell.** Although the passage states that individuals intending to follow a career in surgery or pathology will especially benefit from involving themselves in anatomy demonstrating it is not possible to tell from the passage whether this also applies to the field of Cardiology: *'As there are very few paid medical demonstrator jobs these days, it is likely that your offer of help will be very well received! This is also excellent practice for those of you who intend to become surgeons or pathologists, as the best way to consolidate your knowledge about a subject is to teach it'.*

2 **True.** This statement is true based on the following: *'This is where you have an advantage compared to later on in your career. Although it may not seem it now, you have more time on your hands, as trying to gain teaching experience when working full-time is quite a stretch!'*

3 **False.** The word 'usually' indicates that individuals of other standing may be responsible for running this particular function within a medical school: *'There is usually an Academic Consultant in charge of the medical education of junior medical students'.*

4 **True.** This statement is confirmed by the following in the passage: *'Make sure that you get some feedback for your teaching; this need not be any weighty graphically designed form, just a simple feedback form asking the student to outline the positive aspects of your teaching session and areas for improvement'.*

Example 9

1 **Can't tell.** Although Deaneries in England are indeed responsible for the training of junior doctors the passage does not confirm or contradict this statement.

2 **False.** The passage states that most but not all Deaneries provide 20 minutes for the actual patient simulation exercise and therefore this statement is false. '*The actual time allocated to the consultation may vary between Deaneries. For most, there will be 20 minutes to complete the consultation but you do not have to use all of the time available*'.

3 **Can't tell.** Although OSCE does stand for Objective Structured Clinical Examination the passage does not confirm or contradict this statement.

4 **Can't tell.** The passage states 'most' rather than 'all' Deaneries will give individuals five minutes prior to the commencement of the patient simulated exercise to familiarise themselves with the background to the scenario, which suggests some may give other amounts of time. However the passage does not clarify what these are and therefore it is not possible to confirm whether the statement is true or false: *'For most of the Deaneries you will be given five minutes before the exercise starts to read the brief and information given to you. These five minutes are crucially important and we will explain later how to gain as much information as you can from the brief and use this time to your advantage'*.

Example 10

1 **False.** The passage confirms that although you may believe you are lowering your stress by putting off preparation, in fact the opposite is true: *'When you procrastinate you actually increase your feelings of stress, not diminish them.'*

2 **True.** This is confirmed by the following in the passage: *'This is another common reaction to putting things off and, as is the case with stress, feelings of guilt do not go away until the task is complete'*.

3 **True.** This statement is true based on the following in the passage: *'The word comes from the Latin word procrastinatio: pro- (forward) and crastinus (of tomorrow)'*.

4 **Can't tell.** Although the act of procrastination by an individual may indeed be perceived by others to be unproductive, the passage neither confirms nor contradicts this statement.

Example 11

1. **The correct answer is B.** While Iconic and Echoic Memory have been well researched, there are other types of Sensory Memory, like haptic, olfactory, etc., for which no sophisticated theories exist so far.
2. **The correct answer is D.** Atkinson and Shriffin researched the concepts of Sensory Memory and thought it the same as Iconic Memory. Darwin and others added the concept of Echoic Memory.
3. **The correct answer is D.** As detailed in the passage 'This is due to Iconic Memory. Roughly speaking, we can think of this subtype of memory as a kind of photographic memory, but one which only lasts for a very short time (milliseconds, up to a second)'.
4. **The correct answer is A.** While Iconic and Echoic Memory have been well researched, there are other types of Sensory Memory, like haptic, olfactory, etc.

Example 12

1 **Can't tell.** Although the passage states that a doctor should inform an appropriate person in the case of understaffing, the passage neither confirms nor contradicts that the HR Manager is an appropriate person: '*If you feel patient safety is at risk for any reason, for example by there not being enough doctors on the ward due to illness, then it would be worth saying that you would inform appropriate people to ensure that this is rectified, such as your Consultant or the department lead so that locum cover can be arranged*'.

2 **False.** This statement is false as the passage states: '*It is important to ascertain whether the patient thinks they are obliged to give the present in order to receive good quality healthcare, and you must make sure that they realise that this is not the case*'.

3 **True.** This statement is true based on the following in the passage: '*In general, you would need to look at whether the gift is appropriate, for example, a box of chocolates after a ward stay is more reasonable than giving £200 to a particular doctor. Scenarios involving this situation could come up in any part of the assessment*'.

4 **False.** The passage actually states that patients 'often' (rather than 'always') give gifts to show their appreciation: '*Patients in hospital and in the community often give presents to their doctors, such as chocolates to express their gratitude for help with their treatment*'.

Example 13

1 **False.** This statement is contradicted by the following: *'The primary duty of care is to patients. All applicants to medical schools will be expected to understand the importance of this principle'.*

2 **True.** This statement is confirmed by the following in the passage: *'Doctors must have an understanding of teamwork and respect for the contributions of others. Desirable characteristics include curiosity, creativity, initiative, flexibility and leadership'.*

3 **Can't tell.** Although the passage states that a disability may impede a career in medicine the passage does not specifically define on what grounds a person who is wheelchair bound may or may not be fit to practice. *'The practice of medicine requires the highest standards of professional competence. However, a history of serious ill health or disability will not jeopardise a career in medicine unless the condition impinges upon professional fitness to practise'.*

4 **Can't tell.** Whilst it is clear from the passage that failure to complete the expected period of relevant experience will affect the candidate's chances adversely, it is not clear that it would be enough on its own to make acceptance unlikely. *'Medical schools expect candidates to have had some relevant experience in health or related areas. Indeed, some medical schools stipulate a defined minimum period of relevant work experience'.*

Example 14

1. **The correct answer is C.** Control systems are components that are added to other components, to increase functionality, or to meet a set of design criteria.
2. **The correct answer is A.** From devices as simple as a toaster or a toilet, to complex machines like space shuttles and power steering, control engineering is a part of our everyday life.
3. **The correct answer is D.** Modern methods have been used to great effect more recently, while the Classical methods have been gradually falling out of favour.
4. **The correct answer is B.** From devices as simple as a toaster or a toilet, to complex machines like space shuttles and power steering, control engineering is a part of our everyday life.

Chapter 4

The Quantitative Reasoning subtest

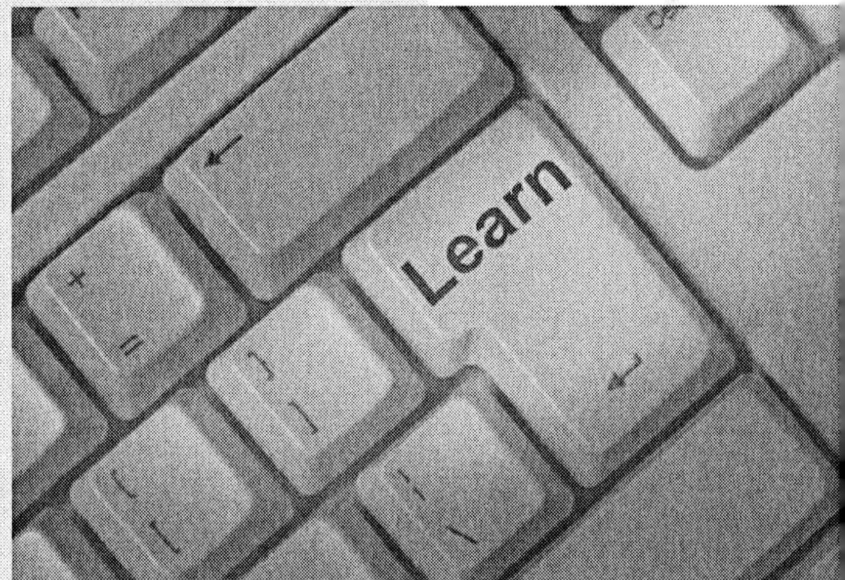

Chapter 4

The Quantitative Reasoning subtest

The Quantitative Reasoning subtest of the UKCAT will test a candidate's ability to solve numerical problems, interpret data and employ basic maths skills in relation to real life scenarios. The aim of this subtest is to assess objectively a candidate's ability to analyse, interpret, and manipulate complex numerical data.

Achieving high scores in the Quantitative Reasoning subtest reflects an ability to manipulate numerical information which is essential for doctors or dentists in their everyday practice.

Before you attempt to answer any Quantitative Reasoning questions it is important that you refresh your basic knowledge of the following topics:

- Addition
- Subtraction
- Multiplication
- Division
- Percentages
- Ratios
- Averages; mean (total value divided by sample number), median (middle value) and mode (most frequent value)
- Fractions
- Decimals

Also, you need to be able to interpret:

- Pie charts
- Line graphs
- Bar graphs
- Tables

The Quantitative Reasoning subtest contains nine stems. There are four questions per stem, making a total of 36 questions. You will have 25 minutes to complete this section, which includes one minute for administration. You will therefore have 40 seconds to spend on each question. This chapter will illustrate the types of numerical questions you will face when you sit your UKCAT.

Summary of Quantitative Reasoning structure

Stem

Stems will consist of various tables, charts and graphs, usually with supporting explanatory text. There will be a total of 9 stems in the UKCAT.

Lead-in question

For each of the stems, there will be four separate lead-in questions. In total there will be 36 lead-in questions which relate to the tables, charts and graphs.

Choices

For each question, you will be given five different answer options which will be in the format of A, B, C, D and E. Only one choice is the correct answer, and the remaining choices are known as *'distracters'*.

When you are working through the UKCAT subtests it can be distracting to monitor exactly how long you spend answering each question, especially when you have the stems to read through. A more useful time management approach is to divide each subtest into four quarters. So, in the case of the Quantitative Reasoning subtest, after approximately six minutes you should be working on the third stem; after approximately 11 minutes you should be completing the fifth stem; and so on. If you find yourself falling behind at these points you know that you need to pick up the pace.

Example of a Quantitative Reasoning question

Below is a dry measures equivalent table, and a recipe for pizza dough. James wants to make pizza but needs to calculate some conversions. James does know that with water, 1 gram is equivalent to 1 millilitre.

3 teaspoons	1 tablespoon	1/2 ounce	14.3 grams
2 tablespoons	1/8 cup	1 ounce	28.3 grams
4 tablespoons	1/4 cup	2 ounces	56.7 grams
5 1/3 tablespoons	1/3 cup	2.6 ounces	75.6 grams
8 tablespoons	1/2 cup	4 ounces	113.4 grams
12 tablespoons	3/4 cup	6 ounces	0.375 pound
32 tablespoons	2 cups	16 ounces	1 pound

Pizza dough recipe

- 1 pound of strong white bread flour
- 1 teaspoon salt
- 1 teaspoon sugar
- 3 teaspoons fast action dried yeast
- 2 cups of water
- 2 tablespoons olive oil

1. How many cups of olive oil are needed?

A 8 cups
B 1/8 cup
C 1/4 cup
D 1 ounce
E 1 cup

Quantitative Reasoning hints and tips

Refresh your memory by working through your GCSE and A level maths books to ensure you are familiar with the following:

- Addition and subtraction
- Multiplication and division
- Fractions and percentages
- Converting fractions, decimals and percentages
- Determining modes, means and medians
- Algebra
- Decimals
- Distance, time and speed triangles
- Calculating area and perimeters
- Analysing charts, bar charts, pie charts, frequency tables, etc
- Square and cube numbers

When working through the questions in this section remember the following:

- As well as the actual data presented, pay particular attention to any accompanying text as this can often effect how the data can be manipulated when calculating the answer.
- **Work through the questions systematically.** You may find that a question refers to your previous answer(s).
- **Work out all your calculations on the whiteboard provided.** If there are errors you may be able to determine from your rough workings at what point you made a mistake.
- Work through the practice mock papers and **identify your strengths and weaknesses** early so you can improve on your weaknesses. For example, you may be better at completing algebra equations rather than fractions. You can then address this weakness.
- When answering questions which involve humans, remember to calculate your final answer to the nearest whole number as people cannot be represented as a decimal or a fraction! This may be an important point to note when converting percentages to actual numbers.
- One major pitfall is to select an option which at first glance you think is nearest to the answer. Often you will find that the majority of the options are very close to each other and may differ in terms of decimal points or a single digit which is either added or removed. Therefore it is very important to evaluate the answer options very carefully. Always answer questions in the correct metric units. For example, a question may ask you to calculate something in centimetres but then give your final answer in metres. Therefore it is important to **read each item very carefully**.
- Some algebra questions may require you to calculate the value of 'x'. Often this will be x on its own, or sometimes the answer may require you to find x^3 or x^2. Therefore it is always important to **look at how the questions require you to give your final answer.**
- Remember to **time yourself as you complete the mock tests**. This will improve your time management skills, ensuring you have adequate time to answer every question.
- Try not to spend too long on one question. All marks are awarded equally in this section.
- If you are unsure of the answer select the best possible answer, flag the question and return to it. By selecting an answer you at least stand a chance of scoring a mark, even if you run out of time and are unable to return to the flagged question.

Four simple steps to Quantitative Reasoning

Step 1

Read the question carefully.

Step 2

Calculate your rough workings step-by-step using the whiteboard provided.

Step 3

Eliminate answers which are obviously incorrect from the five options.

Step 4

Mark the most accurate answer. (Remember to select your answer in the correct units requested by the question.) You will not be penalised for getting an answer wrong, even if you guess. A guess means that you have a 20% chance of getting the mark, so it is better to guess than to leave the question blank! If you really are unsure about a question, eliminate the obvious wrong answers and then make a calculated guess.

Quantitative Reasoning practice examples

Example 1

Below is a dry measures equivalent table, and a recipe for pizza dough. James wants to make pizza but needs to calculate some conversions. James does know that with water, 1 gram is equivalent to 1 millilitre.

3 teaspoons	1 tablespoon	1/2 ounce	14.3 grams
2 tablespoons	1/8 cup	1 ounce	28.3 grams
4 tablespoons	1/4 cup	2 ounces	56.7 grams
5 1/3 tablespoons	1/3 cup	2.6 ounces	75.6 grams
8 tablespoons	1/2 cup	4 ounces	113.4 grams
12 tablespoons	3/4 cup	6 ounces	0.375 pound
32 tablespoons	2 cups	16 ounces	1 pound

Pizza dough recipe

- 1 pound of strong white bread flour
- 1 teaspoon salt
- 1 teaspoon sugar
- 3 teaspoons fast action dried yeast
- 2 cups of water
- 2 tablespoons olive oil

1. **How many cups of olive oil are needed?**
   A 8 cups
   B 1/8 cup
   C 1/4 cup
   D 1 ounce
   E 1 cup

2. **Approximately how many ounces is one teaspoon of salt?**
   A 1/2 ounce
   B 1/8 ounce
   C 1/8 cup
   D 1/6 ounce
   E 1/3 ounce

3. **Approximately how many ml of water are in 2 cups?**
   A 450 ml
   B 500 ml
   C 300 ml
   D 500 g
   E 460 ml

4. **The recipe is for four people. Approximately how much flour in grams would be needed if it were for nine?**
   A 4 cups
   B 800 g
   C 2,050 g
   D 1,020 g
   E 1,100 g

Example 2

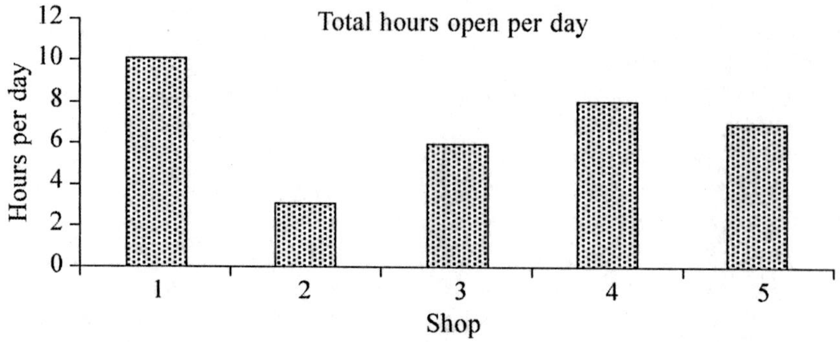

A businessman owns five shops in one town. Shop 1 is open 3 days a week and has 7 employees, Shop 2 is open 5 days a week and has 4 employees, Shop 3 is open 7 days a week and has 3 employees and Shop 4 with 5 employees and Shop 5 with 6 employees are both open 6 days a week. The graph above shows the opening hours of each of the 5 shops.

1. **What are the accumulated total open hours of all the shops in one week?**

   A 200 hours
   B 177 hours
   C 213 hours
   D 184 hours
   E 100 hours

2. **Claire works in Shop 1 earning £9.65 an hour. Her partner Richard works in Shop 4 earning £7.90 an hour. Each works every day their respective shop is open. What is their joint income at the end of the week?**

   A £379.50
   B £772.95
   C £668.70
   D £874.65
   E £549.20

3. **Which shop accumulates the most man hours in a week?**

   A Shop 1
   B Shop 2
   C Shop 3
   D Shop 4
   E Shop 5

4. **On a day when all shops are open, how many man hours are worked in total?**
   A 182 hours
   B 200 hours
   C 164 hours
   D 1,128 hours
   E 211 hours

Example 3

Ian is looking to buy a new computer, and has shortlisted four companies for their offers on the four components he wants. Ian also has a friend who is willing to sell him a processor for £100. He has summarised the information in the table below.

	Monitor	Tower	Processor	Speakers	All 4 group discount	Postage + packaging
Global Computers	£300	£400	£200	£80	0%	£0
Power Computers	£250	£500	£170	£100	30%	£70
Computer World	£180	£600	£210	£110	40%	£100
Electronic Ltd	£270	£490	£150	£100	25%	£10

1. **What is the average price of a tower?**
   A £500.00
   B £500.50
   C £480.00
   D £497.50
   E £495.00

2. **Not including group discount or postage and packaging, what is the cheapest Ian could get all four components for?**
   A £810
   B £980
   C £700
   D £660
   E £1,000

3. **Which company's offer for all four components, including postage and packaging, is the cheapest?**
   A Global Computers
   B Power Computers
   C Computer World
   D Electronic Ltd
   E Can't tell

4. **If Ian takes his friend's offer, which company would be the cheapest to purchase the three remaining components from, excluding postage and packaging?**
   A Global Computers
   B Power Computers
   C Computer World
   D Electronic Ltd
   E Can't tell

Example 4

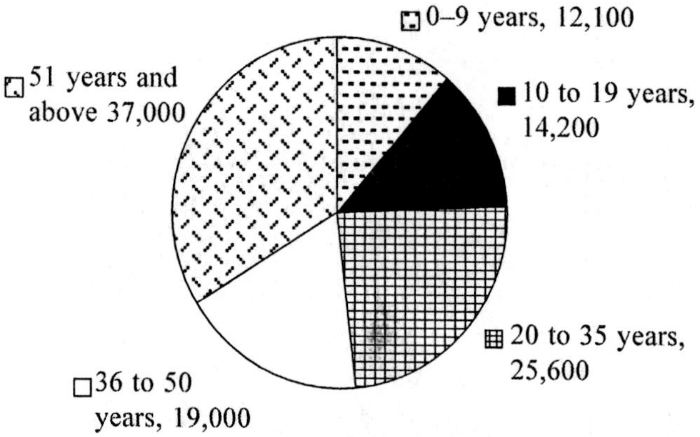

The pie chart above shows the age distribution of males living in the seaside resort of Garside in the year 1989. There are 10% more females than males in all age groups. The population of Garside has tripled since 1970.

1. **What is the percentage of males who are 19 years old or younger living in Garside?**
   A 25%
   B 24%
   C 34%
   D 20%
   E 26%

2. **What is the total population of Garside to the nearest thousand?**
   A 226,000
   B 227,000
   C 220,000
   D 230,000
   E 229,000

3. What is the ratio, to the nearest whole number, of males aged 51 years old and over to males under 51 years?

A 1 in 4
B 1 in 3
C 1:2
D 2:1
E 4:1

4. What is the total number of females aged 35 years or under living in Garside?

A 57,990
B 58,200
C 59,070
D 57,090
E 57,900

Example 5

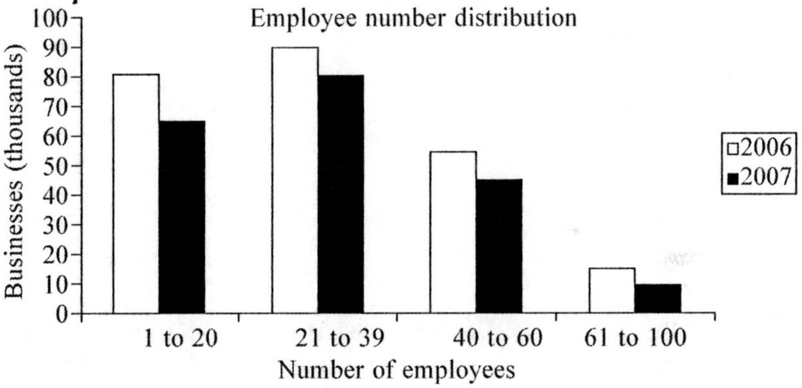

A number of businesses were surveyed over the period of two years to determine the number of employees they had. The data is shown in the graph above.

1. To the nearest whole number, what percentage of the businesses surveyed in 2006 had 39 or fewer employees?

A 61%
B 75%
C 74%
D 17%
E 71%

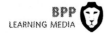

2. **Between the two categories with 39 or fewer employees, what was the mean average of the decrease in numbers of businesses from 2006 to 2007?**
   A 12,500
   B 12.5
   C 13,000
   D 140
   E 200

3. **How many fewer companies were surveyed in 2007 scompared with 2006? (Give your answer as a percentage to the nearest whole number).**
   A 17%
   B 16%
   C 20%
   D 9%
   E 29%

4. **What was the decrease between 2006 and 2007 in the number of companies with 61 to 100 employees?**
   A 30%
   B 1/3
   C 50%
   D Quarter
   E 40%

Example 6

	Mon	Tues	Wed	Thurs	Fri	Sat	Sun
Timber	22	24	25	32	32	27	25
Bamber	18	16	27	27	24	24	25
Syncroy	4	8	5	5	8	2	2
Lambert	41	22	29	31	31	12	12
Tillitia	10	11	6	3	4	3	1
Mangaly	42	40	45	38	38	37	36
Evertop	21	21	23	21	20	20	26
Billerton	5	5	8	5	8	4	7

The table above shows the temperatures (°C) for a number of locations recorded over the course of a week. It was later discovered that the equipment used to record the temperatures in Billerton and Mangaly had been calibrated incorrectly, and was providing readings 20% lower than the actual temperature. Temperature readings can also be expressed in °F which can be calculated (for the purposes of this example) by multiplying the °C reading by 3.

1. **What was the approximate combined mean average daily temperature, in °F, recorded in Bamber, Tillitia and Syncroy over the course of the seven days surveyed?**
   A 36
   B 3.3
   C 33
   D 43
   E 27

2. **What was the median average daily temperature in Billerton in °C?**
   A 7.2
   B 8
   C 5
   D 6
   E 6.5

3. **What was the mean average temperature in °C, to the nearest whole number, across all the locations on Tuesday?**
   A 19
   B 18
   C 20
   D 21
   E 17

4. **Which location showed the greatest range in temperature over the week?**
   A Timber
   B Tillitia
   C Bamber
   D Syncroy
   E Lambert

Example 7

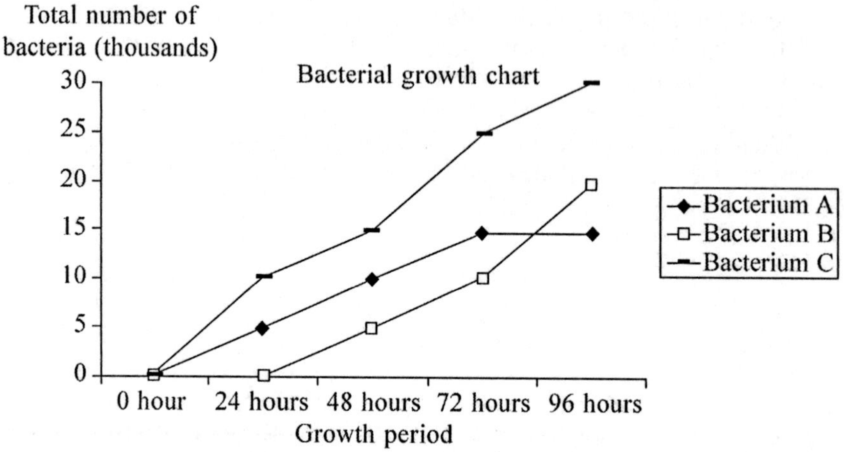

The above chart illustrates the growth of three different bacteria over the course of four days. Bacterium B was grown using standard agar, and Bacteria A and C were grown using an enhanced agar which accelerates growth by 50% over standard agar.

1. **What was the difference in growth of Bacterium B over Bacterium A after four days?**
   A 20
   B 20,000
   C 500
   D 5,000
   E 5

2. **What was the increase in the population of Bacterium B between 72 and 96 hours?**
   A 150%
   B 50%
   C 100%
   D 10%
   E 5%

3. **Which single bacterium showed the greatest growth between 24 hours and 72 hours?**
   A Bacterium A
   B Bacterium B
   C Bacterium C
   D Bacterium A and Bacterium B
   E Bacterium A and Bacterium C

4. What was the total number of bacteria grown by 96 hours?

A 65,000
B 650,000
C 65
D 6.5
E 650

Example 8

	Weekday	Weekend
Suisse Franc	3	2.9
Euro	1.3	1.2
Australian Dollar	4	3.8
US Dollar	1.5	1.35
Canadian Dollar	3	2.8
Egyptian Pound	4	4.5

The above table outlines the various exchange rates, offered by an airport currency conversion agency, to convert £1 in Pounds Sterling into various foreign currencies. The same currency conversion agency will also exchange the foreign currencies back into Pounds Sterling using the same exchange rates outlined in the table but with the addition of a £3 surcharge per currency.

1. What is the difference in Egyptian Pounds when exchanging £120 on a weekday compared to a Saturday or a Sunday?

A 85 more
B 60 more
C 80 more
D 60 less
E 54 less

2. If a traveller wishes to convert two hundred US Dollars and three hundred and fifty Canadian dollars back in to Pounds Sterling on a Monday, how much money in Pounds Sterling in total (rounded to the nearest whole number) will he end up with, after all deductions have been made?

A £250
B £247
C £244
D £243
E £240

3. **How many Euros would £380 be converted to on a Saturday?**
   A 317
   B 300
   C 356
   D 456
   E 465

4. **What is the conversion ratio between Pounds Sterling and Egyptian Pounds on a weekday?**
   A 1:4
   B 4:1
   C 1:2
   D 1:3
   E 5:1

Example 9

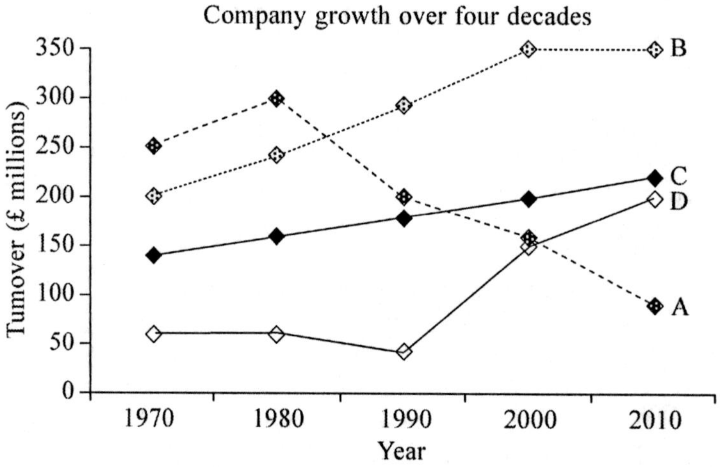

The above bar graph shows the temperature readings recorded at midday in Newburton over the course of a week. For the purposes of this example, the ratio of °C to °F is treated as 1:3.

1. **What was the mean average weekday temperature?**
   A 8°C
   B 12°C
   C 10.9°C
   D 15°C
   E 15.2°C

2. What was the difference in temperature between the hottest and coldest days?

A 10°C
B 22°C
C 14°C
D 8°C
E 9°C

3. What was the mean average temperature (to the nearest whole number) in °F for the entire week?

A 40°F
B 44°F
C 45°C
D 45°F
E 48°F

4. What is the percentage difference in temperature between Saturday and Sunday?

A 60%
B 40%
C 55%
D 43%
E 53%

Example 10

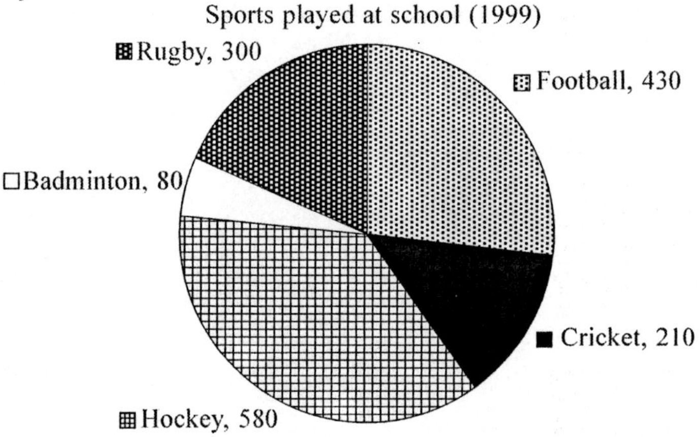

The above pie chart illustrates the results from a questionnaire answered by all students at Pinewood School when they were asked what sports they participated in. The total student number at Pinewood School is 913, although on the day of the survey 37 students were absent or off-site and therefore unable to participate in the survey. Those surveyed were able to name as many sports as they wished in their answers. Sport is not compulsory at Pinewood, but interestingly a survey completed ten years later showed an increased participation in all sports of the order of 20%.

1. **What percentage of students present on the day of the survey played rugby at Pinewood School in 1999?**
   A 32.4%
   B 1:4
   C 34.2%
   D 38%
   E 43.2%

2. **How many individuals played hockey in 2009?**
   A 696
   B 580
   C 480
   D 796
   E 800

3. **What was the mean average participation across all sports in 1999?**
   A 350
   B 340
   C 300
   D 230
   E 320

4. **James plays cricket. In 2009, 25 pupils are to be selected to represent the school in a cricket match. What is the probability that James will be selected? (Give your answer to the nearest whole number).**
   A 11%
   B 10%
   C 15%
   D 25%
   E 12%

Example 11

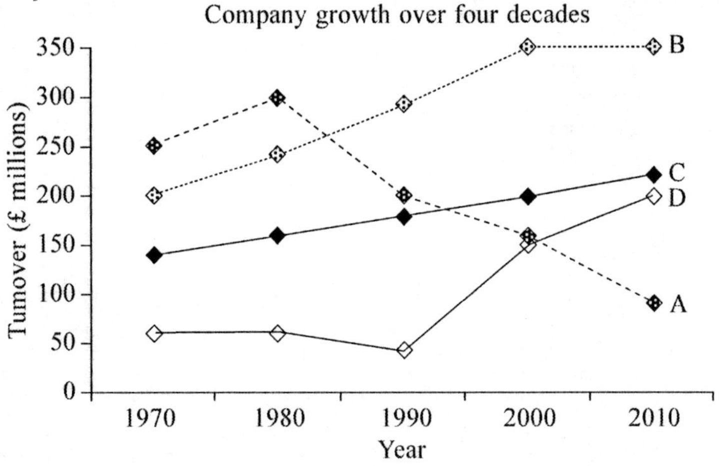

1. **Which company demonstrated the greatest increase in turnover between 1980 and 2000?**
   A Company A
   B Company B
   C Company C
   D Company D
   E Company A and Company C

2. **What was the combined turnover of all four companies in 2010?**
   A £860,000,000
   B £860
   C £368,000,000
   D £6,800
   E £86,000,000

3. **What was the difference between the total turnovers of Company A and Company D between 1970 and 2010?**
   A £490
   B £490,000
   C £490 million
   D £49,000,000
   E £94,000,000

4. In 2010 which company demonstrated the greatest growth compared to 2000?

A Company A
B Company B
C Company C
D Company D
E Company A and B

Example 12

	Mon – Fri	Sat	Sun
Chillwells	8:00 – 18:00	8:00 – 18:00	10:00 – 18:00
Wollards	9:00 – 17:00	10:00 – 16:00	Closed
Simpletons	8:00 – 18:00	6:00 – 20:00	Closed
Multimedia	8:00 – 18:00	Closed	Closed
Gymtastic	8:00 – 16:00	8:00 – 16:00	8:00 – 16:00

The table above shows the opening times of five shops in the town of Gilberston. None of the shops close for lunch except Simpletons and Gymtastic, which close for one hour at 13:00 each weekday but do not close for lunch at weekends.

1. What is the combined number of hours Chillwells, Multimedia and Wollards are open on a Tuesday and Saturday?

A 46 hours
B 44 hours
C 40 hours
D 50 hours
E 38 hours

2. What is the total number of hours Gymtastic is open per week?

A 49 hours
B 56 hours
C 51 hours
D 5,100 minutes
E 60 hours

3. What is the modal average shop opening time during the week?

A 9.00
B 8.00
C 8.30
D 9.30
E 8.45

4. Over the course of a week, how many more hours is Gymtastic open than Multimedia?

A 120 minutes
B 1.5 hours
C 60 minutes
D 600 minutes
E 6 hours

Example 13

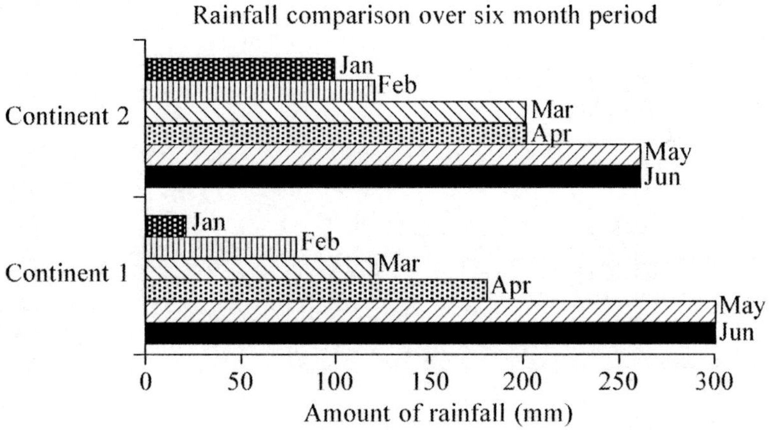

1. When was the highest rainfall recorded on Continent 1?

A May
B June
C May and June
D April
E April and May

2. What was the total rainfall recorded on Continent 1 over the course of the six months?

A 100 mm
B 1,000 cm
C 1 metre
D 10,000 mm
E 1,000,000 m

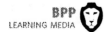

3. **What was the ratio of rainfall between Continent 2 and Continent 1 in the month of March? (Give your answer to two decimal places).**
   A 1.67:1
   B 1:1
   C 2:1
   D 3:1
   E 2.67:1

4. **What was the difference in rainfall between the months of January and April on Continent 2?**
   A 1 cm
   B 10,000 mm
   C 20 cm
   D 1,000 mm
   E 100 mm

Example 14

Smashington	07:00	07:10	07:20	07:30	07:40	07:50	08:00	08:10
Ardefield	07:06	07:16	07:26	07:36	07:46	07:56	08:06	08:16
Jameson	07:12	07:22	07:32	07:42	07:52	08:02	08:12	08:22
Farnsder Outer City Centre	07:19	07:29	07:39	07:49	07:59	08:09	08:19	08:29
Farnsder City Centre	07:28	07:38	07:48	07:58	08:08	08:18	08:28	08:38

The above is an extract from a local tram timetable. The times provided are for trams running Monday to Friday. A reduced service is operated on a Saturday and Sunday, commencing at 08:00.

1. **What is the earliest an individual can arrive in Farnsder City Centre if the earliest they can arrive at Ardefield station is 08:00 on a weekday?**
   A 08:00
   B 08:38
   C 08:18
   D 08:28
   E 08:08

2. **What is the journey time from Jameson to Farnsder City Centre if the 07:22 tram is taken on a weekday?**
   A 16 minutes
   B 28 minutes
   C 30 minutes
   D 17 minutes
   E 9 minutes

3. **If the maximum capacity of all trams operating on a weekday is 48, assuming that one Tuesday morning all trams were operating at capacity upon termination in the City Centre, how many passengers would have alighted by 08:00?**
   A 192
   B 48
   C 96
   D 168
   E 150

4. **How many trams leave Ardefield before 08:00?**
   A 7
   B 3
   C 4
   D 5
   E 6

Example 15

	Present value	Value 12 months ago
Stock 1	23p	16p
Stock 2	35p	43p
Stock 3	12p	12p
Stock 4	18p	7p
Stock 5	43p	99p
Stock 6	21p	18p

1. **Which stock has shown the greatest increase compared to 12 months ago?**
   A Stock 1
   B Stock 2
   C Stock 3
   D Stock 4
   E Stock 5

2. What is the median average value of the stocks 12 months ago?
A 35.4p
B 17p
C 20p
D 16p
E 18p

3. Which stock decreased the most in value compared to 12 months ago?
A Stock 1
B Stock 2
C Stock 3
D Stock 4
E Stock 5

4. What is the mean average value of the present day values of all stocks?
A 25.33p
B 22.66p
C 26.13p
D 24.23p
E 20.21p

Example 16

	Student A	Student B	Student C	Student D
Maths	81	60	75	93
English	56	61	54	65
French	54	34	48	68
Design	70	40	49	85
Art	89	78	54	59
Business Studies	58	32	78	87
Sports Science	89	77	71	76
Geography	67	45	57	54

	A	B	C	D	E	Ungraded
Maths	80–100	70–79	65–69	60–65	50–59	≤49
English	85–100	65–84	55–64	50–54	45–49	≤44
French	90–100	75–89	55–74	51–73	40–50	≤39
Design	75–100	60–74	51–59	45–50	40–44	≤39
Art	80–100	75–79	65–74	50–64	41–49	≤40
Business Studies	85–100	80–84	70–79	60–69	45–59	≤44
Sports Science	90–100	80–89	65–79	55–64	45–54	≤44
Geography	70–100	61–69	50–60	45–49	40–45	≤39

The tables above show the exam marks (%) for various AS level subjects scored by four students and an accompanying table below to determine the applicable exam grades achieved.

1. **What was the mean average grade achieved by the four students in Geography?**
   - A Grade E
   - B Grade D
   - C Grade A
   - D Grade B
   - E Grade C

2. **All of the four students scored Grade C or higher in Art.**
   - A True
   - B False
   - C Can't tell
   - D Maybe
   - E Definitely

3. **In what subjects did Student D score A grades?**
   - A Maths, Design and English
   - B Maths and Design
   - C Maths, Design and Sports Science
   - D Maths, English and Geography
   - E Design, Business Studies and Maths

4. **In what subject was the highest mark scored by any student?**
   - A Maths
   - B English
   - C Design
   - D Geography
   - E Business Studies

Example 17

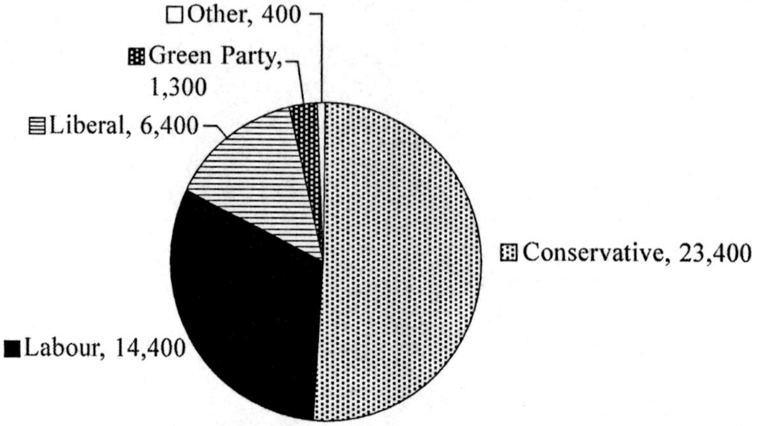

The above chart shows the results from a local by-election for the borough of Digsby in 2002. The total population of this small borough peninsular on the North Coast of England is 136,345, with 72% being eligible to vote. Analysis of the results by a local university showed that the total voter turnout was 8% lower in the previous by-election of 1996 when the population was 129,345.

1. **Of the eligible voters, what percentage actually voted in the 2002 election (to the nearest whole number)?**
   A 38%
   B 44%
   C 47%
   D 48%
   E 58%

2. **What percentage of the votes were for the Green Party in 2002 (to two significant figures)?**
   A 2.80%
   B 3%
   C 2.83%
   D 4%
   E 12%

3. **What was the actual voter turnout in 1996 (to the nearest 1,000)?**
   A 5,000
   B 55,000
   C 42,000
   D 46,000
   E 50,444

4. By what margin did the Conservatives beat their next closest rivals in the 2002 election (to two decimal places)?

A 19.61%
B 19%
C 20.25%
D 50.98%
E 31.37%

Example 18

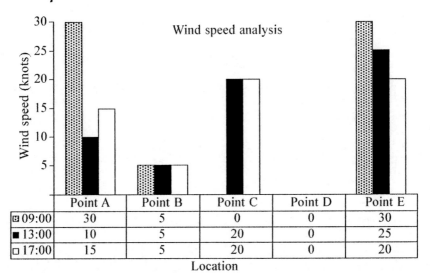

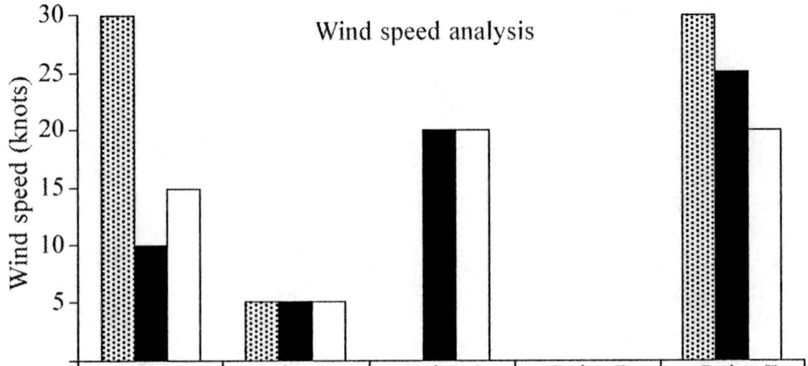

	Point A	Point B	Point C	Point D	Point E
▩ 09:00	30	5	0	0	30
■ 13:00	10	5	20	0	25
□ 17:00	15	5	20	0	20

Location

The data above shows wind speed measurements recorded the previous Tuesday in five locations. Wind speed can also be expressed in metres per second (m/s) for which 1 knot = 25 m/s. Cross-referencing of the data collected showed that the results above were consistently five times greater than the previous Monday for Point A and Point C, but the same for all other points except Point E, which was shown to have decreased by a third on the Tuesday.

1. What was the mean average wind speed at Point E the previous Monday in m/s (to the nearest whole number)?

A 400 m/s
B 25 knots
C 625 m/s
D 937.5 m/s
E 938 m/s

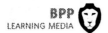

2. **What was the mean average wind speed last Tuesday at Point C, in knots (to two significant figures)?**
   A 13 knots
   B 13 m/s
   C 325 m/s
   D 30 knots
   E 30 m/s

3. **What was the range in wind speeds measured last Tuesday at 17:00?**
   A 375 knots
   B 20 knots
   C 5,000 m/s
   D 500 knots
   E 20 m/s

4. **At which point the previous Tuesday was the highest mean average wind speed recorded?**
   A Point A
   B Point B
   C Point C
   D Point D
   E Point E

Example 19

Location	Average temperature (°C)	Average hours of sunshine (Hours)	Average wind speed (Knots)
Bognor Regis	19	6	17
Brighton	23	7	27
Bournemouth	16	5	35
Plymouth	16	5	33
Portsmouth	24	7	29
Exeter	30	10	15

The table above shows various measurements recorded in the month of July 2009 at various coastal locations (six in total). Further statistical evaluation showed that the month of July experienced consistent increases in all measurements of 12% compared to June 2009, and consistent decreases of 21% when compared to August 2009. The researchers who collected this data have been experimenting with assigning locations a 'Tourism Index' which is calculated using the following formula:

Average temperature (°C) × Average hours of sunshine (Hours) × Average wind speed (Knots)

1. **What was the modal average temperature across the six locations in July?**
   A 61°C
   B 30°C
   C 16°C
   D 16°F
   E 21°C

2. **What was the difference between the windspeeds recorded in Portsmouth and Bognor Regis in July?**
   A 12 m/s
   B 12 knots
   C 21 knots
   D 13 knots
   E 10 knots

3. **What was the Tourism Index for Plymouth in June to the nearest whole number?**
   A 2537
   B 2300
   C 2357.1
   D 3275
   E 2357

4. **Which location demonstrated the second highest Tourism Index in July?**
   A Bognor Regis
   B Portsmouth
   C Bournemouth
   D Exeter
   E Plymouth

Example 20

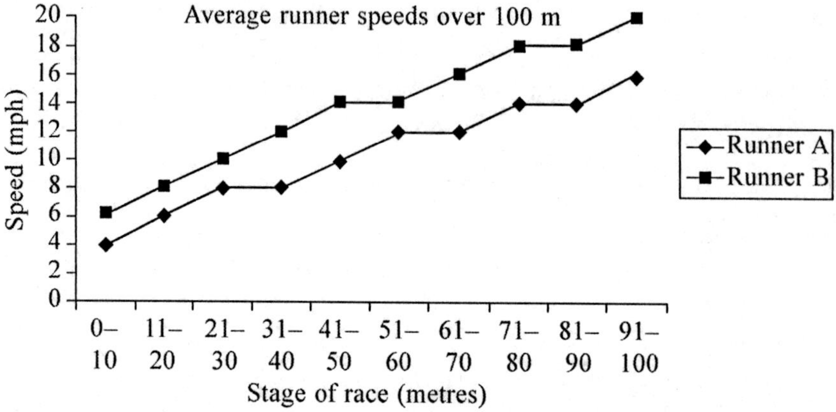

The above graph shows the average speed of two 12-year-old runners at each 10-metre segment of a 100 metres sprint. It is important to note that 1 mph is the equivalent to 5 metres per second (m/s).

1. **What was the difference in peak speeds between Runner A and Runner B?**
   A 4 m/s
   B 60 m/s
   C 40 mph
   D 6 mph
   E 4 mph

2. **What was the average speed of runner A in the 51–60 metre segment of the race?**
   A 12 mph
   B 12 m/s
   C 13 mph
   D 14 mph
   E 10 mph

3. **What is the mean average speed of Runner B over the first 50 metres of the race?**
   A 12 mph
   B 1.0 mph
   C 10 mph
   D 1.5 mph
   E 11 mph

4. **What was the average speed of Runner B during the segment 41–50 metres in m/s?**
   A 70 m/s
   B 14 mph
   C 70 mph
   D 17 m/s
   E 14 m/s

Example 21

Fictional plc operates a daily coach to and from its ball bearing factory for its workers. The coach leaves the town early in the morning, taking the motorway 4 miles south, then takes the exit and follows a dual carriageway 6 miles west. Finally, it follows a single carriageway south for a further 4 miles. The coach follows the same route back to the town at the end of the shift.
The average speed of the coach is 60mph, 40mph and 30mph on the motorway, dual carriageway and single carriageway respectively. The morning shift starts at 7am and workers need to arrive at the location by 6:50am at the latest.

1. **What is the latest time the coach can leave the town and still arrive at the factory on time?**
   A 6:19
   B 6:27
   C 6:29
   D 6:32
   E 6.42

2. **Assuming that the coach fuel consumption rate is 10 miles per gallon, and fuel is priced at £6 per gallon, what is the average weekly fuel bill facing the company, assuming a normal five-day week?**
   A £36
   B £42
   C £64
   D £84
   E £94

3. **If a new dual carriageway were to be built linking the town and the factory directly, how much time will this save on the daily morning commute?**
   A 5 minutes
   B 6 minutes
   C 7 minutes
   D 8 minutes
   E 9 minutes

4. **How much would the company save on their weekly fuel bill after the construction of the new road?**
   A £12
   B £18
   C £24
   D £30
   E £28

Example 22

Item of clothing	Wholesale price (£)	Special discount price (£)	RRP (£)
Jumper	2.83	4.56	6.99
Hat	1.09	1.99	2.99
Scarf	1.37	2.35	3.99
Trousers	5.43	8.76	12.99
Shoes (pair)	8.51	10.34	14.99
Trainers (pair)	9.82	13.42	19.99
Skirts	4.31	6.48	9.99
Baseball caps	0.89	1.45	4.99

The table above displays the various prices for a variety of clothes. Shops can purchase these clothes at either the wholesale price or the special discount price depending on the item in question. Baseball caps, trainers and hats can only be purchased at the special discount price whereas all other items can be purchased at the wholesale price.

1. **How much gross profit would a shop make if they sold 15 trousers, 10 baseball caps and 3 pairs of shoes at the full RRP price (to the nearest pound)?**
   A £120
   B £189
   C £145
   D £158
   E £168

2. **What is the percentage gross profit on a jumper?**
   A 59.5%
   B 40.5%
   C 61.5%
   D 64.5%
   E 52.5%

3. How much would 5 hats and 10 skirts cost for a shop to buy in to sell?

A £63.05
B £53.05
C £45.76
D £45.70
E £45.80

4. What is the difference between the highest and lowest retail price?

A £13
B £14
C £19
D £18
E £17

Example 23

Curriculum (education status)	School year	Number of pupils	
		Female	Male
KS3 (Compulsory)	7	154	161
	8	141	170
	9	122	181
KS4 (Compulsory)	10	80	220
	11	150	150
KS5 (Optional)	12	135	160
	13	177	136

A local mixed secondary school consists of 7 different year groups. The school is going to be undergoing an inspection in the near future, and some statistics about the school need to be calculated by the administration staff beforehand. The table above shows the number of girls and boys in each year in the school, and which curriculum level they are in at present.

1. How many pupils are there in KS3 in total?

A 929
B 417
C 959
D 1,178
E 930

2. **What percentage of pupils in KS4 are girls (to the nearest whole number)?**
   A 38.3%
   B 39%
   C 38%
   D 37%
   E 38.4%

3. **How many pupils are there in compulsory education in total?**
   A 1,530
   B 2,137
   C 1,537
   D 1,648
   E 1,529

4. **What is the ratio of males to females in Year 10?**
   A 1.75:1
   B 3.75:1
   C 0.682
   D 11:4
   E 2:1

Example 24

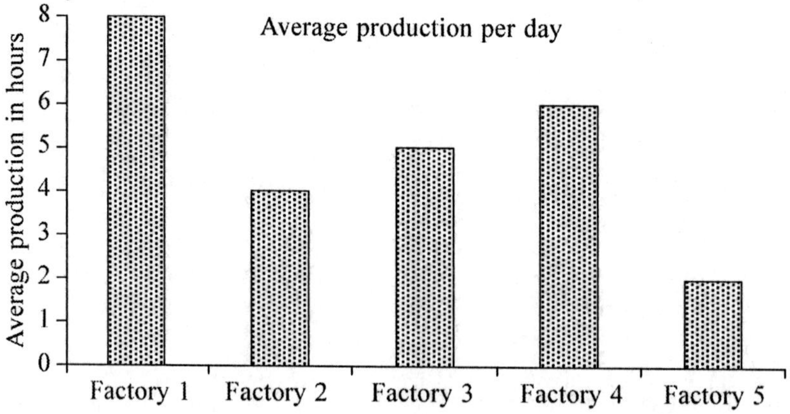

A local business manager owns five factories. The bar chart above shows the average number of hours that each factory is in production on weekdays.

1. **Which factory is the most productive on average?**
   A Factory 1
   B Factory 2
   C Factory 3
   D Factory 4
   E Factory 5

2. **If Ben and Mark both work for this company, Ben in Factory 2 earning £8.60 per hour and Mark in Factory 4 earning £7.50 per hour, what is the difference between their weekly earnings?**
   A £172
   B £225
   C £53
   D £198.50
   E £50

3. **How many hours on average does Factory 3 work on Saturdays?**
   A 6
   B 0
   C Unknown
   D 5
   E 4

4. **Lucy works at different factories on different days of the week. She earns £9.40 per hour and works at Factory 1 on Mondays, Tuesdays, and Fridays and Factory 5 on Wednesdays and Thursdays. How much does she earn per lunar month?**
   A £263.20
   B £1,502.00
   C £940.00
   D £235.00
   E £1,052.80

Example 25

The table below shows the yearly sales and profits made by a large car manufacturer.

	Net profit (millions/£)	Number of vehicles sold
Saloon	101	4,000
Hatchback	98	5,021
Sports convertible	50	1,500
4 × 4	63	2,880
Motorbike	37	1,064

1. **What percentage of total net profit can be accounted for by hatchback sales? (Calculate to 1 decimal place).**
   A 28.1%
   B 27.9%
   C 28.2%
   D 28.0%
   E 28.3%

2. **Which type of vehicle provides the largest net profit per vehicle sold?**
   A Saloon
   B Hatchback
   C Sports convertible
   D 4 × 4
   E Motorbike

3. **The previous year 5,272 hatchbacks were sold. What is the percentage decrease in sales?**
   A 4.76%
   B 5.00%
   C 4.99%
   D 4.54%
   E 5.76%

4. **The following year the motor vehicle company decides to cease the manufacture of motorbikes. How many more 4 × 4's must be sold to cover the loss of net profit?**
   A 1,692
   B 1,783
   C 1,524
   D 1,682
   E 1,674

Example 26

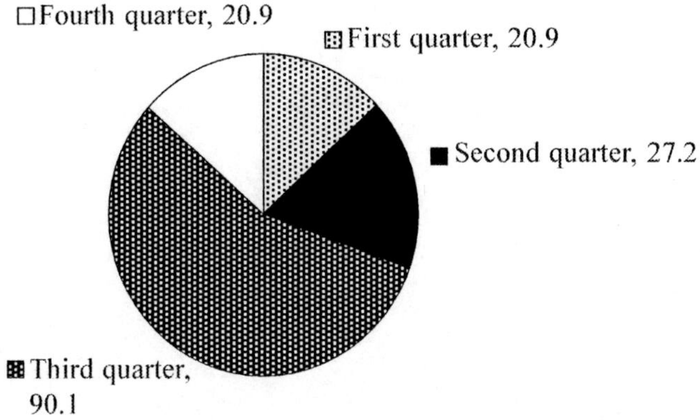

The above pie chart shows the annual turnover (£1,000s) for Baker's Food Factory.

1. **How much revenue did Baker's Food Factory turn over for the middle two quarters?**
   A £1,173
   B £117,300
   C £11,720
   D £118,300
   E £147,800

2. **What was the average revenue for the final three quarters of the year? (Give your answer to the nearest whole number).**
   A £45,966
   B £46,067
   C £3,796.38
   D £46,000.0
   E £46,066.67

3. **By how much did the second quarter revenue exceed the first quarter revenue? (Give your answer as a percentage to 1 decimal place).**
   A 16%
   B 23.2%
   C 30.1%
   D 15.3%
   E 15.9%

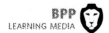

4. **What proportion of turnover was in the fourth quarter (to 2 decimal places)?**
   A 0.576
   B 0.57
   C 0.13
   D 0.567
   E 0.15

Example 27

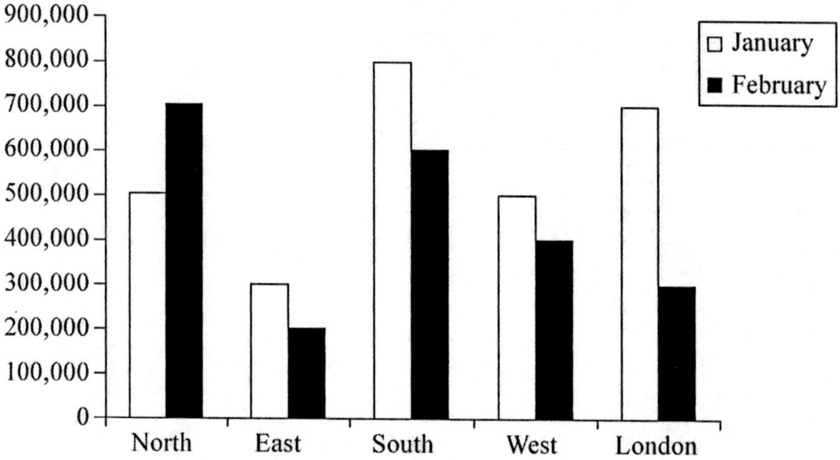

The bar chart above shows the profits (£) for Jones and Sons by geographical area for England.

1. **By what percentage did the profits decrease in the West from January to February?**
   A 25%
   B 80%
   C 20%
   D 33.33%
   E 75%

2. **What was the difference in turnover between the West in February and the East in January?**
   A £1,000,000
   B £100,000
   C £1,000
   D £100
   E £10,000

3. **What was the total turnover in February for all areas away from London?**
   A $160,000
   B £1,900,000
   C £1,600,000
   D £16,000
   E £160,000

4. **Driver A, working for Jones and Sons, travelled a distance of 400 miles at an average speed of 50 miles per hour. Driver B travelled the same distance at an average speed of 80 miles per hour. How many more minutes did driver A take to travel the journey than Driver B?**
   A 180
   B 90
   C 45
   D 240
   E 100

Example 28

Height in centimetres	70–90	91–110	111–130	131–150	151–170	171–190
Number of children	2	7	11	22	6	2

1. **How many children are less than 151 centimetres tall?**
   A 22
   B 6
   C 42
   D 7
   E 50

2. **What fraction of the children are between 70 and 130 centimetres tall?**
   A 2/5
   B 1/4
   C 11/50
   D 3/4
   E 1/2

3. **What percentage of the total number of children surveyed were 131 cm or taller?**
   A 58%
   B 70%
   C 3/5
   D 60%
   E 2/5

4. **The following year the number of children measuring 110 cm or shorter increased by 33%. How many children would there be in total (to the nearest whole number)?**
   A 2
   B 12
   C 3
   D 5
   E 9

Example 29

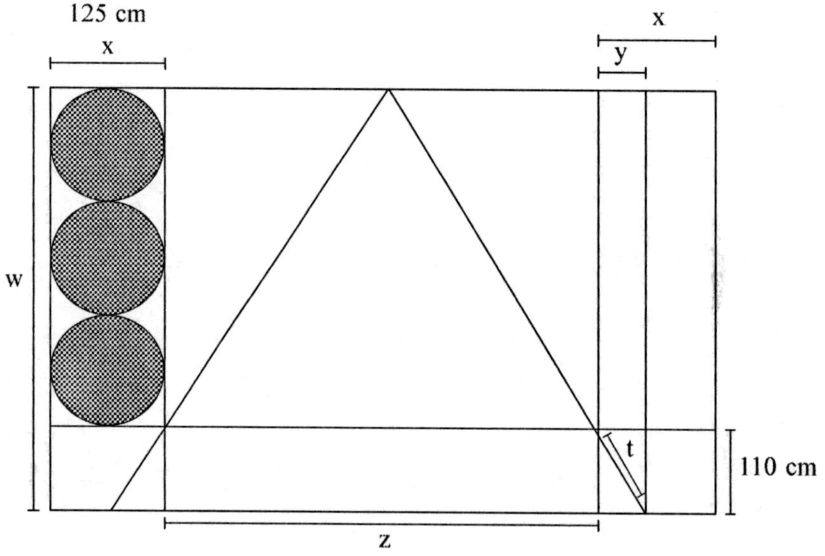

1. **Given that 'x' = 125 cm and 'y' is 35% of 'x', what is the value of 'y'?**
   A 40.375 cm
   B 43.75 cm
   C 35 cm
   D 44.25 cm
   E 47.375 cm

2. What is the total area of the three identical circles shaded in grey, to 2 decimal places?

A 12,271.84 cm^2
B 36,815.53 cm^2
C 12,271.85 cm^2
D 49,087.39 cm^2
E 36,815.54 cm^2

3. What is the correct formula to calculate the area of the large triangle?

A ½ (wz + 2y)
B w(z + 2y)
C ½ zw
D ½ (zw + 2y)
E $\frac{w(z + 2y)}{2}$

4. If y = 40 cm, what is the length of 't' to 2 decimal places?

A 14,014.06 cm
B 118.39 cm
C 119.23 cm
D 119.24 cm
E 117.05 cm

Example 30

	Mon	Tues	Wed	Thurs	Fri
Badminton	85	60	68	89	94
Volleyball	54	37	56	12	24
Squash	102	108	67	156	34
Swimming	56	43	37	38	35
Racketball	54	57	89	90	45
Karate	23	12	34	12	6
Judo	8	9	34	11	19
Kickboxing	4	7	4	6	8

The above table contains data from a survey conducted over the course of a winter week to determine the number of individuals participating in a range of activities at the Springfield Leisure Centre.

1. **Which activity had the highest number of participants over the course of the week?**
   A Badminton
   B Volleyball
   C Squash
   D Swimming
   E Racketball

2. **Which day saw the highest number of participants in total?**
   A Monday
   B Tuesday
   C Wednesday
   D Thursday
   E Friday

3. **What was the difference between Monday and Thursday in the number of individuals who participated in badminton, squash and karate?**
   A 27
   B 28
   C 47
   D 40
   E 257

4. **Which activity had the second lowest number of participants over the course of the week?**
   A Swimming
   B Racketball
   C Karate
   D Judo
   E Kickboxing

Example 31

Colin is looking to develop a small office in London. Floor space in London is £3,000 per square metre. Below is a table which contains length conversions.

1 Inch	2.54 cm
1 Yard	0.91 m
1 Mile	1.61 km

1. **Colin bought a flat screen square TV with a side length of 32 inches. How many cm^2 of wall space will he need to mount it to the nearest whole number?**
   A 5,901 cm^2
   B 8,100 cm^2
   C 7,340 cm^2
   D 6,606 cm^2
   E 6,180 cm^2

2. **Colin's destination is 100 km away. What average speed (in miles per hour) must Colin achieve to reach his destination in one hour?**
   A 62.1 mph
   B 100 mph
   C 59.8 mph
   D 60 mph
   E 65.2 mph

3. **How much would the floor space alone cost to buy a $16m^2$ apartment in London?**
   A £48,500
   B £50,700
   C £48,000
   D £60,000
   E £41,000

4. **Colin's company budgeted £12 million for land, but more was needed and the costs rose to £15 million. How much extra land was needed?**
   A 1,000 m^2
   B 9,000 m^2
   C 10,000 m^2
   D 4,000 m^2
   E 2,500 m^2

Example 32

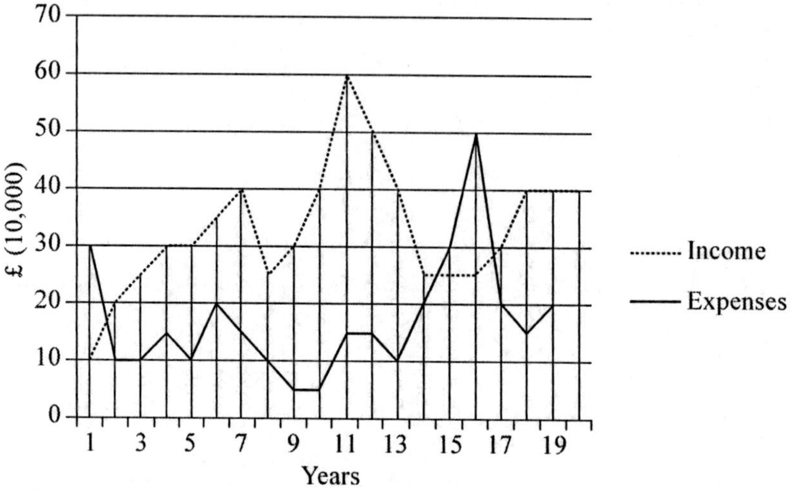

Below is the yearly income and expenses graph for a company in its first 20 years.

1. **What is the average yearly income of the company between its 11th and 20th years?**
   A £478,000
   B £300,000
   C £375,000
   D £278,000
   E £450,000

2. **In year 10, what fraction of the company's income was used up through that year's expenses?**
   A 1/10
   B 1/2
   C 1/6
   D 1/8
   E 3/7

3. **Which year saw the most profit?**
   A Year 10
   B Year 11
   C Year 20
   D Year 7
   E Year 13

4. **In which year did the company stop being in debt and start making genuine profits?**
   A Year 3
   B Year 4
   C Year 7
   D Year 2
   E Year 5

Example 33

Below is a table for 2009 showing the percentage of employees in different employment sectors that took sick days in the respective seasons. Floor has 5,247 employees, Warehouse has 1,184 employees, Management has 900 and Accounting has 1,000 employees.

	Spring	Summer	Autumn	Winter
Floor	5.3	1.6	1.1	3.2
Warehouse	6.2	3.7	0.2	2.1
Management	1.2	2.0	1.3	1.4
Accounting	4.2	3.8	3.7	4.1

1. **How many floor workers took sick days in the spring?**
   A 541
   B 278
   C 379
   D 167
   E 331

2. **How many sick days in 2009 were taken by Management in total?**
   A 42
   B 36
   C 40
   D 29
   E 53

3. **Which sector has the largest percentage of sick days taken in 2009?**
   A Floor
   B Warehouse
   C Management
   D Accounting
   E Can't tell

4. **Which season had the largest number of sick days taken in 2009?**
   A Spring
   B Summer
   C Autumn
   D Winter
   E Can't tell

Example 34

Here are the train times for a return ticket bought for a trip from Nottingham to Bedford and back. The journey length of Nottingham to Bedford is 100 miles, with Leicester lying 47 miles along that journey.

	Depart	Arrive	Stops
Nottingham – Bedford	14:15	15:30	0
Bedford – Nottingham	14:00	16:15	6

1. **What is the average speed of the train travelling from Nottingham to Bedford?**
   A 60 mph
   B 86 mph
   C 39 mph
   D 80 mph
   E 75 mph

2. **If both trains travel at the same speed, what is the duration of a stop?**
   A 10 minutes
   B 5 minutes
   C 20 minutes
   D 60 minutes
   E 15 minutes

3. **If the return journey did not have any stops, but had the same departure and arrival times, what would be the train's average speed?**
   A 40 mph
   B 44.44 mph
   C 38.65 mph
   D 29 mph
   E 33.25 mph

4. **On the outward journey, at what time does the train pass through Leicester?**
   - A 14:35
   - B 14:50
   - C 15:15
   - D 15:00
   - E 14:20

Example 35

Dale School is a school which encourages its students to study at least two languages. Below is a table showing the number of students studying one or two languages. There are also 50 students not accounted for on the table, who study three languages: French, German and Spanish.

	Only	French	Spanish	German	Italian
French	20		103	132	97
Spanish	30	103		140	82
German	15	132	140		73
Italian	10	97	82	73	

1. **Which language is most popular?**
   - A French
   - B Spanish
   - C German
   - D Italian
   - E Can't tell

2. **How many students study two languages?**
   - A 627
   - B 712
   - C 1,300
   - D 993
   - E 1,286

3. **How many students study at Dale School?**
   - A 1,450
   - B 679
   - C 1,286
   - D 752
   - E 543

4. **What percentage of students study both German and Spanish alone?**
   A 22.4%
   B 12.0%
   C 18.6%
   D 33.9%
   E 20.0%

Example 36

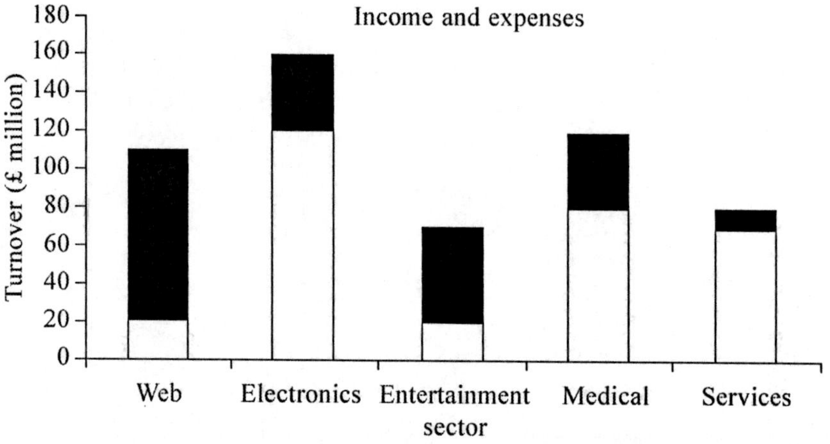

Below is a bar chart showing the income of sectors of the Globo.inc Company. The lower segment of each bar shows the proportion of that income needed for the expenses of running the sector.

1. **What is the total income of these Globo.inc sectors?**
   A £320 million
   B £650 million
   C £625 million
   D £510 million
   E £540 million

2. **Which sector has the largest profit?**
   A Web
   B Electronics
   C Entertainment
   D Medical
   E Services

3. **What are the total expenses of these Globo.inc sectors?**
   A £270 million
   B £400 million
   C £370 million
   D £310 million
   E £350 million

4. **What percentage of the Electronics sector income is used up by expenses?**
   A 0%
   B 25%
   C 50%
   D 75%
   E 100%

Example 37

Below are the results of a survey of 1,500 people asking whether car, motorcycle, bus or walking / cycling was their most used form of transport. It is known that for every kilometre travelled the average car produces 145 grams of CO_2 and the average motorcycle produces 85 grams of CO_2.

Transport type	% using it most
Bus	5
Walk / cycle	3
Cars	64
Motorcycle	28

1. **What number of those asked normally drove a car?**
   A 870
   B 1,000
   C 200
   D 960
   E 820

2. **If the motorcyclists drove an average of 18 km a day each, what would be their total CO_2 output for the week?**
   A 4.5 million grams
   B 1.2 million grams
   C 3.5 million grams
   D 6.6 million grams
   E 5.0 million grams

3. **How many times larger is the number of people that use a motorcycle than the number that take the bus?**
   A 4.3
   B 5.6
   C 3.2
   D 4.8
   E 5.3

4. **What is the difference in the number of people that take the bus to those that walk / cycle?**
   A 30
   B 100
   C 12
   D 86
   E 50

Example 38

Below are two equations. Equation 1 is for converting Fahrenheit to Celsius. Equation 2 is for converting Celsius to Kelvin.

(Eq °1)°C = $\frac{5 \times (°F - 32)}{9}$	(Eq^n 2) K = °C + 272

1. **Rearrange equation 1 to make °F the subject.**
   A °F = (°C × 5/9) – 32
   B °F = (5 × 9/°C) – 32
   C K = 5 × (°C – 32)/9
   D °F = (°C × 9/5) + 32
   E °F = (9 × 5/32) + °C

2. **Rearrange equation 2 to make °C the subject.**
   A °C = K + 272
   B °C = K – 272
   C °C = K × 272
   D °C = K/272
   E Can't be done

3. **What is 164°F in °C?**
   A 42.9 °C
   B 83.4 °C
   C 93.1 °C
   D 67.4 °C
   E 73.3 °C

4. What is 150°F in K?

A 821.7 K
B 496.1 K
C 333.3 K
D 784.6 K
E 337.6 K

Example 39

Equation 1 gives the final velocity of an object, where V is the final velocity, U is the initial velocity, a is the acceleration and S is the distance.

Equation 1: $V^2 = U^2 + 2aS$

1. What is V when U = 6, a = 8 and S = 4?

A 5
B 10
C 15
D 20
E 25

2. Rearrange the equation to make a the subject.

A $a = 2S - U + V^3$
B $a = (U^2 - V^2) \times 2S$
C $a = (V^2 - U^2)/2S$
D $a = (V^2/U^2) \times 4S$
E $a = 46$

3. Rearrange the equation to make S the subject.

A $S = 2a - U + V^3$
B $S = (U^2 - V^2) \times 2a$
C $S = (V^2 - U^2)/2a$
D $S = (V^2/U^2) \times 4a$
E $S = 75$

4. If V = 12, U = 8 and a = 8, what is S?

A 5
B 10
C 15
D 20
E 25

Example 40

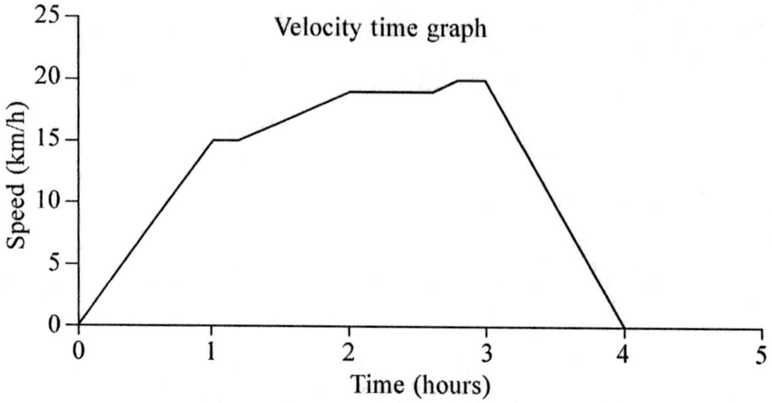

The graph below is a velocity time graph. The formula $S = ½at^2$ indicates the distance an accelerating object has moved if it started from a standstill, where S = distance, a = acceleration and t = time.

1. **How many times was the acceleration zero?**
   A 1
   B 2
   C 3
   D 4
   E 5

2. **What is the acceleration of the object for the first hour?**
   A 10 km/h^2
   B 15 km/h^2
   C 20 km/h^2
   D 25 km/h^2
   E 30 km/h^2

3. **What distance was travelled in the first hour of the graph?**
   A 15 km
   B 7.5 km
   C 14 km
   D 6.5 km
   E 5 km

4. **What is the acceleration shown by the graph between hours 3 and 4?**
   A -15 km/h^2
   B 15 km/h^2
   C -20 km/h^2
   D -10 km/h^2
   E Can't tell

Example 41

Below is an equation. It is known that raising something to the power of a half is the same as square rooting it.

$$X = \frac{(Y^2 + 9)}{A}$$

1. **Make Y the subject of the equation.**
   A $Y = (XA - 9)^{½}$
   B $Y = (X - A9)^2$
   C $Y = 9^2 - XA$
   D $Y = 9 - X^2A$
   E $Y = (X - 9A)^{½}$

2. **Make A the subject of the equation.**
   A $A = 9^2 - XY$
   B $A = 9 - X^2Y$
   C $A = (X - Y9)^2$
   D $A = (Y^2 + 9)/X$
   E $A = 9 - X^2Y^2$

3. **If X = 7, and A = 4, what is the value of Y?**
   A 15
   B 5.54
   C 8
   D 4.36
   E 19

4. **What is the value of X if Y = 13 and A = 16?**
   A 15
   B 12.15
   C 11.13
   D 8.20
   E 5

Example 42

A survey of 136,000 people in Bromham was taken, to understand what percentages of the population lived in which property type.

Type of property in Bromham	%
Flat	13
Terraced	23
Semi-detached	38
Detached	15
Bungalow	11

1. **How many people live in semi-detached properties in Bromham?**
   A 25,805
   B 51,680
   C 32,870
   D 18,632
   E 9,724

2. **How many people live in flats and terraced properties in Bromham?**
   A 25,805
   B 48,960
   C 32,870
   D 18,632
   E 9,724

3. **65% of people that live in bungalows are retired. How many people is that?**
   A 25,805
   B 51,680
   C 32,870
   D 18,632
   E 9,724

4. **70% of the people that live in flats and 20% of people that live in terraced properties are students. How many students is that?**
   A 25,805
   B 51,680
   C 32,870
   D 18,632
   E 9,724

Justifications of Quantitative Reasoning practice examples

Example 1

1. **The correct answer is B.**
   The recipe states that 2 tablespoons of olive oil are needed. The equivalent value in cups can be found in the table: **1/8 cup**.

2. **The correct answer is D.**
   The table shows that 3 teaspoons are 1/2 ounce. Dividing this by three will give the value for just one teaspoon.

   Ie (1/2) ÷ 3 = **1/6 ounce**.

3. **The correct answer is A.**
   We are told that a gram of water equals 1 millilitre. The table shows that 1/2 a cup is 113.4g, which is equivalent to 113.4ml. Therefore 2 cups = (1/2 cup) × 4 = 113.4ml × 4 = **453.6ml**. Answer A is the closest to this value.

4. **The correct answer is D.**
   The recipe given is for four people. 9 ÷ 4 = 2.25, so amounts must be multiplied by 2.25 to find the quantity required for nine people. 1 pound of flour × 2.25 = 2.25 pounds of flour required.

   To convert this into grams: the table shows that 1 pound = 2 cups. It also shows that ½ cup = 113.4g. So 1 pound = 113.4 × 4 = 453.6g.

   Therefore the total grams needed are 453.6 × 2.25 = **1,020.6g**. Answer D is the closest to this value.

Example 2

1. **The correct answer is B.**
   Multiply the number of hours per day each shop is open by the number of days each shop is open and add them all together.
   Ie (10 × 3) + (3 × 5) + (6 × 7) + (8 × 6) + (7 × 6) = **177 hours**

2. **The correct answer is C.**
   Multiply Claire's hourly rate by Shop 1's total open hours per day and number of open days per week. Do the same for Richard, then add the two values together.
   Ie £9.65 × 10 × 3 = £289.50
   £7.90 × 8 × 6 = £379.20
   £289.50 + £379.20 = **£668.70**

3. **The correct answer is E.**
   Multiply the number of hours each shop is open by its total number of employees, and then by the number of days the shop is open each week.
   Ie Shop 1 10 × 3 × 7 = 210 hours
   Shop 2 3 × 5 × 4 = 60 hours
   Shop 3 6 × 7 × 3 = 126 hours
   Shop 4 8 × 5 × 6 = 240 hours
   Shop 5 7 × 6 × 6 = **252 hours**

4. **The correct answer is A.**
   Multiply each shop's open hours by their respective number of workers, and then add them all together.
   Ie (10 × 7) + (3 × 4) + (6 × 3) + (8 × 5) + (7 × 6) = **182 hours**

Example 3

1. **The correct answer is D.**
   Find the average by adding up the possible prices, then dividing that by the number of prices.

   Ie (£400 + £500 + £600 + £490) ÷ 4 = **£497.50**

2. **The correct answer is A.**
   When excluding company group discount and postage and packaging, the cheapest option is to mix and match the cheapest items from each company or his friend.

   Ie (£180 + £400 + £150 + £80) = **£810**

3. **The correct answer is C.**
   To find the total price of each company's offer, first add the respective prices of each of the components together. Then apply the percentage discount. Then add on postage and packaging.

Ie Global Computers	((£300 + £400 + £200 + £80) × 1) + 0 = £980.00
Power Computers	((£250 + £500 + £170 + £100) × 0.7) + £70 = £784.00
Computer World	**((£180 + £600 + £210 + £110) × 0.6) + £100 = £760.00**
Electronic Ltd	((£270 + £490 + £150 + £100) × 0.75) + £10 = £767.50

4. **The correct answer is A.**
   Add the respective prices of each of the components together excluding the price of the processor to find the cheapest option.

Ie **Global Computers**	**£300 + £400 + £80 = £780**
Power Computers	£250 + £500 + £100 = £850
Computer World	£180 + £600 + £110 = £890
Electronic Ltd	£270 + £490 + £100 = £860

Example 4

1. **The correct answer is B.**
   First the total number of males needs to be calculated:

   12,100 + 14,200 + 25,600 + 19,000 + 37,000 = 107,900
   The number of males aged 19 or younger is:

   12,100 + 14,200 = 26,300

   The % of males aged 19 or younger is:

   (26,300 ÷ 107,900) × 100 = **24%** (to the nearest whole number)

2. **The correct answer is B.**
   From question 1, we already know the total number of males:

   12,100 + 25,600 + 14,200 + 19,000 + 37,000 = 107,900

   As there are 10% more females than males, the total number of females can be calculated as:

   107,900 × 1.1 = 118,690

   Therefore the total population is:
   107,900 + 118,690 = 226,590 = **227,000** (to the nearest thousand)

3. **The correct answer is C.**

   Males aged 51 and over: 37,000

   Males aged under 51:

   19,000 + 25,600 + 14,200 + 12,100 = 70,900

   Calculate the ratio as follows:

   70,900 ÷ 37,000 = 1.92

   There are almost twice as many males under 51 as over 51. Therefore the ratio of males over 51 to males under 51 is **1:2** (to the nearest whole number).

4. **The correct answer is D.**
Number of males aged 35 or under:

25,600 + 14,200 + 12,100 = 51,900

As there are 10% more females, the number of females aged 35 or under is:

51,900 × 1.1 = **57,090**

Example 5

1. **The correct answer is E.**
Companies with 39 employees or fewer in 2006 are:

80 + 90 = 170,000

Calculate all companies in 2006 as:

80 + 90 + 55 + 15 = 240,000

The percentage of companies with 39 or fewer in 2006 is therefore:
(170 ÷ 240) × 100 = **71%** (to the nearest whole number)

2. **The correct answer is A.**
Companies with 1 to 20 employees decreased by 15, whereas companies with 21 to 39 employees decreased by 10. Therefore:
(15 + 10) ÷ 2 = 12.5, or **12,500** as the data is given in thousands.

3. **The correct answer is A.**
The total number of companies in 2006 is 240,000, as we know from question 1.
Calculate the total number of companies surveyed in 2007 as:

65 + 80 + 45 + 10 = 200,000

Calculate how many fewer companies were surveyed in 2007:

240,000 – 200,000 = 40,000

The percentage decrease is therefore:

(40,000 ÷ 240,000) × 100 = **17%** (to the nearest whole number)

4. **The correct answer is B.**
Subtract 2007 from 2006, and calculate the difference as a fraction of the 2006 figure:
(15 – 10 = 5) ÷ 15 = **1/3**

Example 6

1. **The correct answer is C.**
   Bamber: 18 + 16 + 27 + 27 + 24 + 24 + 25 = 161 ÷ 7 = 23
   Tillitia: 10 + 11 + 6 + 3 + 4 + 3 + 1 = 38 ÷ 7 = 5.4
   Syncroy: 4 + 8 + 5 + 5 + 8 + 2 + 2 = 34 ÷ 7 = 4.9
   Calculate the mean average daily temperature between the three locations as:

   (23 + 5.4 + 4.9 = 33.3) ÷ 3 = 11.1°C

   As 1°C = 3°F, the average temperature in °F is:
   11.1 × 3 = **33.3°F**, which is closest to answer C.

2. **The correct answer is D.**
   The middle value of the sequence is 5: (4, 5, 5, **5**, 7, 8, 8).
   But Billerton's readings must be increased by 20% to correct for the calibration error mentioned in the question:

   5 × 1.2 = **6 °C**

3. **The correct answer is C.**
   The total of all temperatures on Tuesday, with calibration adjustments shown, is:

   24 + 16 + 8 + 22 + 11 + 48 (40 + 20%) + 21 + 6 (5 + 20%) = 156

   Divide by 8 locations to obtain the mean average: 19.5, or **20** to the nearest whole number.

4. **The correct answer is E.**
   The range is calculated by subtracting the lowest value from the highest value:

   Timber = 32 – 22 = 10

   Tillitia = 11 – 1 = 10

   Bamber = 27 – 16 = 11

   Syncroy = 8 – 2 = 6

   Lambert = 41 – 12 = 29

Example 7

1. **The correct answer is D.**
   The population of Bacterium B at 96 hours is 20,000. The population of Bacterium A at 96 hours is 15,000. The difference at 96 hours is therefore **5,000**.

2. **The correct answer is C.**
   From the graph, the population change in Bacterium B over the period is from 10,000 to 20,000, ie a 10,000 increase.
   The percentage growth therefore = (10,000 increase ÷ 10,000) × 100 = **100%**

3. **The correct answer is C.**
   Bacterium A: difference in growth = 10,000
   Bacterium B: difference in growth = 10,000
   Bacterium C: difference in growth = **15,000**

4. **The correct answer is A.**
   15,000 + 20,000 + 30,000 = **65,000** bacteria in total.

Example 8

1. **The correct answer is D.**
   £120 × 4 = 480 Egyptian Pounds on a weekday
   £120 × 4.5 = 540 Egyptian Pounds on a weekend
   The difference = **60 less**

2. **The correct answer is C.**
   200 US Dollars ÷ 1.5 = 133.33 – £3 surcharge = £130.33
   350 Canadian Dollars ÷ 3 = 116.67 – £3 surcharge = £113.67
   £130.33 + £113.67 = **£244** (to the nearest whole number)

3. **The correct answer is D.**
   £380 × 1.2 Euros = **456 Euros**

4. **The correct answer is A.**
   £1 converts to 4 Egyptian Pounds on a weekday. The ratio is therefore **1:4**

Example 9

1. **The correct answer is E.**
   Calculate:

   10°C (Monday) + 14 °C (Tuesday) + 12 °C (Wednesday) + 18 °C (Thursday) + 22 °C (Friday) = 76

   Then divide 76 by 5 (days) to reach the answer of: **15.2**

2. **The correct answer is C.**
Friday was the warmest day at 22 °C. Sunday was the coldest day at 8 °C.
The difference is therefore:

22 °C – 8 °C = **14 °C**

3. **The correct answer is D.**
From question 1, we know that Monday to Friday temperatures totalled 76. Therefore:

76 + 20 (Sat) + 8 (Sun) = 104 as a total for the week.

Divide by 7 to arrive at a daily average of 14.9 °C.

To convert to °F:

14.9 × 3 = 44.57, or **45 °F** to the nearest whole number.

4. **The correct answer is A.**
The difference in temperature between Saturday and Sunday is 20 – 8 = 12°C.
To calculate the difference as a percentage:

(12 ÷ 20) × 100 = **60%**

Example 10

1. **The correct answer is C.**
The total number of students is 913. There were 37 absent students, making 876 who took part in the survey. 300 students played rugby. Calculate the percentage who played rugby as follows:

(300 ÷ 876) × 100 = **34.2%**

2. **The correct answer is A.**
580 students played hockey in 1999. 2009 saw a 20% increase in participation, so:

(580 × 1.2) = **696**

3. **The correct answer is E.**
Add the participation in each sport:
430 (football) + 210 (cricket) + 580 (hockey) + 80 (badminton) + 300 (rugby) = 1,600.
Divide 1,600 by 5 to arrive at the average of **320**

4. **The correct answer is B.**
The number of pupils playing cricket in 2009 is an increase of 20% since 1999. Therefore:

$210 \times 1.2 = 252$ players

25 out of those 252 will be selected, which to the nearest whole number gives a **10% chance.**

Example 11

1. **The correct answer is B.**
Company A: 1980 turnover = £300 million. 2000 turnover = £160 million. Difference = –£140 million.
Company B: 1980 turnover = £240 million. 2000 turnover = £350 million. Difference = **£110 million.**
Company C: 1980 turnover = £160 million. 2000 turnover = £200 million. Difference = £40 million.
Company D: 1980 turnover = £60 million. 2000 turnover = £150 million. Difference = £90 million.

2. **The correct answer is A.**
Company A: 2010 turnover = £90 million
Company B: 2010 turnover = £350 million
Company C: 2010 turnover = £220 million
Company D: 2010 turnover = £200 million
The total is therefore £860 million or **£860,000,000**

3. **The correct answer is C.**
For Company A:
£250m + £300m + £200m + £160m + £90m = £1,000 million
For Company D:
£60m + £60m + £40m + £150m + £200m = £510 million
Therefore: £1000m – £510m = **£490 million**

4. **The correct answer is D.**
Company D showed the greatest growth (£50 million) in the period.

Example 12

1. **The correct answer is B.**
Calculate as follows:
Chillwells: 10 hours (Tuesday) + 10 hours (Saturday) = 20 hours
Multimedia: 10 hours (Tuesday) + 0 hours (Saturday) = 10 hours
Wollards: 8 hours (Tuesday) + 6 hours (Saturday) = 14 hours
Total hours open are therefore: 20 + 10 + 14 = **44 hours**

2. **The correct answer is C.**
   Calculate as follows:
   Weekday = (8 hours – 1 hour = 7 hours) × 5 days = 35 hours
   Saturday = 8 hours
   Sunday = 8 hours
   Therefore the total is 35 + 8 + 8 = **51 hours** per week

3. **The correct answer is B.**
   The most frequent opening time is **8.00.**

4. **The correct answer is C.**
   From question 2, we know that Gymtastic is open for 51 hours per week.
   Multimedia is open for: 10 hours × 5 days = 50 hours
   Gymtastic is therefore open for 1 hour (**60 minutes**) more than Multimedia each week.

Example 13

1. **The correct answer is C.**
   The months with the highest recorded rainfall on Continent 1 were in May and June with 300 mm.

2. **The correct answer is C.**
   Add the figures for each month:
   20 mm + 80 mm + 120 mm + 180 mm + 300 mm + 300 mm = 1,000 mm or **1 metre**.

3. **The correct answer is A.**
   Continent 2 had 200 mm of rain in March, whereas Continent 1 had 120 mm.
   Divide 200 by 120 to arrive at 1.666. To two decimal places, the ratio is therefore **1.67:1**.

4. **The correct answer is E.**
   April's rainfall was 200 mm, January's 100 mm. The difference is therefore **100 mm**.

Example 14

1. **The correct answer is D.**
   The earliest tram that can be taken is the 08.06 from Ardefield which arrives in the City Centre at **08:28**.

2. **The correct answer is A.**
   Starting in Jameson at 07:22, arriving at the City Centre at 07:38, is a journey of **16 minutes.**

3. **The correct answer is A.**
   Four trams would have successfully terminated at the City Centre, therefore 4 × 48 = **192 passengers.**

4. **The correct answer is E.**
   Six trams leave Ardefield before 08:00 on a weekday. (Since 0 is not one of the possible answers, it can be assumed that the question does not refer to weekends.)

Example 15

1. **The correct answer is D.**
   Stock 4: 18p – 7p = an **11p increase** in value.

2. **The correct answer is B.**
   The relevant values in order are: 7p, 12p, **16p, 18p,** 43p, 99p.
   The median value lies between 16 and 18, and is therefore **17p.**

3. **The correct answer is E.**
   Stock 5: 99p – 43p = a **56p decrease** in value.

4. **The correct answer is A.**
   Add the values of present day stocks: 23p + 35p + 12p + 18p + 43p + 21p = 152
   Divide by 6, giving **25.33p.**

Example 16

1. **The correct answer is E.**
   Add together the fours students' marks in Geography and divide by 4:

   (67 + 45 + 57 + 54 = 223) ÷ 4 = 55.75

   From the second table, it can be seen that this is equivalent to **Grade C.**

2. **The correct answer is B.**
   While students A and B scored marks that were equivalent to A and B grades, Students C and D scored 54 and 59 respectively, both equivalent to **D Grades** and therefore the answer is false.

3. **The correct answer is E.**
   Student D scored A grades in **Maths, Design and Business Studies**.

4. **The correct answer is A.**
   Student D scored 93% in **Maths**.

Example 17

1. **The correct answer is C.**
   Calculate the total actual voters:

   23,400 (Conservative) + 14,400 (Labour) + 6,400 (Liberal) + 1,300 (Green Party) + 400 (Other) = 45,900 voters in 2002.
   Calculate the total number of eligible voters (72% of the total population):
   136,345 × 0.72 = 98,168.4

   Calculate the percentage of the eligible voters who did vote:
   (45,900 ÷ 98,168.4) × 100 = 46.8 or **47% voter turnout** (to the nearest whole number).

2. **The correct answer is C.**
   From question 1, we know that there were 45,900 voters in 2002. Calculate 1,300 Green Party votes as a percentage of 45,900.
   (1,300 ÷ 45,900) × 100 = **2.83%**

3. **The correct answer is C.**
   From 1, we know total actual voters were 45,900 in 2002. The question states that the total voter turnout was 8% lower in 1996.
   Therefore:

   1996 turnout = 45,900 × (100% – 8%)

   1996 turnout = 45,900 × 0.92 = 42,228, or **42,000** (to the nearest 1,000).

4. **The correct answer is A.**
   As we know, there were 45,900 voters in 2002. Calculate the Conservative percentage of the vote:

   (23,400 ÷ 45,900) × 100 = 50.98%.

   Calculate the Labour percentage of the vote:

   (14,400 ÷ 45,900) × 100 = 31.37%

   Therefore the margin between the parties was:

   50.98% – 31.37% = **19.61%**

Example 18

1. **The correct answer is E.**
   Point E Tuesday average measurement: 30 + 25 + 20 = 75 ÷ 3 = 25 knots.
   Convert knots to m/s:

   25 × 25 = 625 m/s

   Tuesday's wind speed is 1/3 lower, hence:

   Tuesday w/s = 2 ÷ 3 × Monday w/s

   So Monday = 3 ÷ 2 × 625 = 937.5 = **937** (to the nearest whole number)

2. **The correct answer is A.**
   Point C: (0 + 20 + 20) ÷ 3 = **13 knots (to 2 significant figures).**

3. **The correct answer is D.**
   Quickest wind speed = 20 knots
   Slowest wind speed = 0 knots
   20 knots × 25 = **500 knots**

4. **The correct answer is E.**
   The highest average wind speed was recorded at Point E.
   30 + 25 + 20 = 75 ÷ 3 = **25 knots**

Example 19

1. **The correct answer is C.**
   The most frequent temperature was 16°C:
   16, 16, 19, 23, 24, 30

2. **The correct answer is B.**
   29 knots (Portsmouth) – 17 knots (Bognor Regis) = **12 knots**

3. **The correct answer is E.**
   Tourism Index for Plymouth: 16 × 5 × 33 = 2640.
   July temperature is 12% more than June, hence:
   June = 2640 ÷ 1.12 = **2357 (to the nearest whole number).**

4. **The correct answer is D.**
   Bognor Regis: 19 × 6 × 17 = 1938
   Brighton: 23 × 7 × 27 = 4347
   Bournemouth: 16 × 5 × 35 = 2800
   Plymouth: 16 × 5 × 33 = 2640
   Portsmouth: 24 × 7 × 29 = 4872
   Exeter: 30 × 10 × 15 = 4500

Example 20

1. **The correct answer is E.**
   Runner B 20 mph – Runner A 16 mph = **4 mph**

2. **The correct answer is A.**
   The average speed of Runner A in the 51–60 metre segment of the race was **12 mph.**

3. **The correct answer is C.**
   6 + 8 + 10 + 12 + 14 = 50 ÷ 5 = **10 mph**

4. **The correct answer is A.**
   14 mph × 5 = **70 m/s**

Example 21

1. **The correct answer is C.**
   Calculate the time it takes to drive 1 mile at the applicable speed for each of the various road sections, and then multiply by the corresponding number of miles:

   For the motorway: 60 mins ÷ 60 mph = 1 minute per mile × 4 minutes = 4 minutes

   For the double carriageway: 60 mins ÷ 40 mph = 1.5 minutes per mile × 6 miles = 9 minutes

   For the single carriageway: 60 mins ÷ 30 mph = 2 minutes per mile × 4 miles = 8 minutes.

   Therefore: 06:50 – 4 – 9 – 8 = **06.29 am** is the latest the coach can leave.

2. **The correct answer is D.**
   Each one-way trip is 14 miles long, and the coach makes 10 trips per week, thus the amount of fuel consumed per week is:

   (14 miles × 10 trips = 140 miles) ÷ 10 mpg = 14 gallons

   14 gallons × £6 = **£84**

3. **The correct answer is B.**
   Think of the question in terms of trigonometry. The town and the factory are two of the corners of a right-angled triangle, and the direct road between the two will follow the hypotenuse. The length of the road can be calculated using Pythagoras' Theorem:

   $\sqrt{(x^2 + y^2)} = z$

   The total distance travelled south (x) = 4 + 4 = 8 miles. The total distance travelled west (y) = 6 miles.
   The length of a direct carriageway would therefore be:

   $\sqrt{(8^2 + 6^2)} = \sqrt{100} = 10$ miles

   We know that the average speed on a dual carriageway is 40 mph, thus the time of the commute is:

   60 ÷ 40 × 10 miles = 15 minutes

   The time saved on each trip will thus be 21 minutes (see first question) – 15 minutes = **6 mins.**

4. **The correct answer is C.**
   The journey is now 4 miles shorter, giving a saving of:
   4 (miles) ÷ 10 (mpg) × 10 (journeys per week) × £6 (per gallon) = **£24** per week

Example 22

1. **The correct answer is E.**
   Trousers: (£12.99 × 15) – (£5.43 × 15) = £113.40
   Baseball caps: (£4.99 × 10) – (£1.45 × 10) = £35.40
   Shoes: (£14.99 × 3) – (£8.51 × 3) = £19.44
   Now calculate total gross profit:
   £113.40 + £35.40 + £19.44 = £168.24 = **£168** (to the nearest pound)

2. **The correct answer is A.**
   £6.99 – £2.83 = £4.16 ÷ £6.99 × 100 = **59.5%**

3. **The correct answer is B.**
   Hat: £1.99 × 5 = £9.95
   Skirt: £4.31 × 10 = £43.10
   5 hats and 10 skirts:
   £9.95 + £43.10 = **£53.05**

4. **The correct answer is E.**
   Trainers: £19.99
   Hat: £2.99
   Difference = **£17**

Example 23

1. **The correct answer is A.**
   KS3 comprises Years 7, 8, and 9.
   The total number of pupils refers to both boys and girls:

   154 + 161 + 141 + 170 + 122 + 181 = **929**

2. **The correct answer is C.**
   Percentage of girls in KS4 = (total no. girls in KS4 ÷ total no. pupils in KS4) × 100:
   [(80 + 150) ÷ (80 + 150 + 220 + 150)] × 100 = 38.333 = **38** to the nearest whole number

3. **The correct answer is E.**
   Compulsory education refers to KS3 and KS4.
   Total pupils refers to both boys and girls.
   Therefore:

   154 + 161 + 141 + 170 + 122 + 181 + 80 + 220 + 150 + 150 = **1,529**

4. **The correct answer is D.**
   Ratio of males to females = No. males : No. females:
   220:80 = **11:4**

Example 24

1. **The correct answer is A.**
   Each bar represents the number of hours worked on average per day in each factory. **Factory 1** has the highest bar with 8 hours per day.

2. **The correct answer is C.**
   Ben: 4 hours per day × £8.60 × 5 days per week = £172
   Mark: 6 hours per day × £7.50 × 5 days per week = £225
   Calculate the difference between Ben's wages and Mark's wages:

   £225 – £172 = **£53**

3. **The correct answer is C.**
   The data only refers to weekdays, therefore we are unable to answer the question for weekends.

4. **The correct answer is E.**
   8 hours at Factory 1 × 3 days per week = 24 hours. 2 hours at Factory 5 × 2 days per week = 4 hours. Total hours are therefore 28.
   Multiply by £9.40, and then by 4 weeks in the lunar month:

   28 × £9.40 × 4 = **£1,052.80**

Example 25

1. **The correct answer is A.**
   Calculate total net profit:

   101 + 98 + 50 + 63 + 37 = £349 million

   Find what percentage 98 million is of 349 million. This is calculated by:

   (98 ÷ 349) × 100 = **28.1%**

2. **The correct answer is E.**
   For each vehicle we must calculate the profit gained per vehicle sold. This is calculated by dividing the net profit for that type of vehicle by the number of vehicles sold.

   Once this has been calculated for each category we can see that motorbikes provide the highest profit per unit, which is equal to **£34,774.40.**

3. **The correct answer is A.**
   The difference in sales = 5,272 – 5,021 = 251
   % decrease = (251 ÷ 5,272) × 100 = **4.76%**

4. **The correct answer is A.**
   In order to arrive at this we must calculate how many 4 × 4's must be sold to produce £37 million. We must first calculate how much profit is made by the sale of one 4 × 4.

   63,000,000 ÷ 2,880 = £21,875 per 4 × 4

   We then divide 37 million by this number to arrive at the answer.
   £37,000,000 ÷ £21,875 = 1,691.43 or **1,692** to cover the loss.

Example 26

1. **The correct answer is B.**
   Sum the revenue from the middle two quarters:

   £27,200 + £90,100 = **£117,300**

2. **The correct answer is B.**
   To calculate the average of the final three quarters, first sum the revenue from the final three quarters:

   £27,200 + £90,100 + £20,900 = £138,200

   Then divide the total amount by three to calculate the mean average for the three quarters:

   £138,200 ÷ 3 = **£46,067** (to the nearest pound)

3. **The correct answer is C.**
To find the percentage increase we first find the difference in revenue between quarters 1 and 2, which is:

£27,200 – £20,900 = £6,300

We then calculate the % increase:

(£6,300 ÷ £20,900) × 100 = **30.1%** (to 1 decimal place)

4. **The correct answer is C.**
To find the proportion of the revenue earned in the fourth quarter, we first find the total revenue earned over the four quarters, which is:

£27,200 + £20,900 + £20,900 + £90,100 = £159,100

Then we divide the revenue from the fourth quarter by the total revenue for all four quarters, which is:

£20,900 ÷ £159,100 = **0.13** (to 2 decimal places)

Example 27

1. **The correct answer is C.**
Decrease in profits = £500,000 – £400,000 = £100,000
Decrease as a percentage = (100,000 ÷ 500,000) × 100 = **20%**

2. **The correct answer is B.**
£400,000 – £300,000 = **£100,000**

3. **The correct answer is B.**
£700,000 + £200,000 + £600,000 + £400,000 = **£1,900,000**

4. **The correct answer is A.**
The question does not require information from the graph provided.
Time = Distance/Speed:
Driver A: 400 ÷ 50 = 8 hours
Driver B: 400 ÷ 80 = 5 hours
The difference between the two is 3 hours, which equals **180 minutes**

Example 28

1. **The correct answer is C.**
2 + 7 + 11 + 22 = **42**

2. **The correct answer is A.**
Number of children 70–130cm:

2 + 7 + 11 = 20

Total number of children = 50

20 ÷ 50 = **2/5**

3. **The correct answer is D.**
Number of children 131 cm or taller:

22 + 6 + 2 = 30

Total number of children = 50

(30 ÷ 50) × 100 = **60%**

4. **The correct answer is B.**
Number of pupils 110cm or taller: 2 + 7 = 9
A 33% increase is 9 × 1.33 = 3
Therefore total number of pupils =
9 + 3 = **12**

Example 29

1. **The correct answer is B.**
125 × 35 ÷ 100 = **43.75cm**

2. **The correct answer is E.**
The diameter of the circles is equal to x = 125 cm. The radius = 62.5 cm.
The area of the 3 circles is therefore:

$(\pi \times r^2) \times 3 = \mathbf{36,815.54\ cm^2}$

3. **The correct answer is E.**
Area of triangle = ½(base × height)
Base = z + 2y, height = w
Area = ½((z +2y)w)

$$\text{Area} = \frac{w(z + 2y)}{2}$$

4. **The correct answer is E.**
The length of t can be calculated using Pythagoras' theorem:

$t^2 = y^2 + v^2$

$t^2 = 110^2 + 40^2$

$t^2 = 13{,}700$

t = **117.05** (to 2 decimal places)

Example 30

1. **The correct answer is C.**
Squash is the activity with the highest number of participants, a total of **467.**

2. **The correct answer is D.**
Thursday saw the highest number of individuals participating in all activities: **414.**

3. **The correct answer is C.**
Monday: 85 (badminton) + 102 (squash) + 23 (karate) = 210
Thursday: 89 (badminton) + 156 (squash) + 12 (karate) = 257
Difference between Monday and Thursday:

257 – 210 = **47**

4. **The correct answer is D.**
The activity of judo saw the second lowest number of participants over the course of the week: **81.**

Example 31

1. **The correct answer is D.**
First convert 32 inches into cm then square it:

32 inches × 2.54 = 81.28cm

$81.28^2 = 6{,}606.4\text{cm}^{2.}$

6,606cm^2 is therefore the closest answer.

2. **The correct answer is A.**
Convert the distance from km to miles, then divide by one hour:

100 km/1.61 = 62.1 miles

62.1 miles/1 hour = **62.1mph**

3. **The correct answer is C.**
   Multiply $16m^2$ by £3,000/m^2:
   $16m^2$ × £3,000/m^2 = **£48,000**

4. **The correct answer is A.**
   Divide the difference in the two prices by the cost of one metre squared:

   (£15,000,000 – £12,000,000)/(£3,000/m^2) = **1,000m^2**

Example 32

1. **The correct answer is C.**
   Add up the income from years 11 to 20, and then divide by 10 to find the average income:
   (60 + 50 + 40 + 25 + 25 + 25 + 30 + 40 + 40 + 40) × £10,000 = £3,750,000
   £3,750,000/10 = **£375,000**

2. **The correct answer is D.**
   Read off the graph the income and expenses for year 10. Then find the fraction by dividing the expense by the income:
   eg £50,000/£400,000 = **1/8**

3. **The correct answer is B.**
   The single year with the most profit is that with the biggest positive difference between income and expenses. From the graph, this is **year 11** (income £600,000, expenses £150,000) with a profit of £450,000.

4. **The correct answer is A.**
   Add up the income and expenses of each year until the total income is greater than the total expense.

Year	1	2	3	4
Total income	10	30	***55***	85
Total expense	30	40	***50***	65

Example 33

1. **The correct answer is B.**
   Divide the number of floor workers by 100 to find 1% of employees, then multiply by the percentage of sick days taken in spring.
   5,247 ÷ 100 = 52.47
   52.47 × 5.3 = **278.091**, to which B is the closest available answer.

2. **The correct answer is E.**
Divide the number of floor workers by 100 then multiply by the percentage of sick days taken in spring. Repeat this for summer, winter and autumn. Then add all together.
900 ÷ 100 = 9
For spring = 9 × 1.2 = 10.8
For summer = 9 × 2.0 = 18
For autumn = 9 × 1.3 = 11.7
For winter = 9 × 1.4 = 12.6
Total = 10.8 + 18 + 11.7 + 12.6 = **53.1**, to which E is the closest available answer.

3. **The correct answer is D.**
Add the percentages for each sector over the whole year and divide by 4 to find the sector with the highest average percentage:
For **Accounting**:

4.2 + 3.8 + 3.7 + 4.1 = 15.8

15.8 ÷ 4 = 3.95%

4. **The correct answer is A.**
Find the number of sick days for each sector in each season. Add up for a season total.
For **Spring:**

Floor (5,247 ÷ 100) × 5.3 = 278.1

Warehouse (1,184 ÷ 100) × 6.2 = 73.4

Management (900 ÷ 100) × 1.2 = 10.8

Accounting (1,000 ÷ 100) 4.2 = 42

Total = 278.1 + 73.4 + 10.8 + 42 = 404.3

Example 34

1. **The correct answer is D.**
Divide the distance by the number of hours taken to find the speed in mph:
The journey time is 75 minutes = 1.25 hours
Distance is 100 miles.
100 miles ÷ 1.25 hours = **80mph**

2. **The correct answer is A.**
   Find the time difference in the two journeys, then divide that by the number of stops.
   135 minutes – 75 minutes = 60 minutes
   60 minutes ÷ 6 = **10 minutes**

3. **The correct answer is B.**
   Divide the distance by the number of hours taken to find the speed in mph:
   The journey time is 135 minutes = 2.25 hours
   Distance is 100 miles.
   Speed = 100 ÷ 2.25 = **44.44mph**

4. **The correct answer is B.**
   Find the time it takes for the train to travel 47 miles, then add that time to the departure time:

   Time = distance ÷ speed

   47 miles ÷ 80mph = 0.5875 hours (× 60 to convert into minutes) = 35.25 minutes, which is treated as 35 minutes.

   14:15 + 35 minutes = **14:50**

Example 35

1. **The correct answer is C.**
   Find the sum of all students studying a particular language, ignoring repeats. Then compare each language.

   For German:
   15 (German alone) + 132 (German and French) + 140 (German and Spanish) + 73 (German and Italian) + 50 (French, German and Spanish) = **410**

2. **The correct answer is A.**
   Find the sum of the values in the table that represent a class of students studying 2 languages making sure to ignore repeats.

   103 (French and Spanish) + 132 (French and German) + 140 (Spanish and German) + 97 (French and Italian) + 82 (Spanish and Italian) + 73 (German and Italian) = **627**

3. **The correct answer is D.**
   Find the sum of all students that study one language with the students that study two and three languages.

   One language = (20 + 30 + 15 + 10) = 75
   Two languages = (103 + 132 + 140 + 97 + 82 + 73) = 627
   Three languages = 50
   Total = 75 + 627 + 50 = **752**

4. **The correct answer is C.**
   Find the number of students that study only German and Spanish, ignoring the repeat. Divide this by the number of students in total, then multiply by 100 to find the percentage.
   Number of pupils who study German and Spanish = 140
   Number of students in total = 752
   (140 ÷ 752) × 100 = **18.6%**

Example 36

1. **The correct answer is E.**
   Add up the income from each sector.
   £110m + £160m + £70m + £120m + £80m = **£540 million**

2. **The correct answer is A.**
   The bar chart shows that Web has the largest profit.

3. **The correct answer is D.**
   Add up the expenses of each sector.
   £20 million + £120 million + £20 million + £80 million + £70 million = **£310 million**

4. **The correct answer is D.**
   Divide the expenses by the income and multiply by 100 to find the percentage.
   (120 ÷ 160) × 100 = **75%**

Example 37

1. **The correct answer is D.**
   Divide the total number of people that were surveyed by 100 and then multiply by 64.
   (1,500 ÷ 100) × 64 = **960**

2. **The correct answer is A.**
   Find the output of one motorcyclist for the week. Then multiply it by the number of motorcyclists surveyed.
   CO_2 output for one motorcyclist for a week = 18 × 85 × 7 = 10,710 grams
   Total number of motorcyclists = (1,500 ÷ 100) × 28 = 420
   Total CO_2 output for week = 420 × 10,710 = **4.5 million grams**

3. **The correct answer is B.**
   Divide the percentage of motorcyclists by the percentage of those that take the bus.
   28 ÷ 5 = **5.6**

4. **The correct answer is A.**
   Find the percentage difference between the two. Divide this number by 100 and multiply by the number of people surveyed.
   5% – 3% = 2%.
   (2 ÷ 100) × 1,500 = **30**

Example 38

1. **The correct answer is D.**
   Multiply both sides by 9; divide both sides by 5; and then finally add 32 to both sides.

   °C = (5 × (°F – 32))/9

   °C × 9 = 5 × (°F – 32)

   °C × 9/5 = °F – 32

   (°C × 9/5) + 32 = °F

2. **The correct answer is B.**
   Take 272 from both sides.

   K = °C + 272.

   K – 272 = °C

3. **The correct answer is E.**
   Substitute given values into equation 1 and calculate.
   5/9 × (164 – 32) = **73.3 °C**

4. **The correct answer is E.**
   Substitute the given value into equation 1 and calculate the value in °C. Then substitute this value into equation 2 and calculate.
   To convert °F to °C: 5/9 × (150 – 32) = 65.6 °C.
   Substitute °C into equation 2: 65.6 °C + 272 = **337.6 K**

Example 39

1. **The correct answer is B.**
   Substitute the values given into the equation and calculate:

   $V^2 = 6^2 + (2 \times 8 \times 4)$

   $V^2 = 100$

   $\mathbf{V = 10}$

2. **The correct answer is C.**
   Minus U^2 then divide by 2S.

   $V^2 = U^2 + 2aS$

   $V^2 - U^2 = 2aS$

   $\mathbf{(V^2 - U^2)/2S = a}$

3. **The correct answer is C.**
   Minus U^2 then divide by 2a.

   $V^2 = U^2 + 2aS$

   $V^2 - U^2 = 2aS$

   $\mathbf{(V^2 - U^2)/2a = S}$

4. **The correct answer is A.**
   Rearrange the equation to make S the subject then substitute in the given values and calculate.

   $S = (V^2 - U^2)/2a$

   $S = (12^2 - 8^2) \div (2 \times 8)$

   $\mathbf{S = 5}$

Example 40

1. **The correct answer is C.**
   Simply count the number of times the graph is horizontal (where there is no change in speed).

2. **The correct answer is B.**
   Acceleration is the change in speed over the change in time.
   15 km/h ÷ 1 hour = **15 km/h**$^{\mathbf{2}}$

3. **The correct answer is B.**
Use the graph to gather values and substitute them into the equation given and calculate.

$S = 0.5 \times 15 \times 1^2$

$S = \mathbf{7.5\ km}$

4. **The correct answer is C.**
Acceleration is the change is speed over the change in time:

$-20\ \text{km/h} \div 1\ \text{hour} = \mathbf{-20\ km/h^2}$

Example 41

1. **The correct answer is A.**
First multiply both sides by A, then take 9 from both sides, finally square root both sides:

$X = (Y^2 + 9)/A$

$XA = Y^2 + 9$

$XA - 9 = Y^2$

$\mathbf{(XA - 9)^{1/2} = Y}$

2. **The correct answer is D.**
Multiply both sides by A, then divide both sides by X:

$X = (Y^2 + 9)/A$

$XA = (Y^2 + 9)$

$\mathbf{A = (Y^2 + 9)/X}$

3. **The correct answer is D.**
Rearrange to make **Y** the subject, then substitute in the given values and calculate:

$Y = (XA - 9)^{1/2}$

$Y = ((7 \times 4) - 9)^{1/2} = (19)^{1/2} = \mathbf{4.36}$

4. **The correct answer is C.**
Substitute in the given values and calculate:

$X = (13^2 + 9) \div 16 = (178) \div 16 = \mathbf{11.13}$

Example 42

1. **The correct answer is B.**
   Find 38% of the total population.
   (38 ÷ 100) × 136,000 = **51,680**

2. **The correct answer is B.**
   Add the two percentages together. Then find this percentage of the total population:

   13% + 23% = 36%

   (36 ÷ 100) × 136,000 = **48,960**

3. **The correct answer is E.**
   Find the number of people that live in a bungalow. Then find 65% of this value:

   (11 ÷ 100) × 136,000 = 14,960 people live in bungalows.

   (65 ÷ 100) × 14,960 × 65 = **9,724**

4. **The correct answer is D.**
   Find the number of people that live in flats and the number of people that live in terraced houses. Then find the number in each which are students and add the two student populations together.
   For flats:

   Total number of people = (13 ÷ 100) × 136,000 = 17,680

   Number of students = (70 ÷ 100) × 17,680 = 12,376

   For terraced:

   Total number of people = (23 ÷ 100) × 136,000 = 31,280

   Number of students = (20 ÷ 100) × 31,280 = 6,256

   Total number of students living in flats and terraces = 12,376 + 6,256 = **18,632**

Chapter 5

The Abstract Reasoning subtest

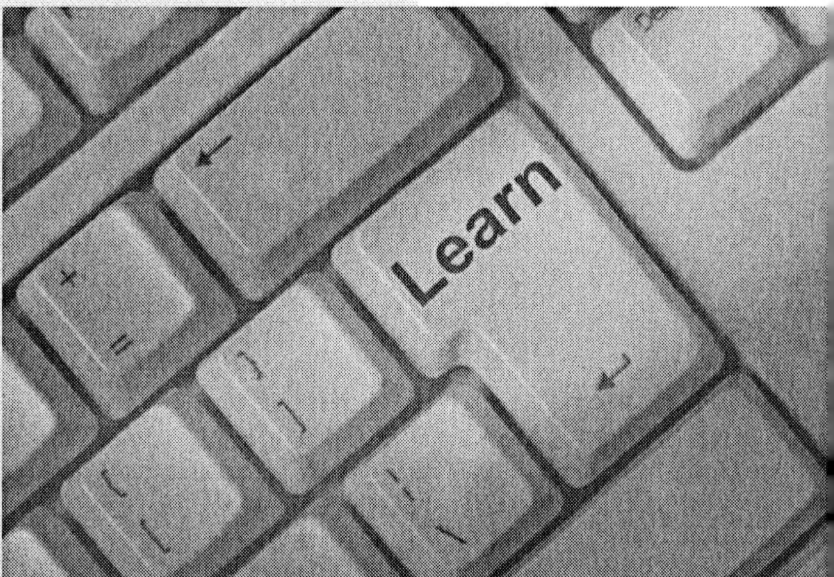

Chapter 5

The Abstract Reasoning subtest

This section of the UKCAT explores a candidate's ability to infer relationships using divergent and convergent thinking. This specific type of test will explore your ability to solve abstract logical problems and requires no prior knowledge or educational experience. As such, these specific tests are the least affected by the candidate's educational experience, and high performance in this subtest is arguably the best indication of pure intelligence or innate reasoning ability.

Divergent thinking encompasses the ability to generate many different ideas about a topic in a short period of time. Convergent thinking is related to reasoning that combines information focusing on solving a problem (especially solving problems that have a single correct solution). Convergent thinking involves combining or joining different ideas together based on common elements.

Achieving high scores in the Abstract Reasoning subtest reflects a candidate's ability to process multiple visual images and identify patterns and relationships between the information provided, which is an essential skill required of a healthcare professional. Abstract Reasoning tests are usually presented in sequences and patterns, which involve symbols and shapes.

When attempting such questions, we need to understand the following concepts:

- Symmetry – are the shapes in a symmetrical format?
- Number patterns – is there a common pattern in the sequence of numbers, eg 2, 4, 6, 8 and so on?
- Size – do the shapes vary in size?
- Shapes – are there specific shapes being used?
- Characteristics – are the symbols and shapes curved; do they have straight lines or angles?
- Rotation – are the shapes or symbols rotated clockwise or anticlockwise?
- Direction – are the symbols or shapes in any specific direction, ie are they aligned diagonally, horizontally or vertically?
- Lines – are they continuous or dashed?

The Abstract Reasoning subtest consists of 11 stems. There are four different item types in the UKCAT exam. You may come across one or two of them.

Type 1: You will be presented with two sets (Set A and Set B) which each contain six shape formations. You will then be presented with five further shape options which are the lead-in questions. You will be expected to identify whether each lead-in question belongs to 'Set A', 'Set B' or 'Neither'.

Type 2: You will be presented with a series of shapes and be asked to select the next shape in the series.

Type 3: You will be presented with a statement involving a group of shapes and will be asked to determine which shape completes the statement.

Type 4: You will be presented with two sets of shapes - Set A and Set B and will be asked to select which of the response options belongs to Set A or Set B.

You will be allocated a time limit of 14 minutes for the Abstract Reasoning subtest, which equates to approximately 14 seconds for each answer. This time allocation includes one minute for administration purposes.

Summary of Abstract Reasoning structure

Stem

The stem will consist of a pair of shapes known as 'Set A' and 'Set B.' Each set will contain a total of six shapes, all of which will have common themes. There will be a total of 11 stems.

Lead-in question

For each stem there will be a total of five shapes which act as the lead-in questions. There will be a total of 55 lead-in questions.

Choices

Your task will either be to decide whether the test shapes are part of 'Set A', 'Set B' or 'Neither' or select the correct answer from a number of possible options.

In each case only one of the choices will be correct. The time limit is 14 minutes. Therefore you will have approximately 14 seconds per question.

When you are working through the UKCAT subtests it can be distracting to monitor exactly how long you spend on answering each question, especially when you have a stem to read through. Therefore, a more useful time management approach is to divide each subtest into four quarters. So, in the case of the Abstract Reasoning subtest, after approximately four minutes you should be working on the fourth stem, after approximately eight minutes you should be commencing the seventh stem, and so on. If you find yourself falling behind at these points you know that you need to pick up the pace.

Example of an Abstract Reasoning question

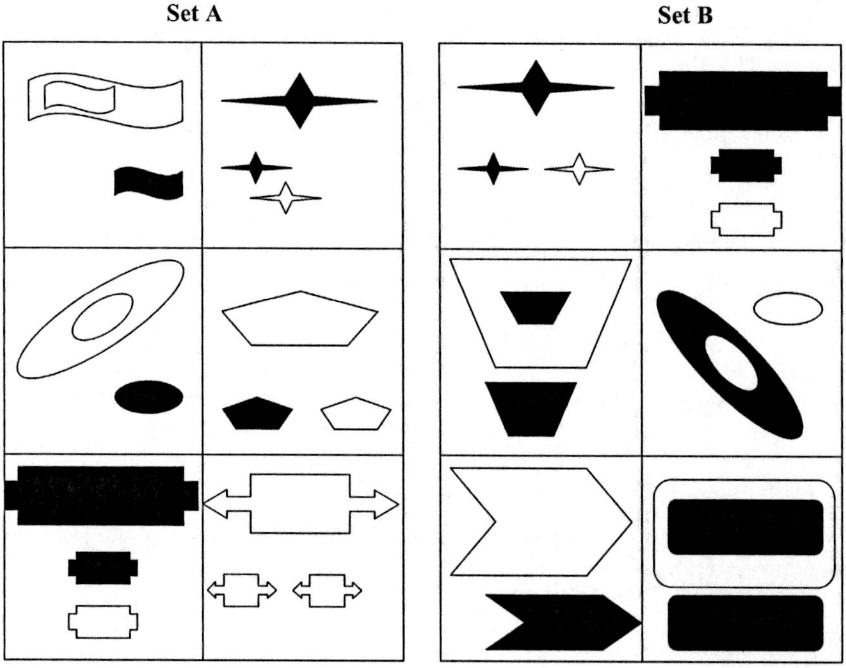

Test Shape 1

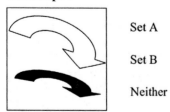

Set A

Set B

Neither

Abstract Reasoning hints and tips

Throughout the Abstract Reasoning subtest the shapes can be ordered in a variety of ways. The various patterns that can be used to distinguish between the shapes include:

- Symmetry
- Number patterns
- Size
- Shapes
- Characteristics
- Rotation
- Direction
- Lines of shapes

Symmetrical characteristics

- Some of the larger symmetrical shapes may be replicated among smaller '*distracter*' shapes.
- Some shapes may seem symmetrical at first glance but are in fact asymmetrical, such as a parallelogram.
- Some sets contain shapes which are symmetrical and are only made up of straight lines while asymmetrical shapes may be curved, or vice versa.
- Some symmetrical shapes may have a dotted or dashed outline while asymmetrical shapes may have a solid outline, or vice versa.
- Some sets may have symmetrical shapes which are shaded in black, while asymmetrical shapes may be white or vice versa.

Number patterns

- Certain number patterns may be symbolised by specific shapes. For example, if a set contained shapes in sets of 2, 4 and 6 they may be represented by (say) small triangles.
- Some number patterns are often replicated in both sets; however the accommodating shapes may differ from one set to another. For example, in Set A, if there are small triangles in groups of 2, 4 and 6 and small circles in groups of 3, 6 and 9, this pattern may be reversed in Set B, whereby there will be small circles in groups of 2, 4 and 6 and small triangles in groups of 3, 6 and 9.
- Some number patterns may be represented with various types of shading, eg black or white shading, or different outlines, eg dotted, dashed or solid outlines.

Size

- Do the shapes vary in size?
- Are shapes of a certain size positioned in specific areas in a set?
- Often shapes of the same size are used in both sets, although they are positioned differently. For example in Set A, there could be three different-sized circular shapes – small, medium and large. The smallest shape could always be positioned within the largest shape. The same-sized shapes may also be used in Set B; however, the rules change slightly and instead the medium sized circular shape could be positioned within the largest shape.
- Shapes may be shaded or unshaded. For example, curved shapes are shaded in black and shapes with straight lines are left white.

Characteristics

- Some sets may contain curved or straight-lined shapes.
- A common method of causing confusion is to combine a mixture of curved and straight lines within a shape.
- Other sets may contain shapes which possess a dashed or solid outline or even a mixture of both.
- Some shapes may be present in differing quantities.

Rotation and direction

- Shapes can be positioned horizontally or vertically, and towards the middle, top, bottom, right or left of the test box.
- Shapes can be positioned in either a clockwise or anticlockwise position.

Three simple steps to Abstract Reasoning

Once you acknowledge the various ways in which the shapes can be presented, you will find it easier to apply this knowledge if you follow the three simple steps below:

Step 1

First identify the different shapes and symbols used within each stem. Look for characteristics such as size, number and colour.

Step 2

Try to identify any patterns which the shapes or symbols form, such as recurring number patterns, rotation and positioning of shapes, symmetry and direction of shapes.

Step 3

Try to identify the next part of the sequence for each lead-in question, and relate them to either 'Set A', 'Set B' or 'Neither'. If you really are unsure of the answer, go with your gut instinct rather than leaving a blank.

In the next section you will find some examples of the types of Abstract Reasoning questions you will face when you attempt the UKCAT.

Abstract Reasoning practice examples

Example 1

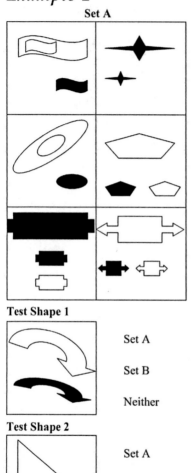

Set A

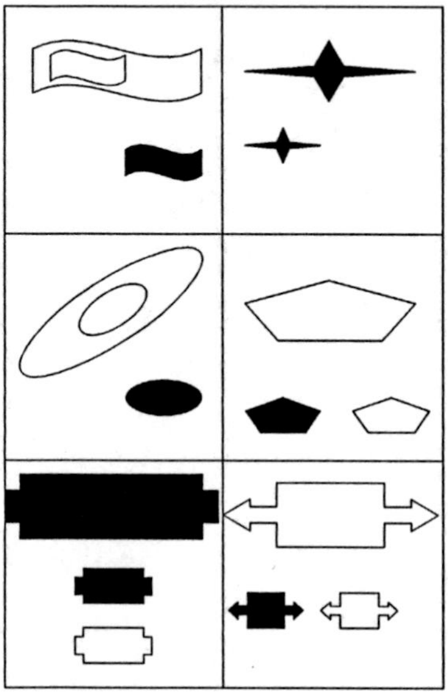

Set B

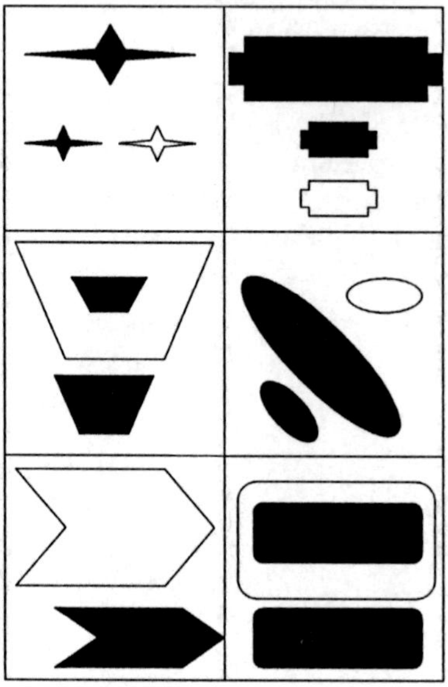

Test Shape 1

Set A

Set B

Neither

Test Shape 2

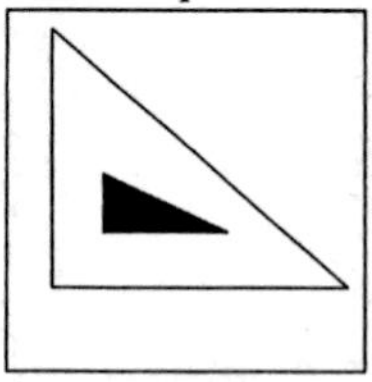

Set A

Set B

Neither

Test Shape 3

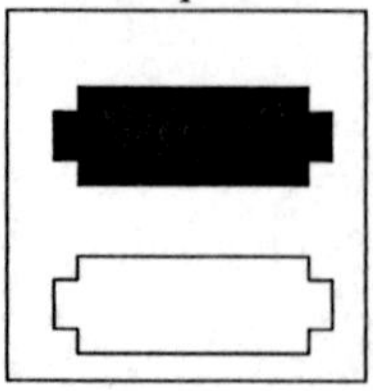

Set A

Set B

Neither

Test Shape 4

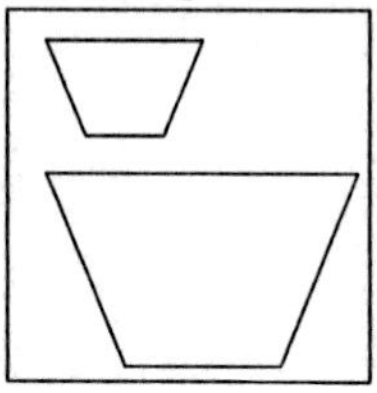

Set A

Set B

Neither

Test Shape 5

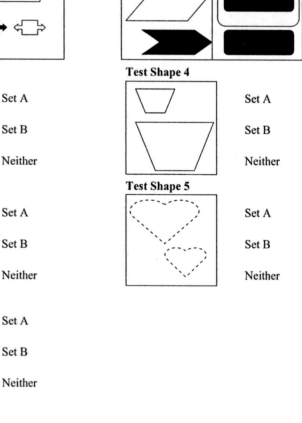

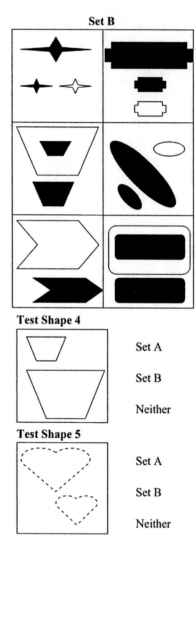

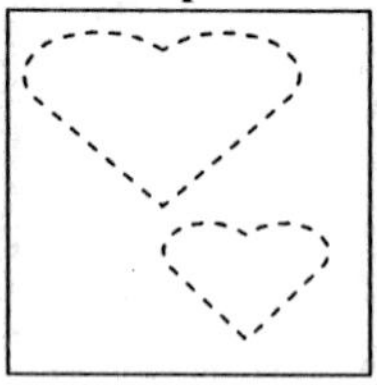

Set A

Set B

Neither

Example 2

Set A **Set B**

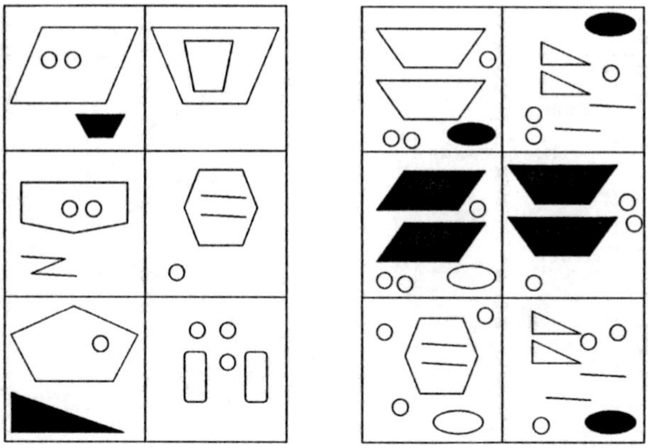

1. Which of the following belong to Set A?

A B C D E

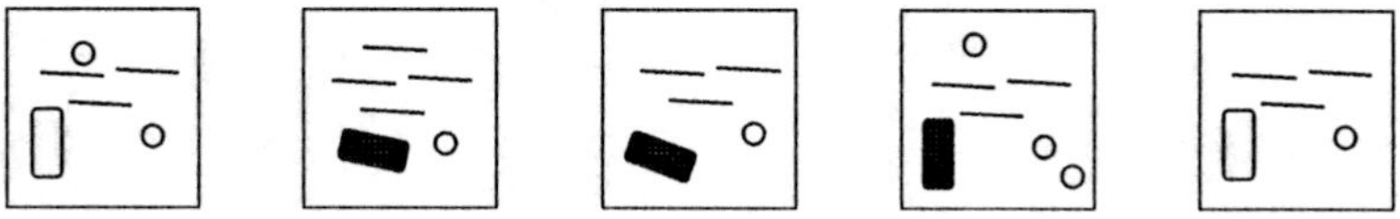

2. Which of the following belong to Set A?

A B C D E

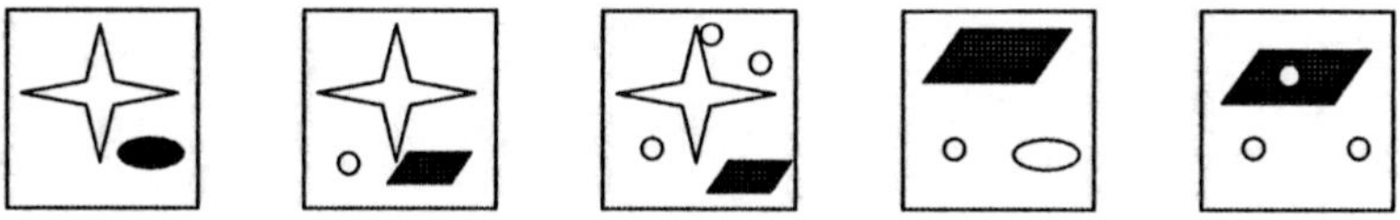

3. Which of the following belong to Set A?

A B C D E

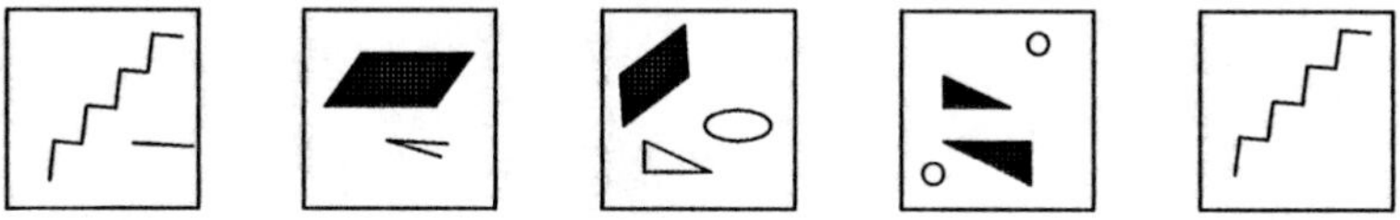

4. Which of the following belong to Set B?

A B C D E

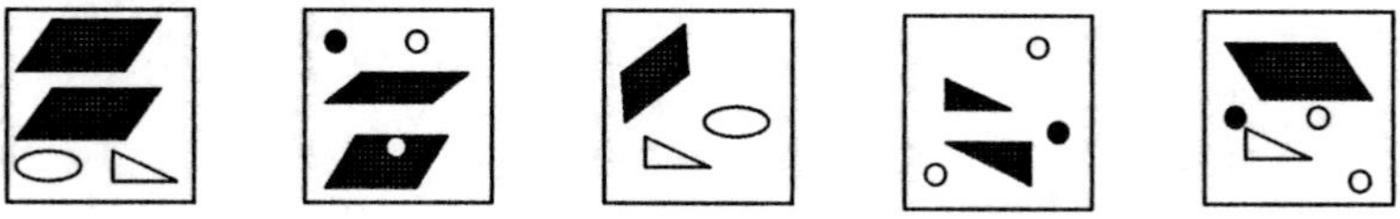

5. Which of the following belong to Set B?

A B C D E

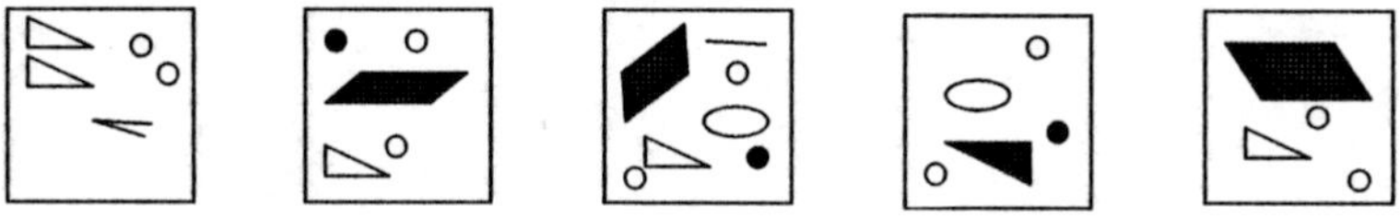

Example 3

Set A

Set B

Test Shape 1

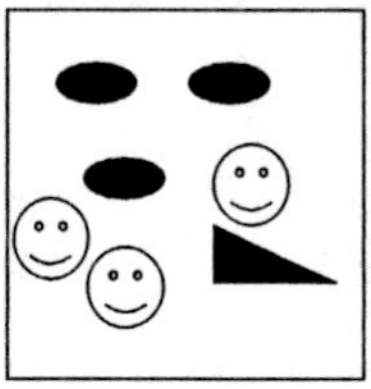

Set A

Set B

Neither

Test Shape 2

Set A

Set B

Neither

Test Shape 3

Set A

Set B

Neither

Test Shape 4

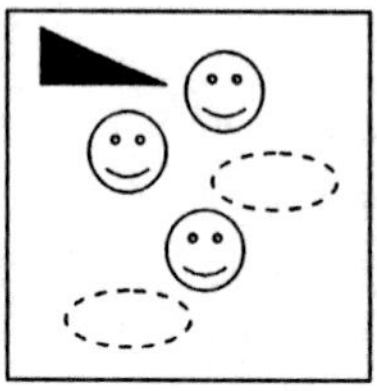

Set A

Set B

Neither

Test Shape 5

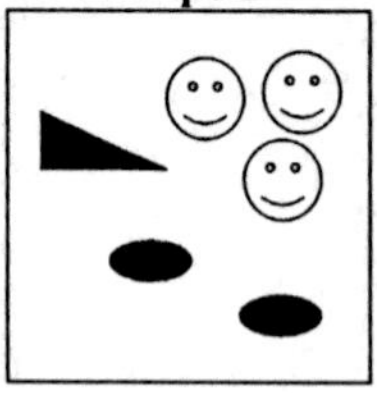

Set A

Set B

Neither

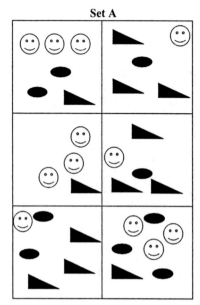

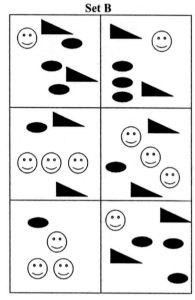

Example 4

Set A

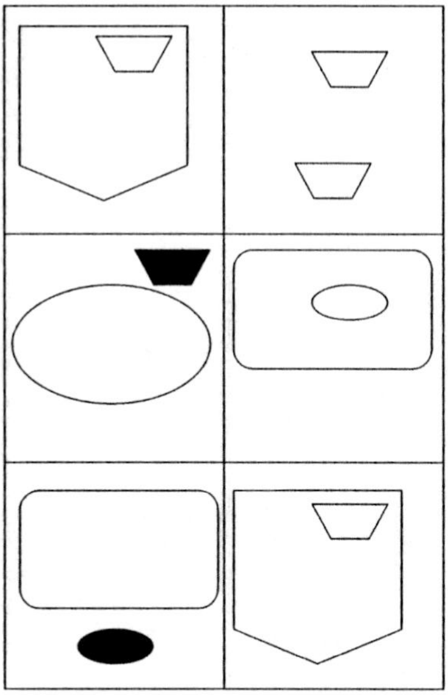

Set B

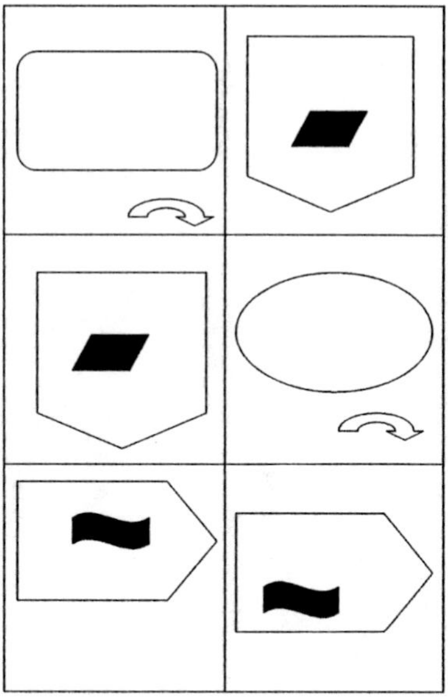

Test Shape 1

Set A

Set B

Neither

Test Shape 2

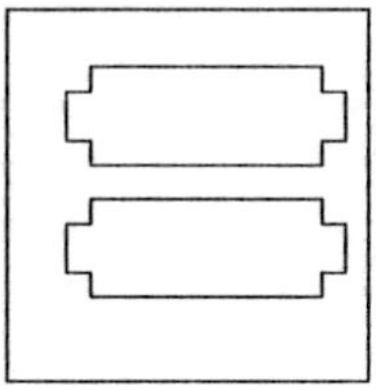

Set A

Set B

Neither

Test Shape 3

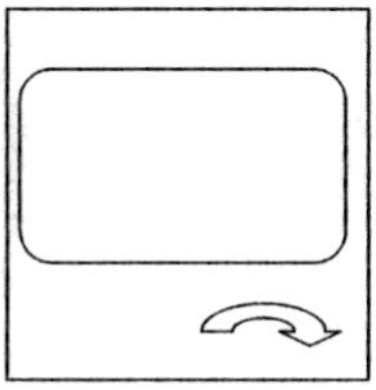

Set A

Set B

Neither

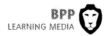

Test Shape 4

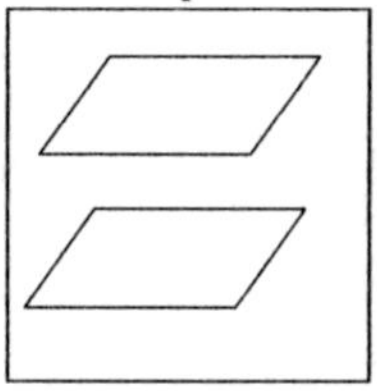

Set A

Set B

Neither

Test Shape 5

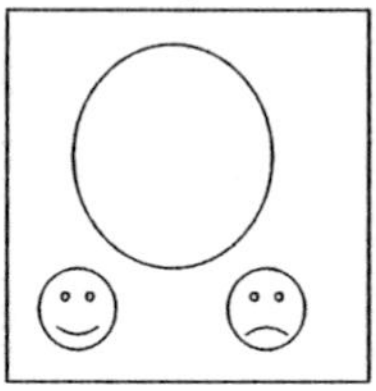

Set A

Set B

Neither

Example 5

Set A

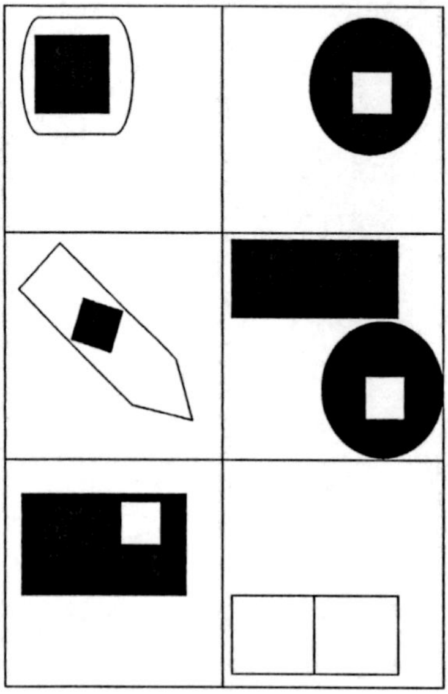

Set B

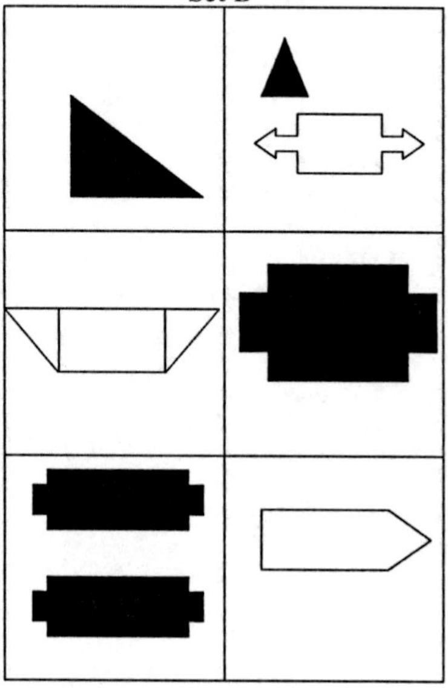

Test Shape 1

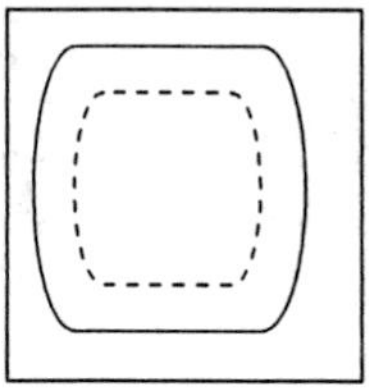

Set A

Set B

Neither

Test Shape 2

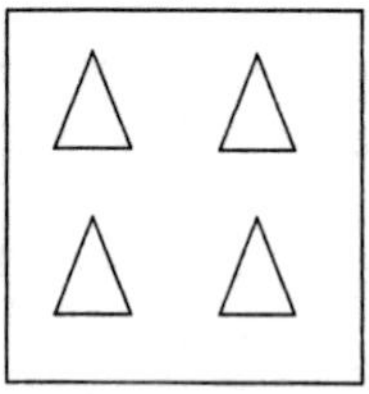

Set A

Set B

Neither

Test Shape 3

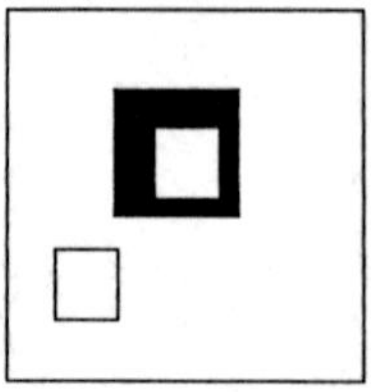

Set A

Set B

Neither

Test Shape 4

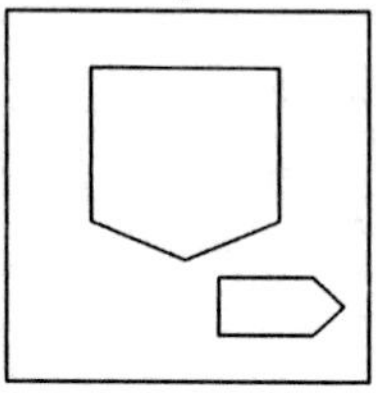

Set A

Set B

Neither

Test Shape 5

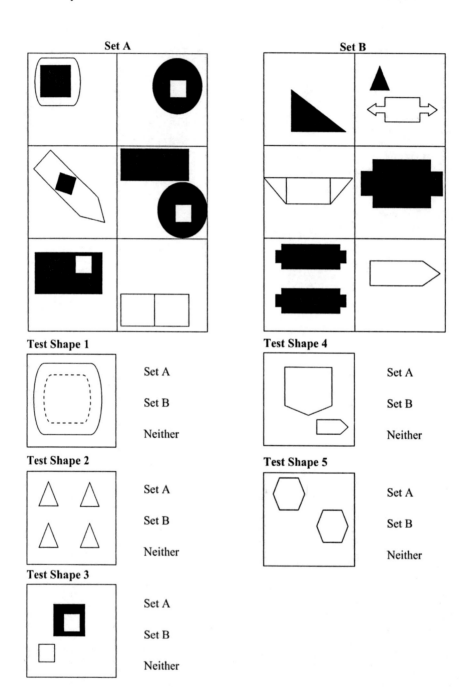

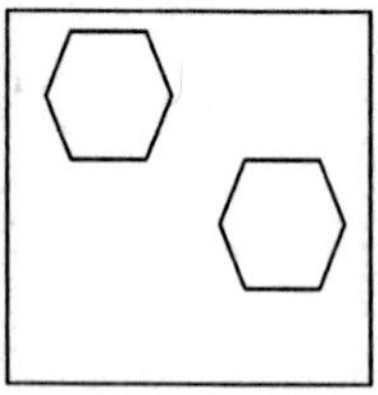

Set A

Set B

Neither

Example 6

Set A

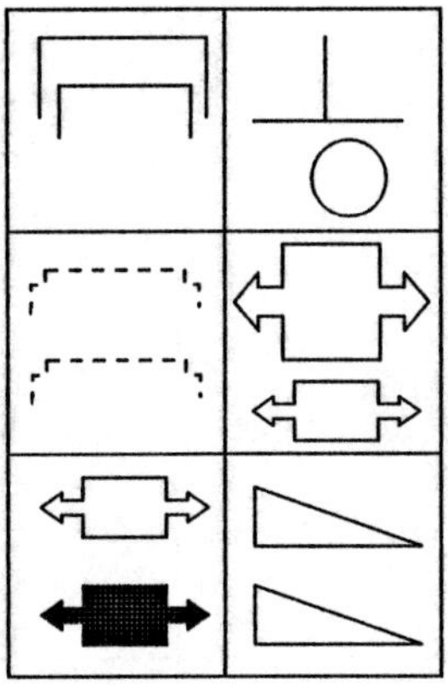

Set B

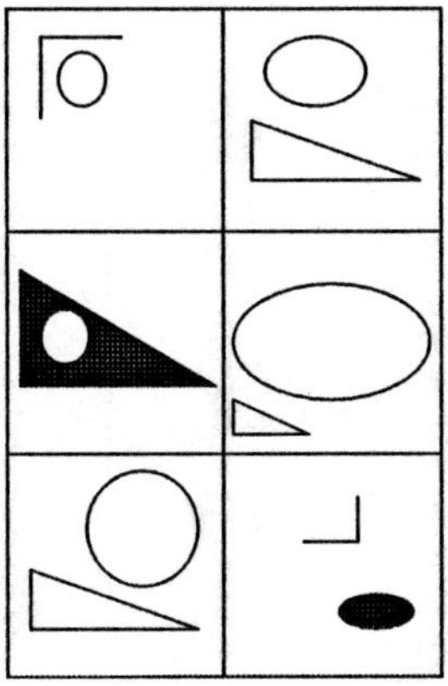

1. Which of the following belong to Set A?

A B C D E

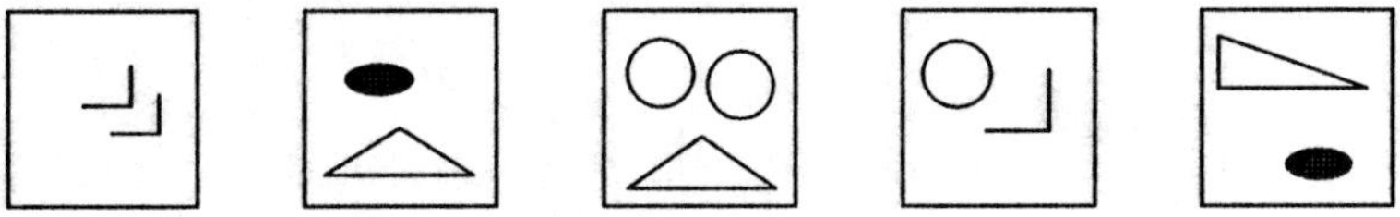

2. Which of the following belong to Set A?

A B C D E

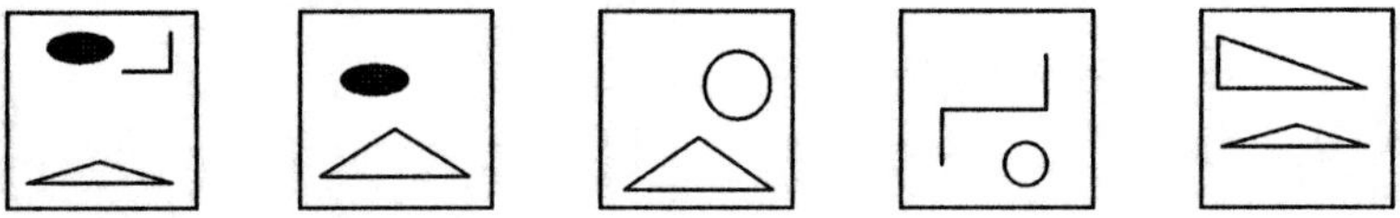

3. Which of the following belong to Set A?

A B C D E

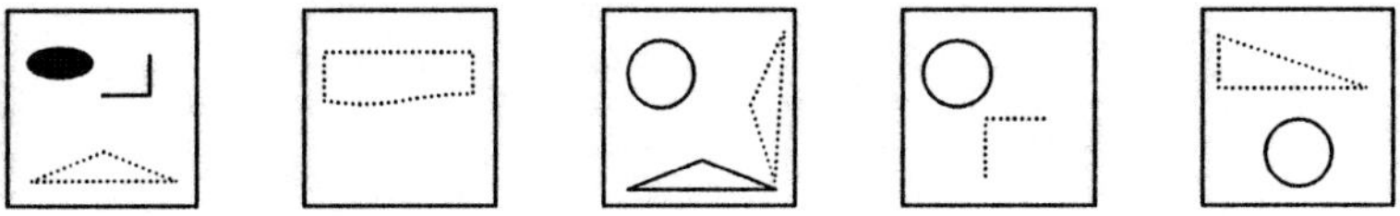

4. Which of the following belong to Set B?

A B C D E

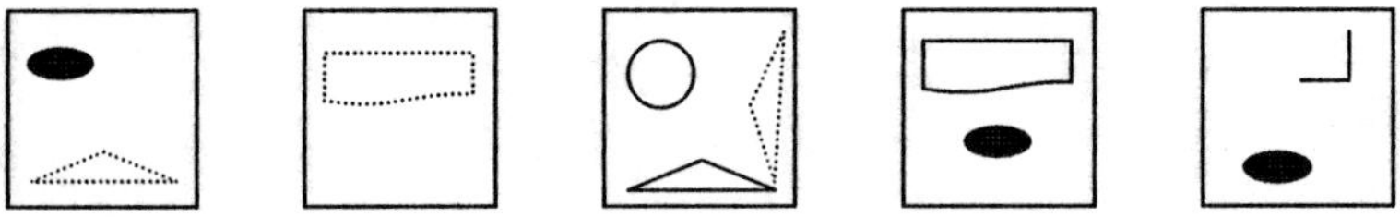

5. Which of the following belong to Set B?

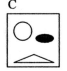

A B C D E

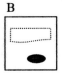

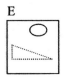

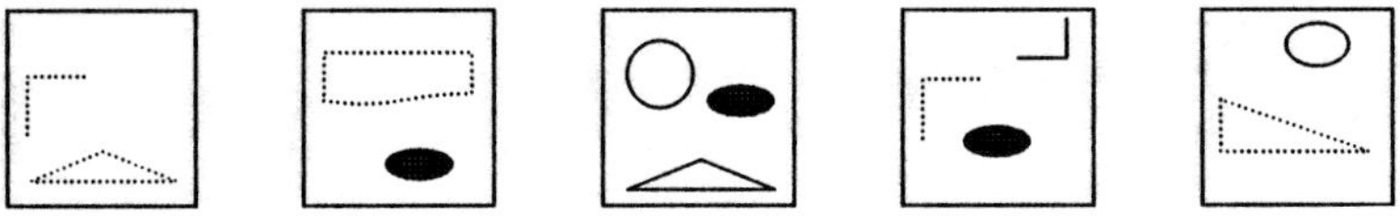

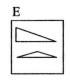

Example 7

Set A

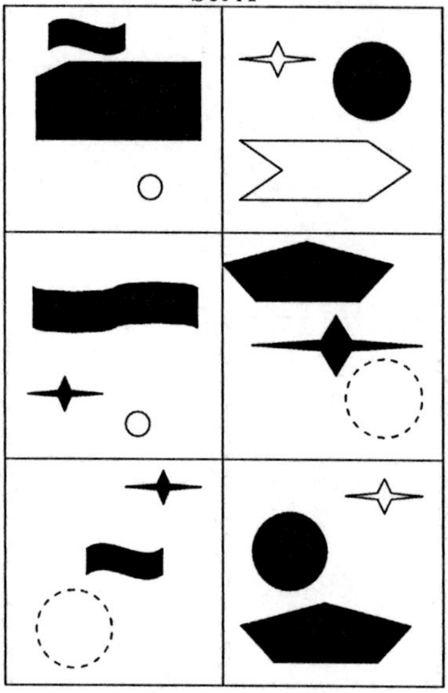

Set B

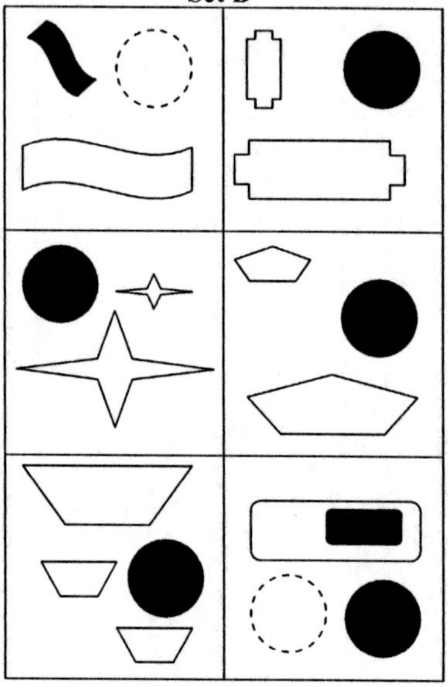

Test Shape 1

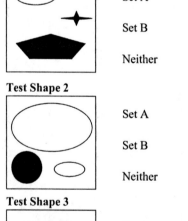

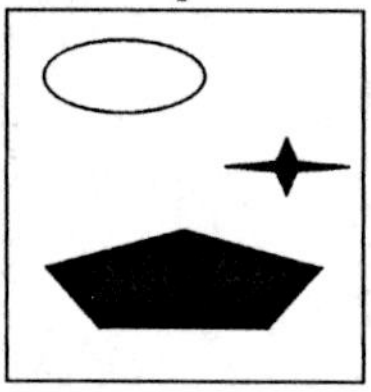

Set A

Set B

Neither

Test Shape 2

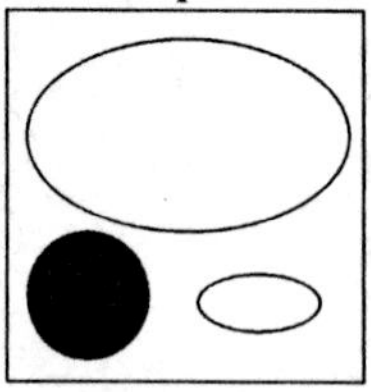

Set A

Set B

Neither

Test Shape 3

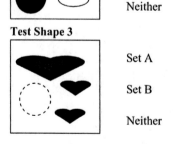

Set A

Set B

Neither

Test Shape 4

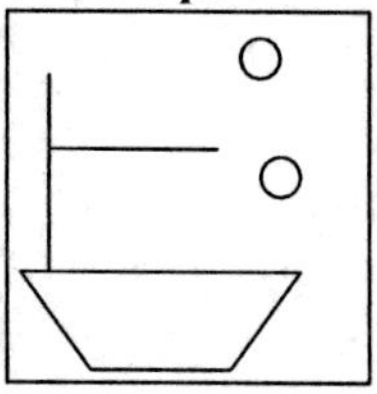

Set A

Set B

Neither

Test Shape 5

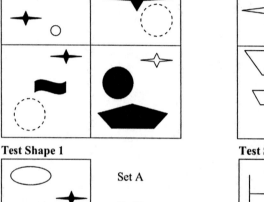

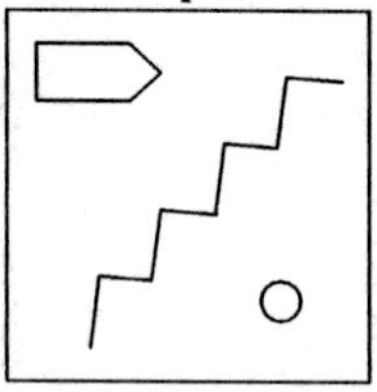

Set A

Set B

Neither

Example 8

Set A **Set B**

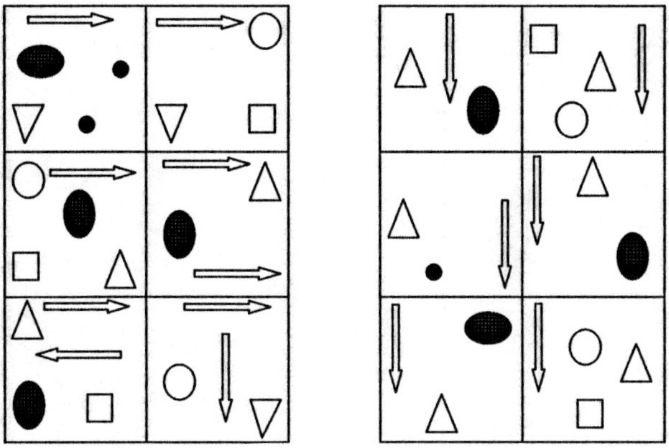

1. Which of the following belong to Set A?

A B C D E

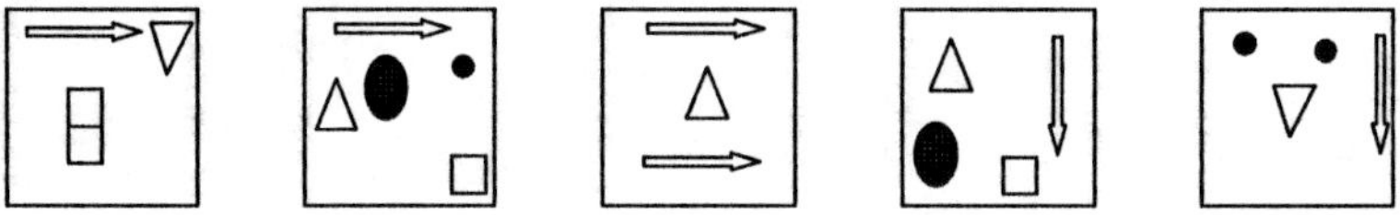

2. Which of the following belong to Set A?

A B C D E

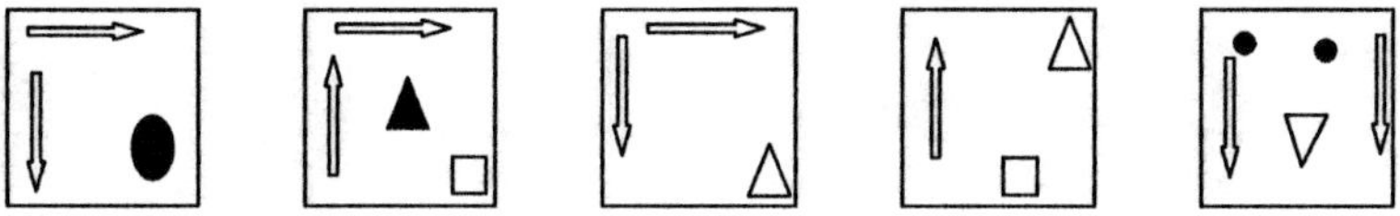

3. Which of the following belong to Set B?

A B C D E

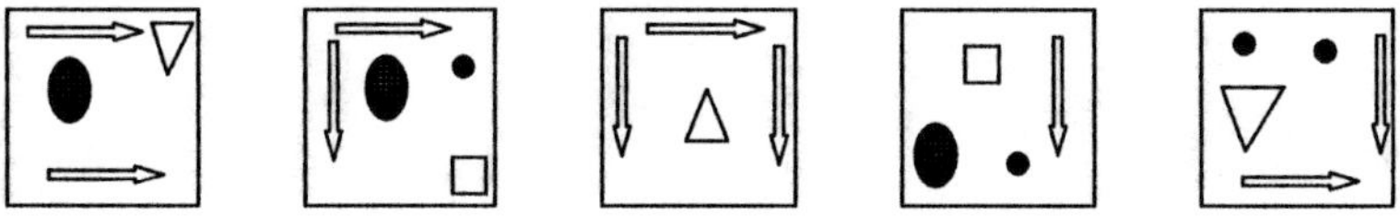

4. Which of the following belong to Set B?

A B C D E

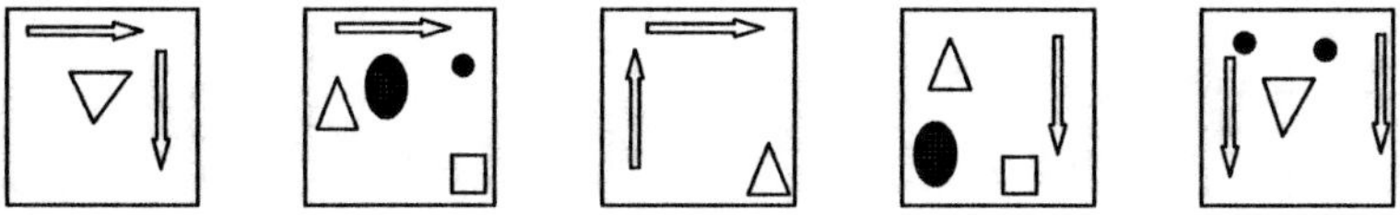

5. Which of the following belong to Set B?

A B C D E

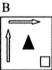

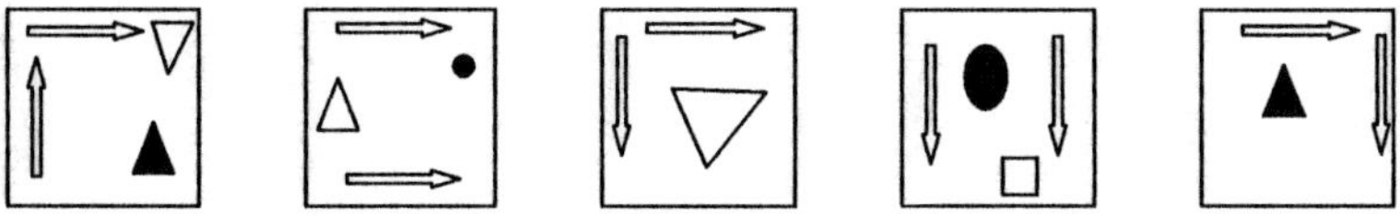

Example 9

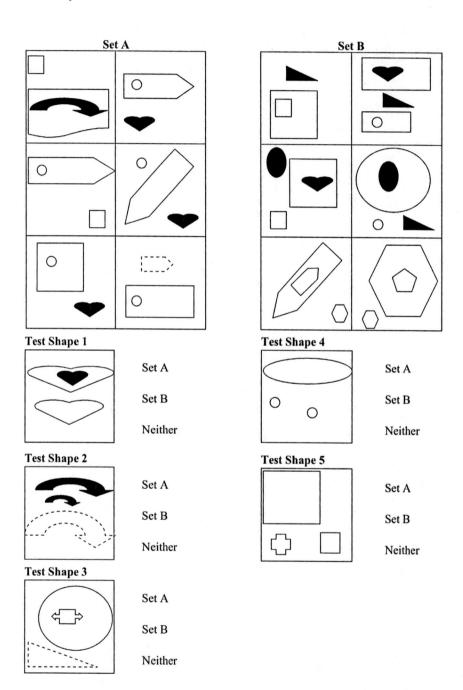

Set A

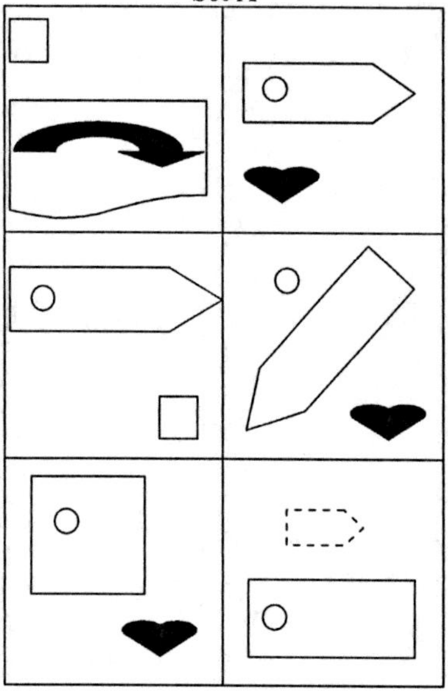

Set B

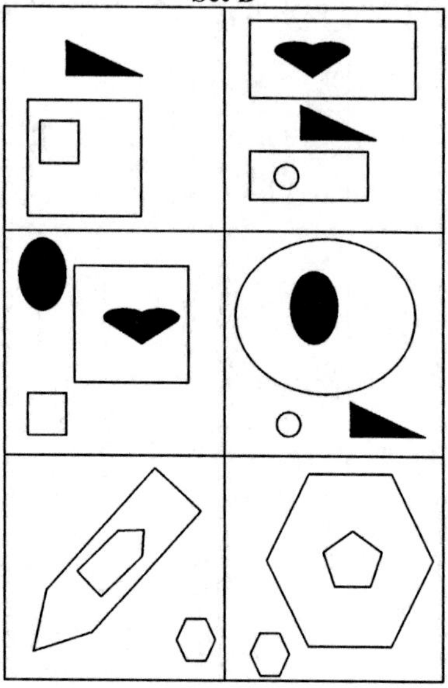

Test Shape 1

Set A

Set B

Neither

Test Shape 2

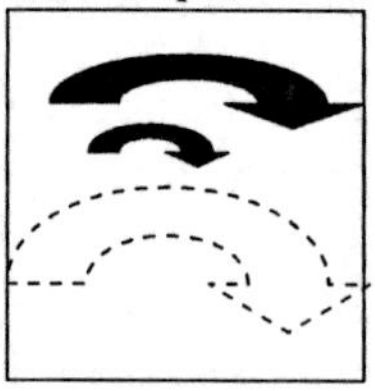

Set A

Set B

Neither

Test Shape 3

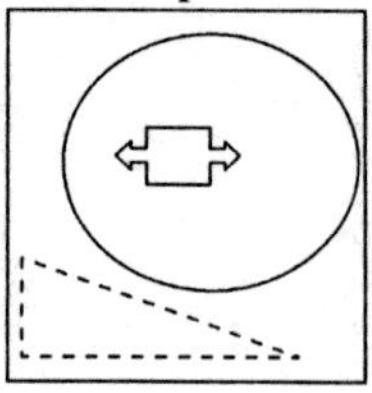

Set A

Set B

Neither

Test Shape 4

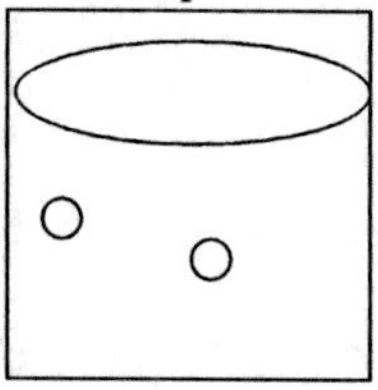

Set A

Set B

Neither

Test Shape 5

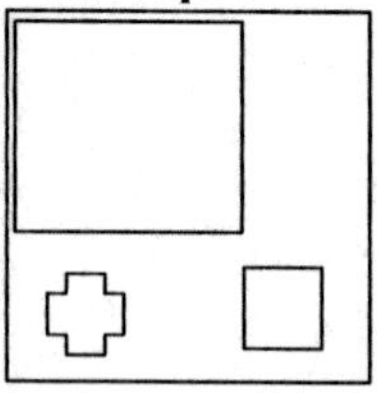

Set A

Set B

Neither

Example 10

Set A

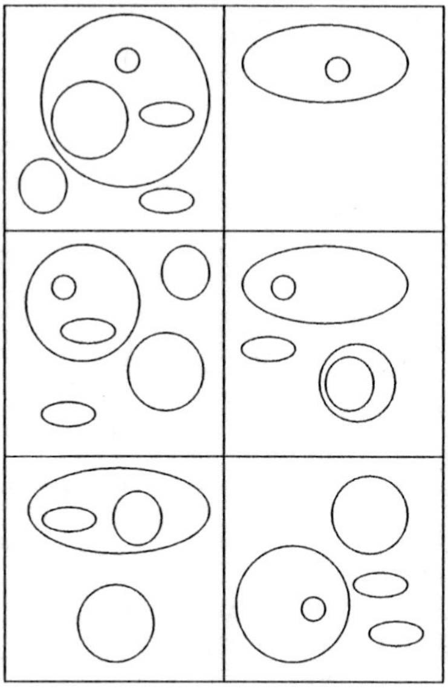

Set B

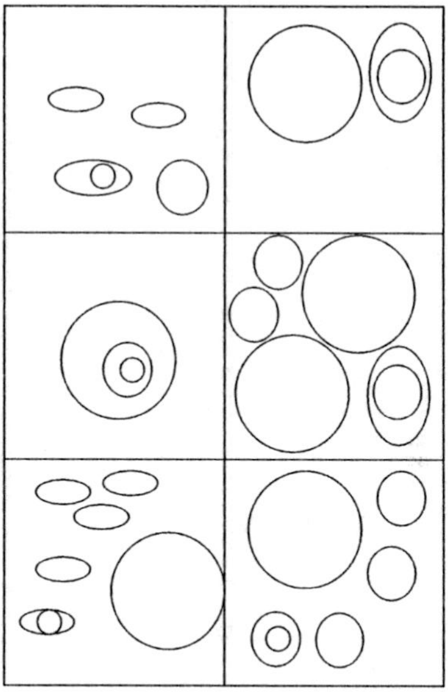

Test Shape 1

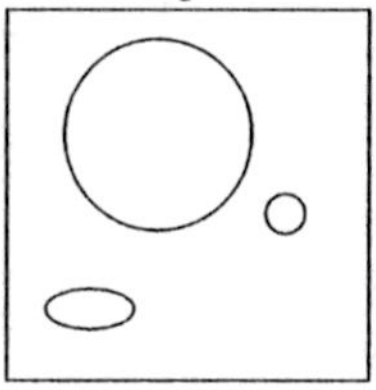

Set A

Set B

Neither

Test Shape 2

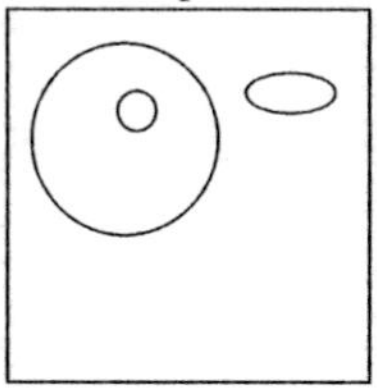

Set A

Set B

Neither

Test Shape 3

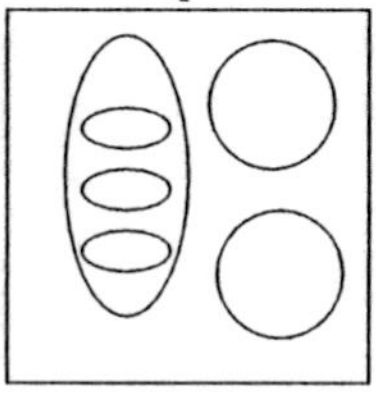

Set A

Set B

Neither

Test Shape 4

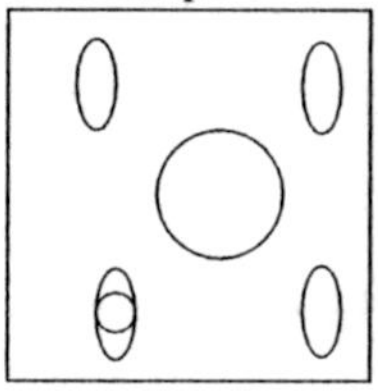

Set A

Set B

Neither

Test Shape 5

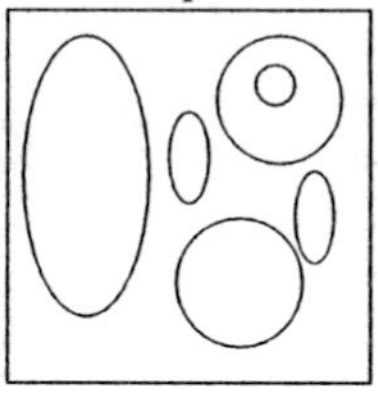

Set A

Set B

Neither

Example 11

Set A

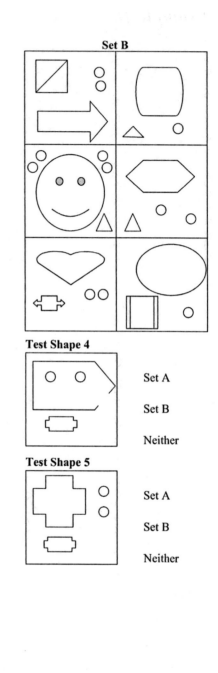

Set B

Test Shape 1

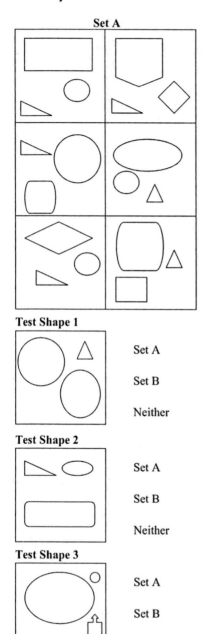

Set A

Set B

Neither

Test Shape 2

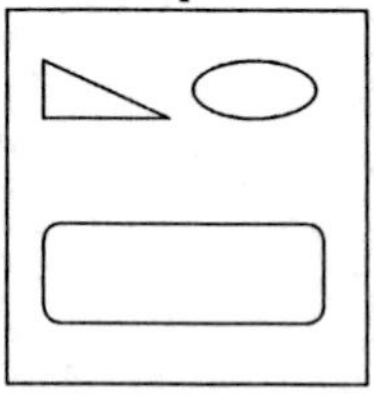

Set A

Set B

Neither

Test Shape 3

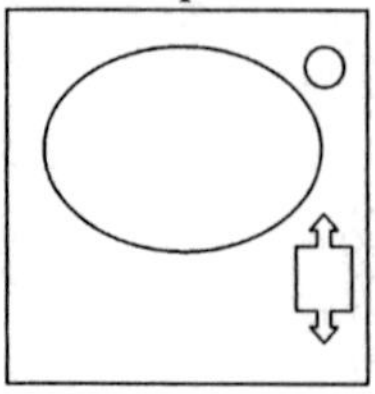

Set A

Set B

Neither

Test Shape 4

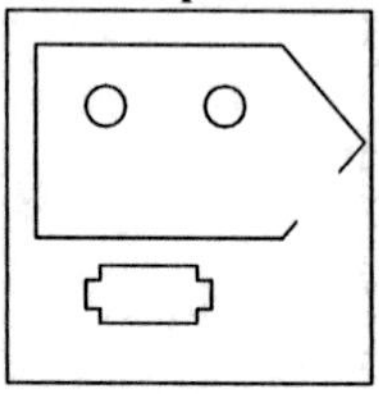

Set A

Set B

Neither

Test Shape 5

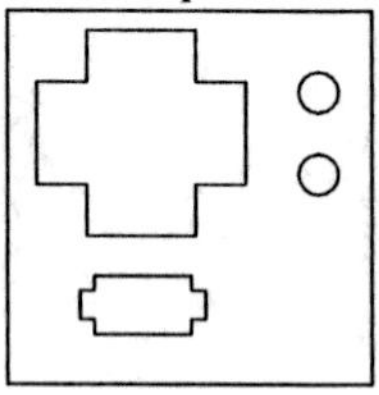

Set A

Set B

Neither

Example 12

Set A

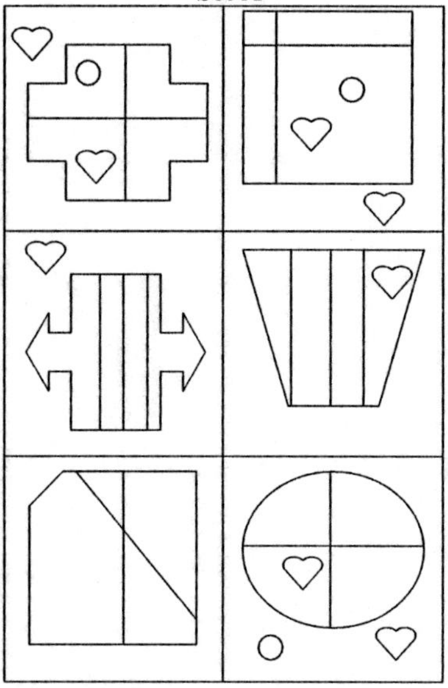

Set B

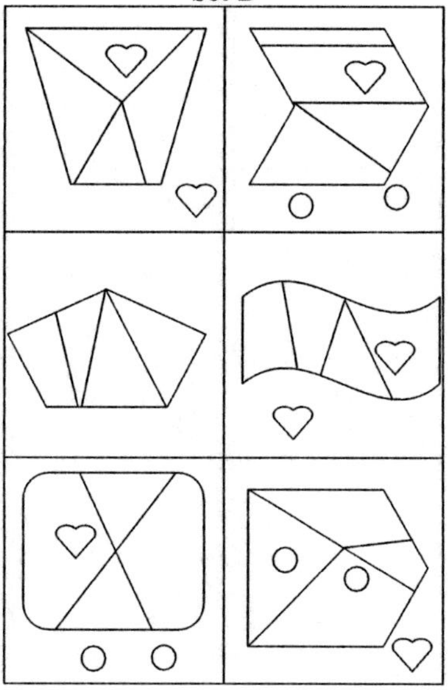

Test Shape 1

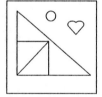

Set A

Set B

Neither

Test Shape 2

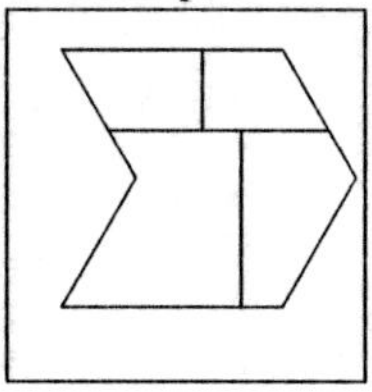

Set A

Set B

Neither

Test Shape 3

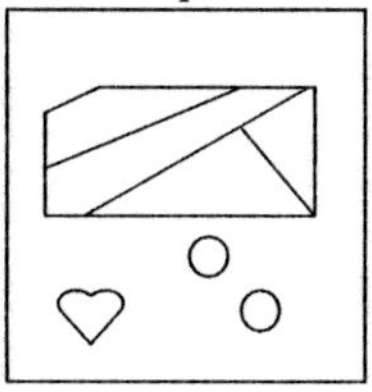

Set A

Set B

Neither

Test Shape 4

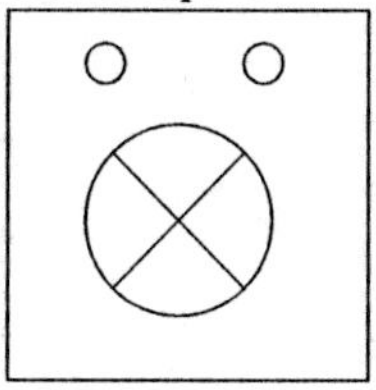

Set A

Set B

Neither

Test Shape 5

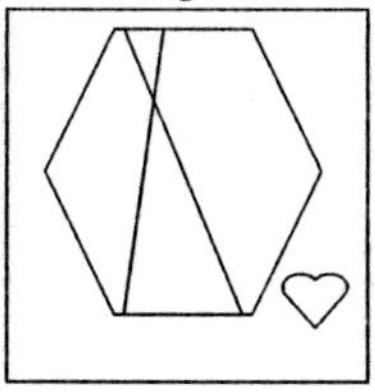

Set A

Set B

Neither

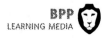

Example 13

Set A

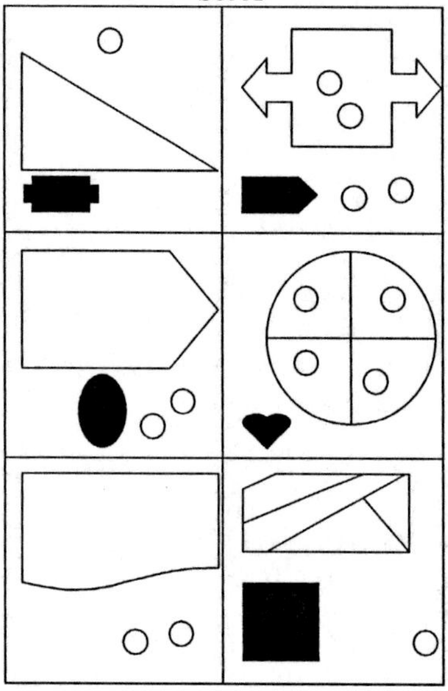

Set B

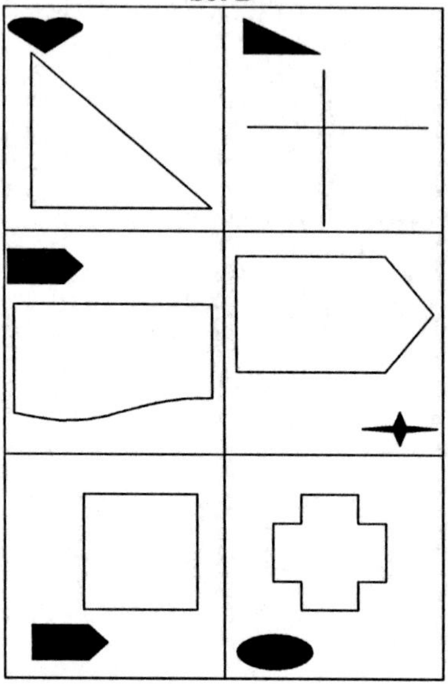

Test Shape 1

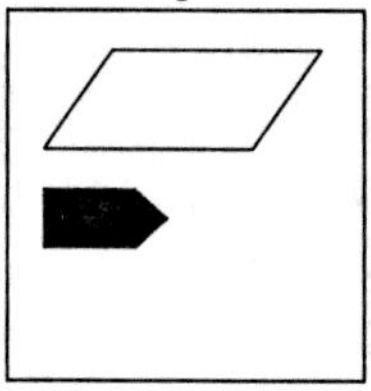

Set A

Set B

Neither

Test Shape 2

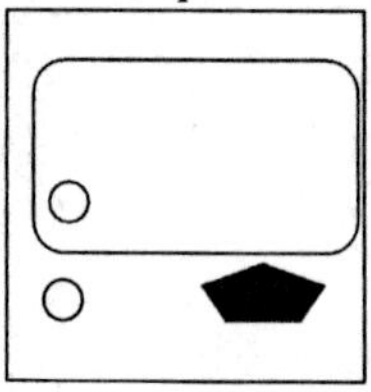

Set A

Set B

Neither

Test Shape 3

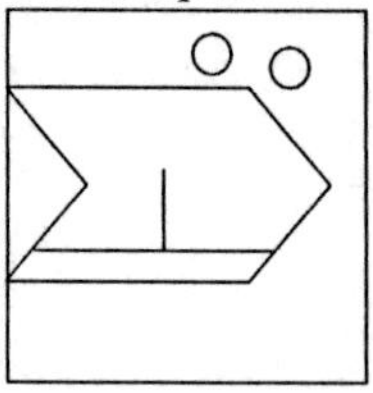

Set A

Set B

Neither

Test Shape 4

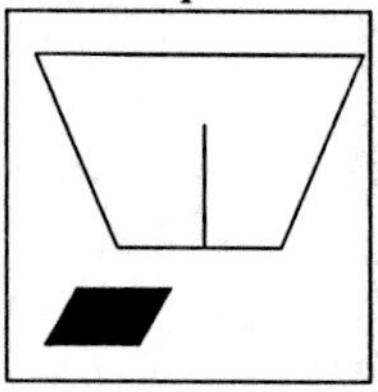

Set A

Set B

Neither

Test Shape 5

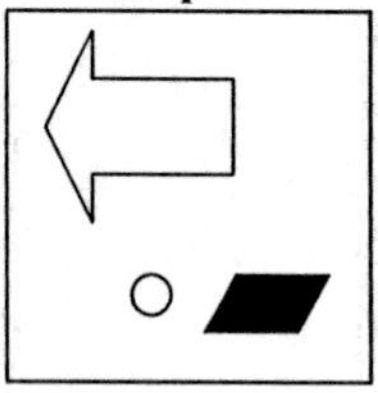

Set A

Set B

Neither

Example 14

Set A **Set B**

1. Which of the following shapes belong to Set A?

A B C D E

2. Which of the following shapes belong to Set A?

A B C D E

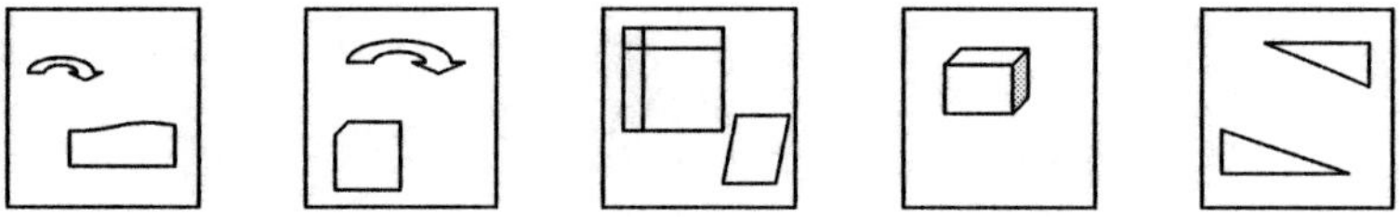

3. Which of the following shapes belong to Set B?

A B C D E

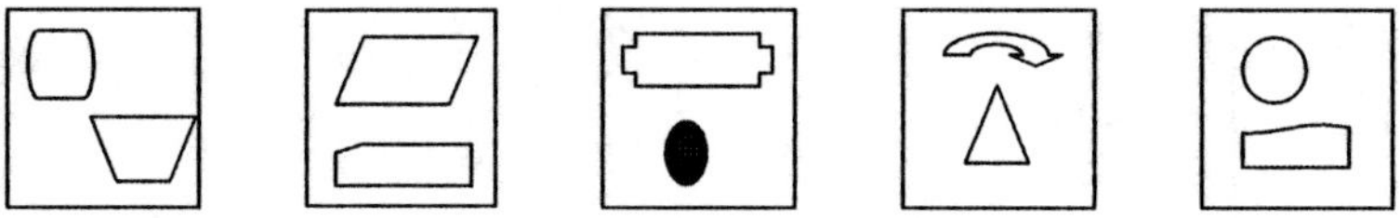

4. Which of the following shapes belong to Set B?

A B C D E

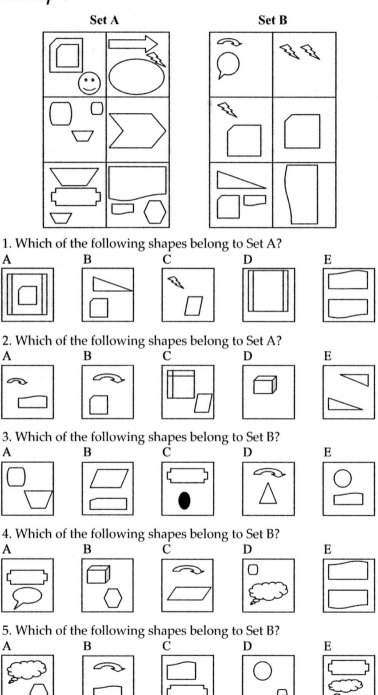

5. Which of the following shapes belong to Set B?

A B C D E

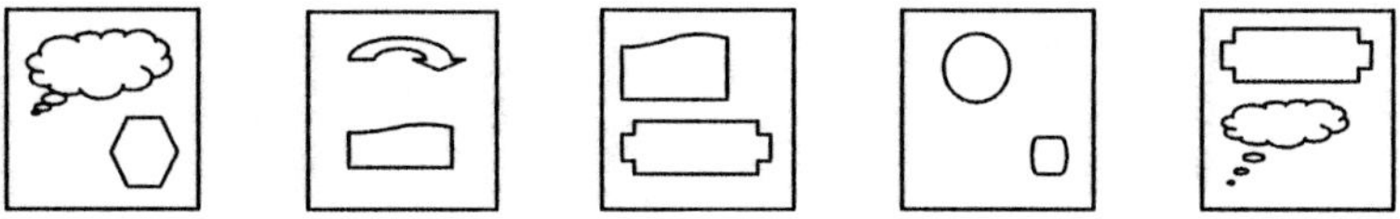

Example 15

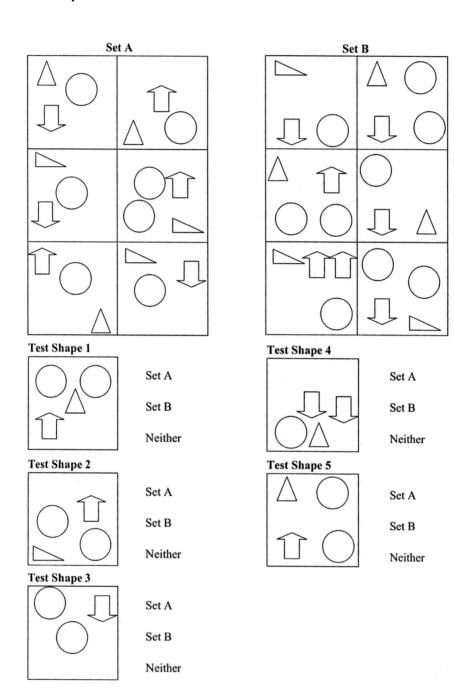

Set A

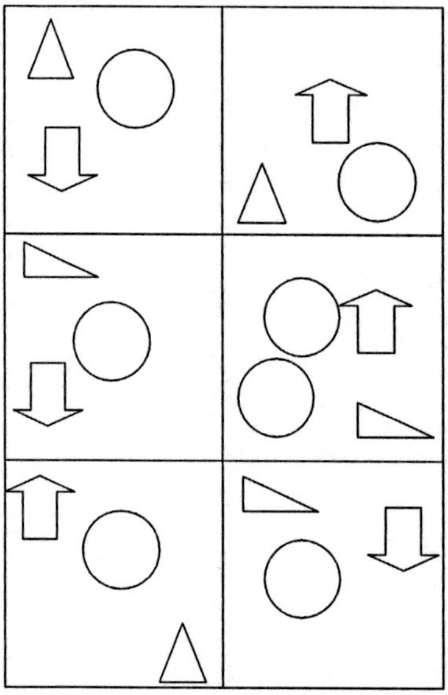

Set B

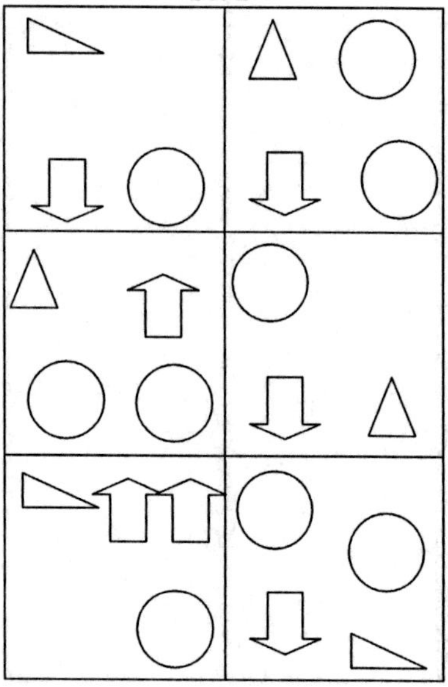

Test Shape 1

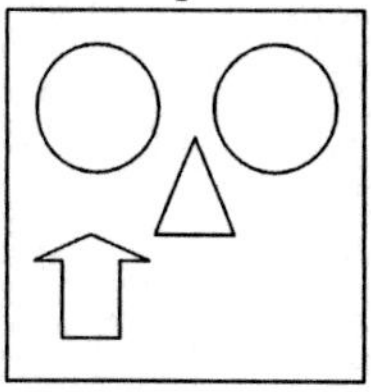

Set A

Set B

Neither

Test Shape 2

Set A

Set B

Neither

Test Shape 3

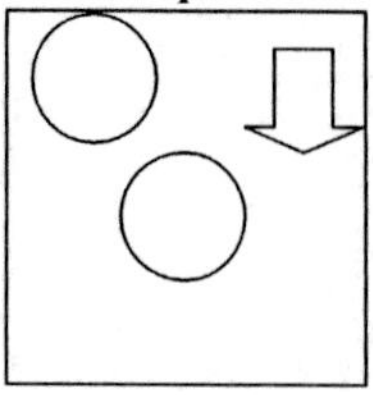

Set A

Set B

Neither

Test Shape 4

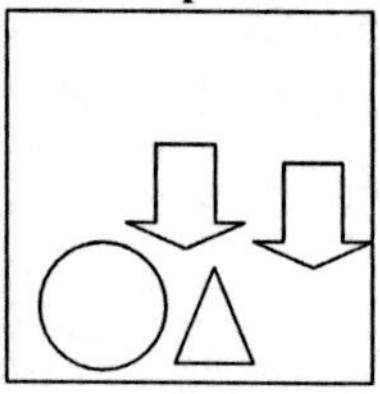

Set A

Set B

Neither

Test Shape 5

Set A

Set B

Neither

Example 16

Set A

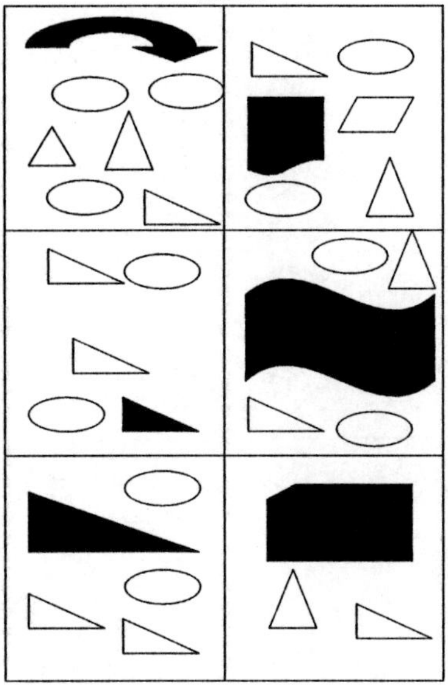

Set B

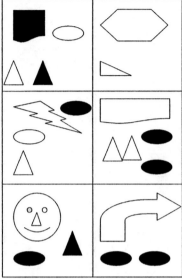

Test Shape 1

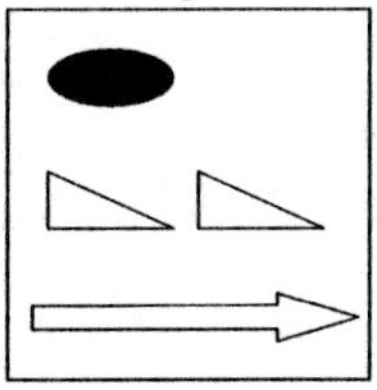

Set A

Set B

Neither

Test Shape 2

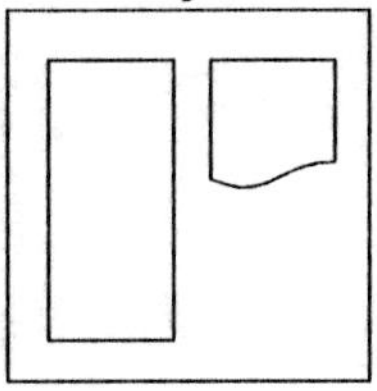

Set A

Set B

Neither

Test Shape 3

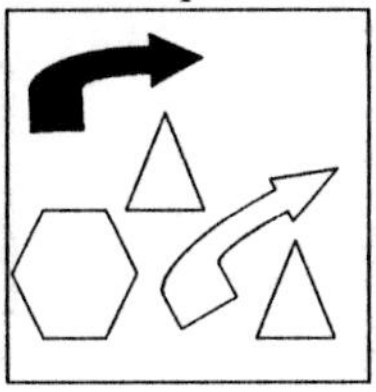

Set A

Set B

Neither

Test Shape 4

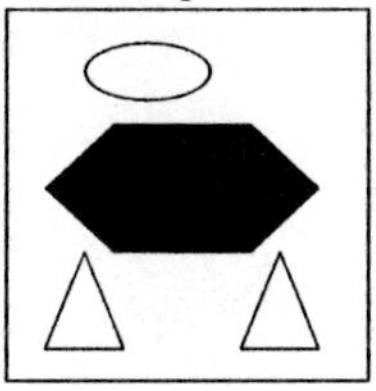

Set A

Set B

Neither

Test Shape 5

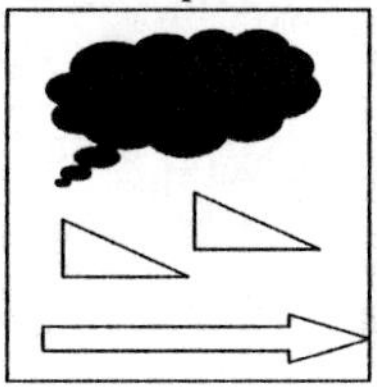

Set A

Set B

Neither

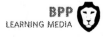

Example 17

Set A

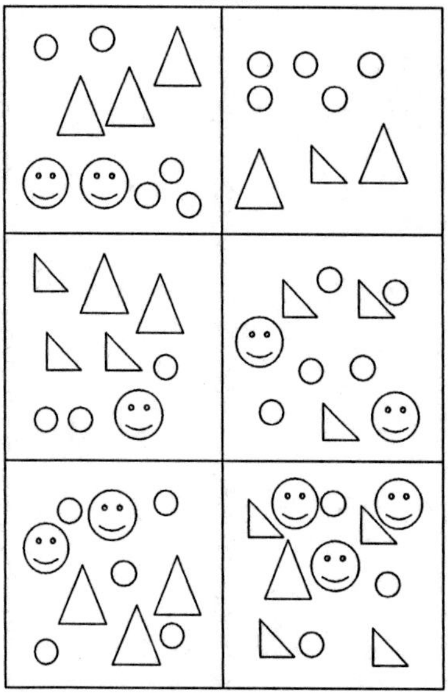

Set B

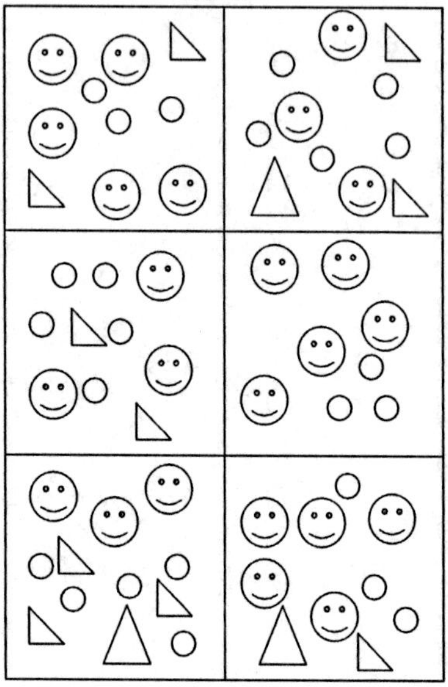

Test Shape 1

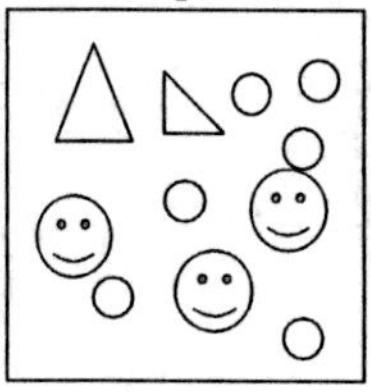

Set A

Set B

Neither

Test Shape 2

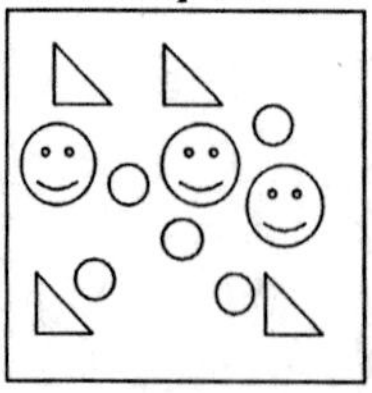

Set A

Set B

Neither

Test Shape 3

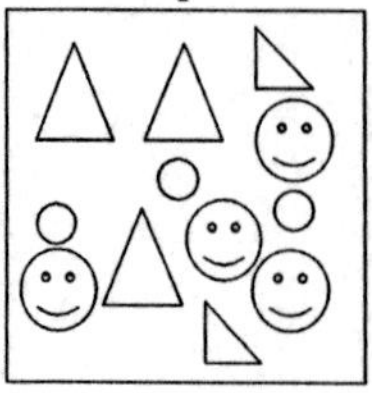

Set A

Set B

Neither

Test Shape 4

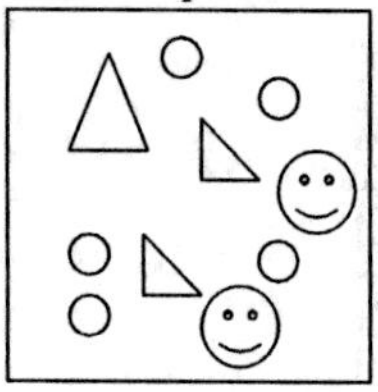

Set A

Set B

Neither

Test Shape 5

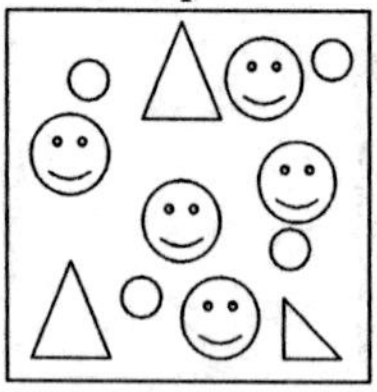

Set A

Set B

Neither

Example 18

Set A **Set B**

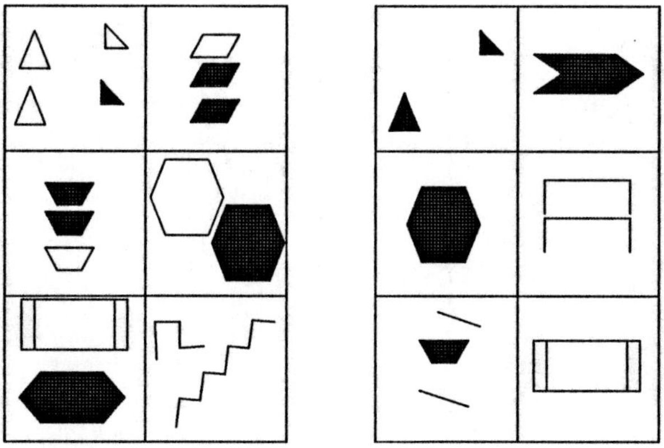

1. Which of the following shapes belong to Set A?

A B C D E

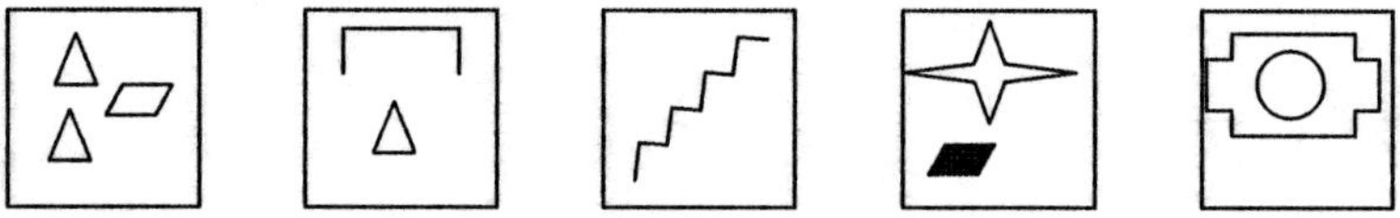

2. Which of the following shapes belong to Set A?

A B C D E

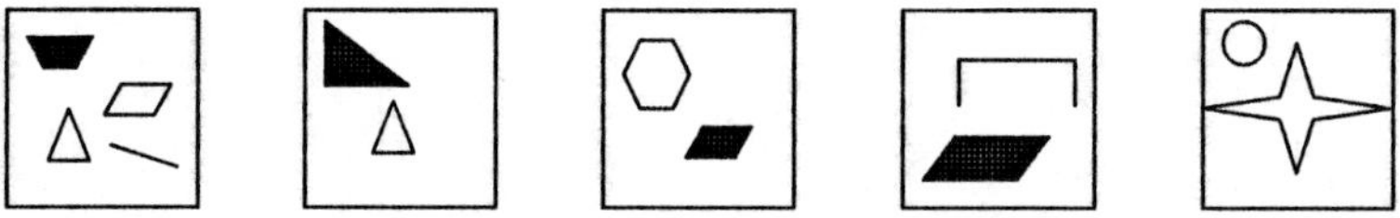

3. Which of the following shapes belong to Set A?

A B C D E

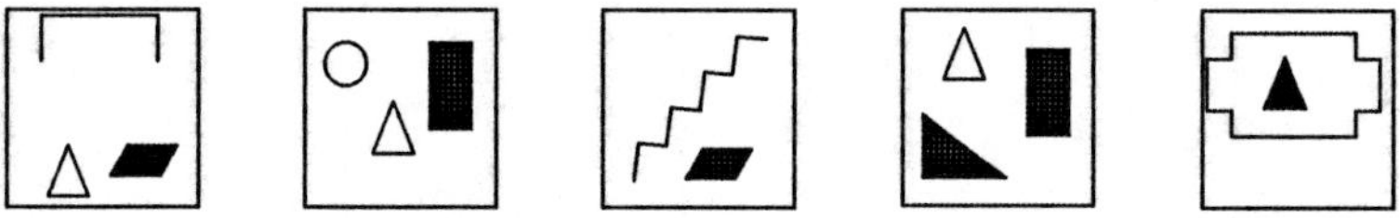

4. Which of the following shapes belong to Set B?

A B C D E

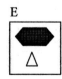

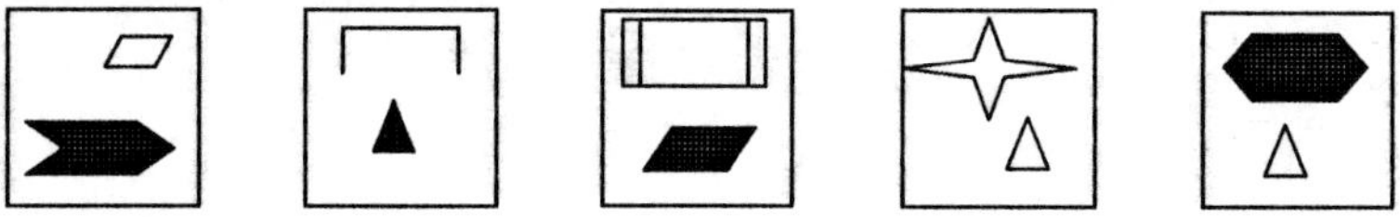

5. Which of the following shapes belong to Set A?

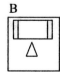

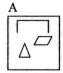

A B C D E

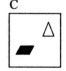

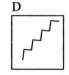

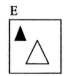

Example 19

Set A

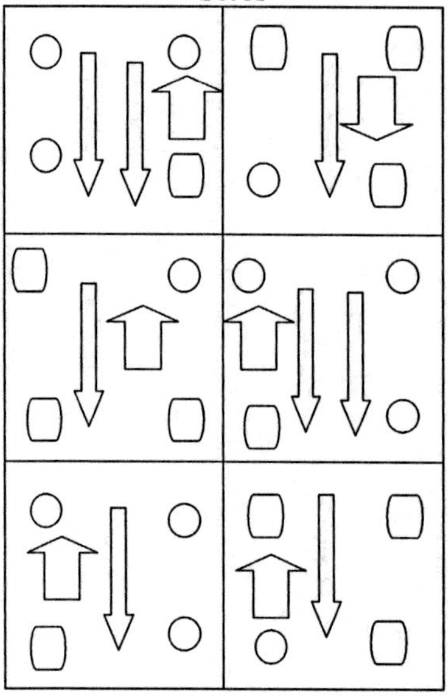

Set B

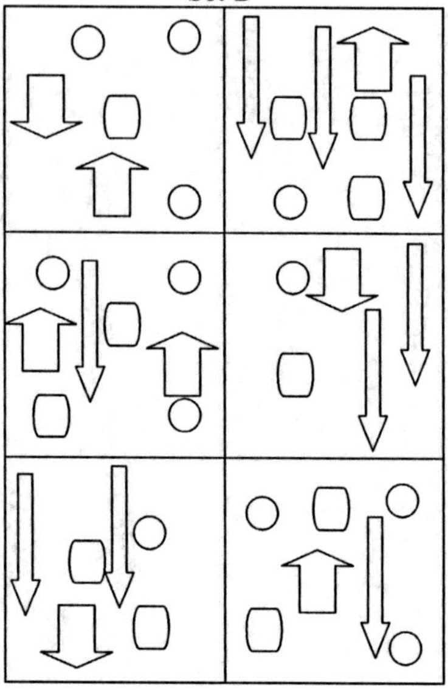

Test Shape 1

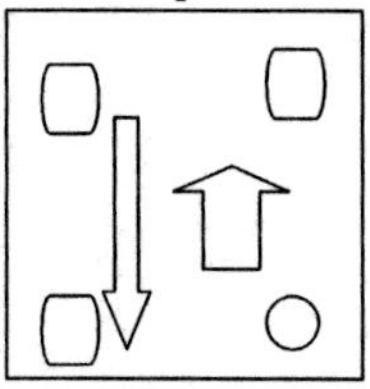

Set A

Set B

Neither

Test Shape 2

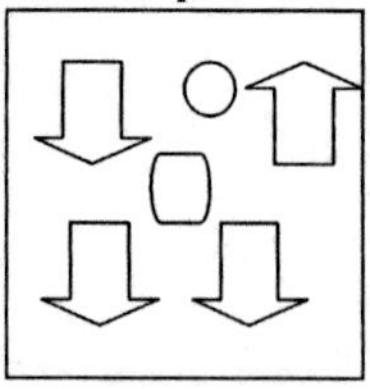

Set A

Set B

Neither

Test Shape 3

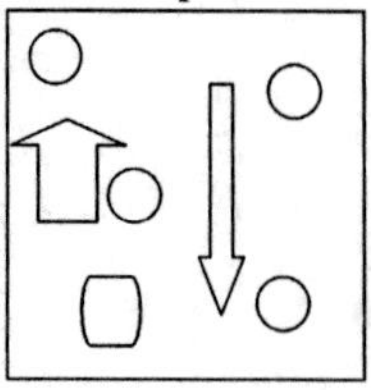

Set A

Set B

Neither

Test Shape 4

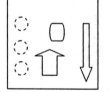

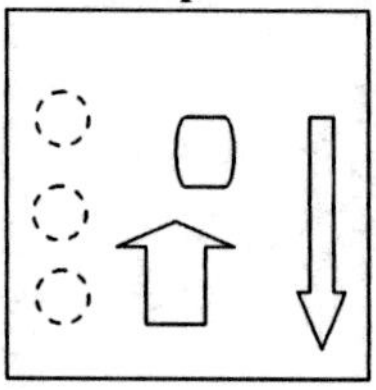

Set A

Set B

Neither

Test Shape 5

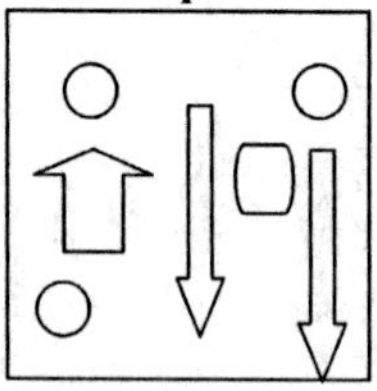

Set A

Set B

Neither

Example 20

Set A

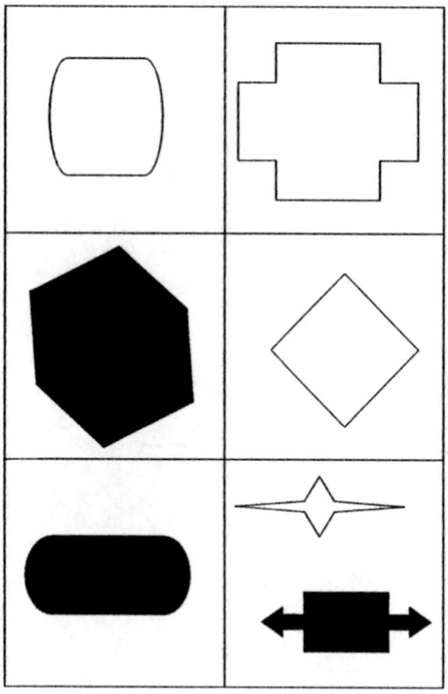

Set B

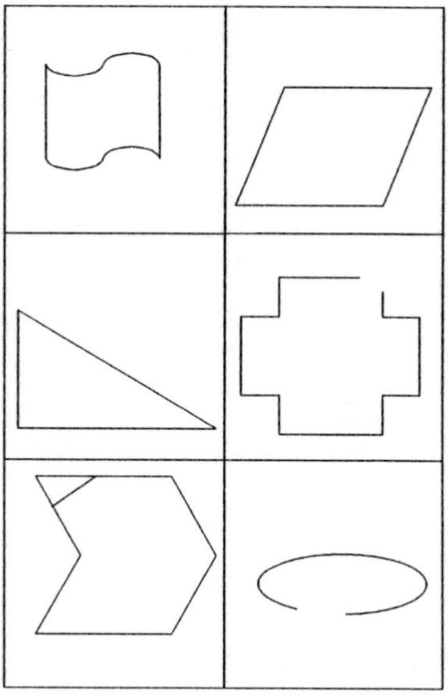

Test Shape 1

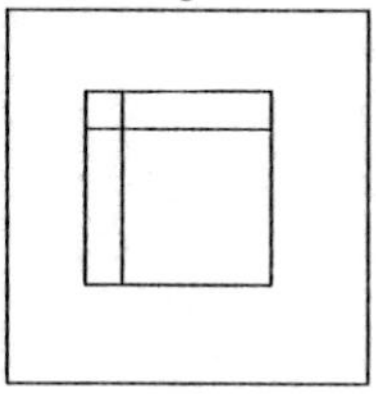

Set A

Set B

Neither

Test Shape 2

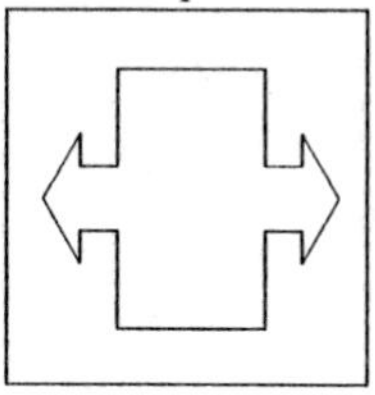

Set A

Set B

Neither

Test Shape 3

Set A

Set B

Neither

Test Shape 4

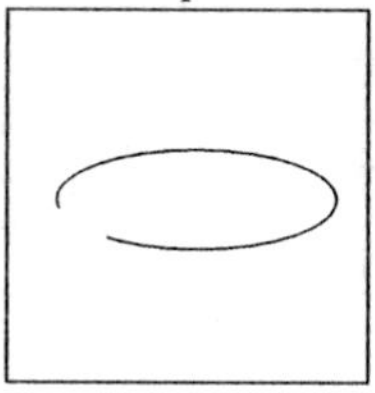

Set A

Set B

Neither

Test Shape 5

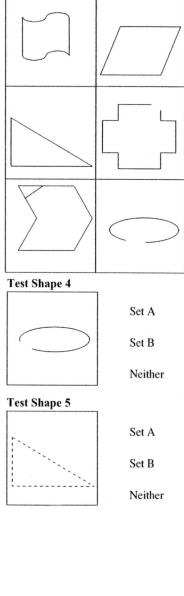

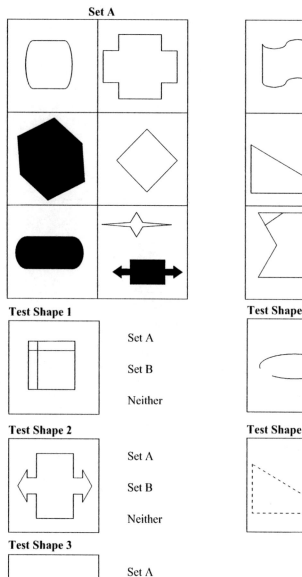

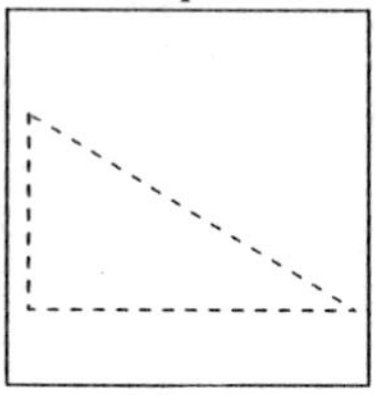

Set A

Set B

Neither

Example 21

Set A

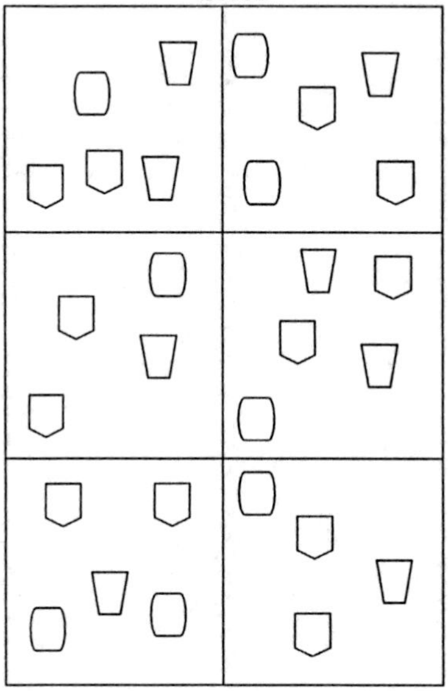

Set B

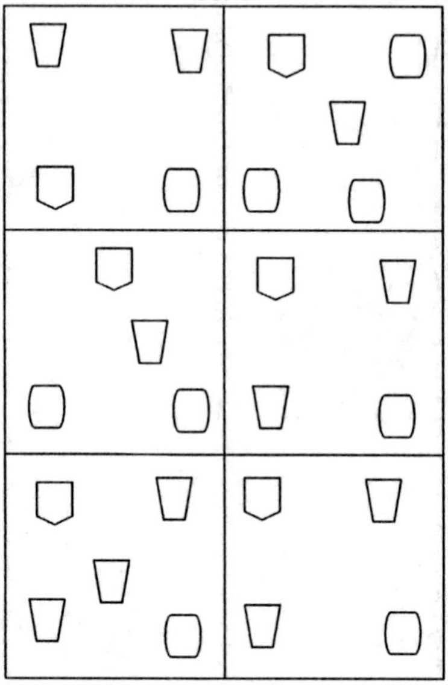

Test Shape 1

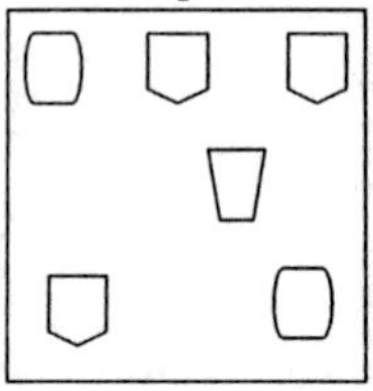

Set A

Set B

Neither

Test Shape 2

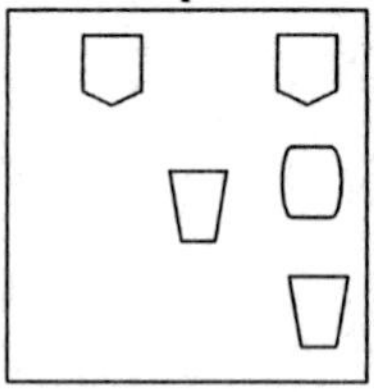

Set A

Set B

Neither

Test Shape 3

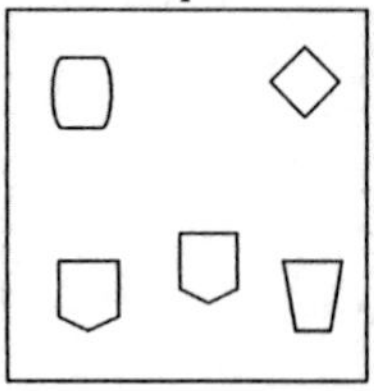

Set A

Set B

Neither

Test Shape 4

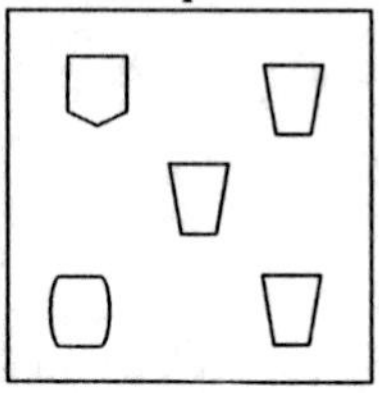

Set A

Set B

Neither

Test Shape 5

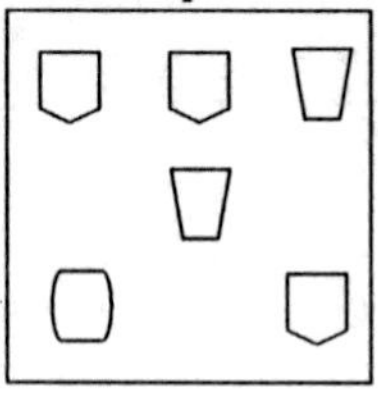

Set A

Set B

Neither

Example 22

Set A

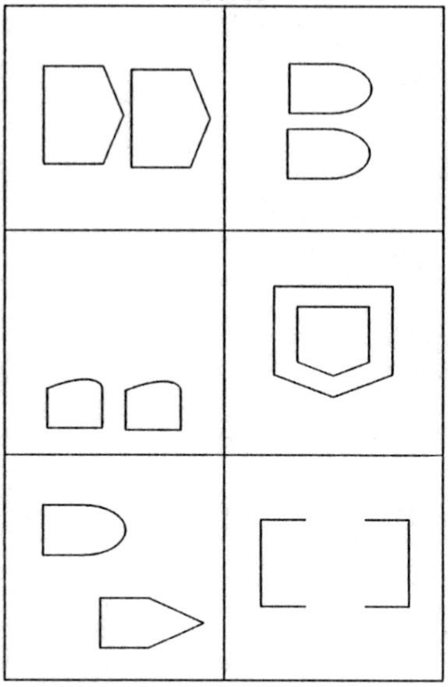

Set B

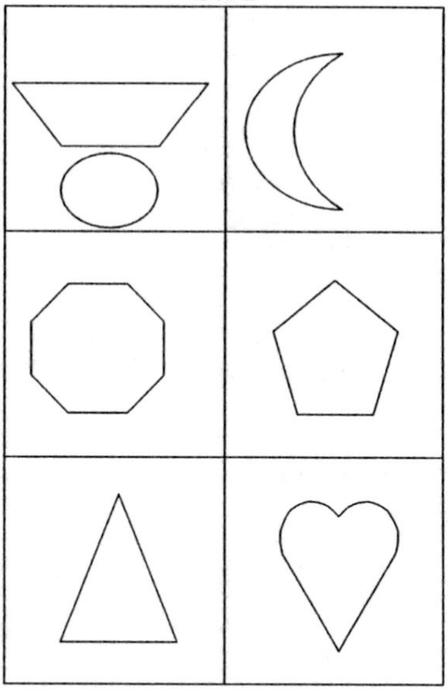

Test Shape 1

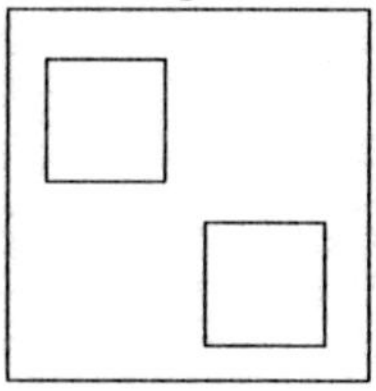

Set A

Set B

Neither

Test Shape 2

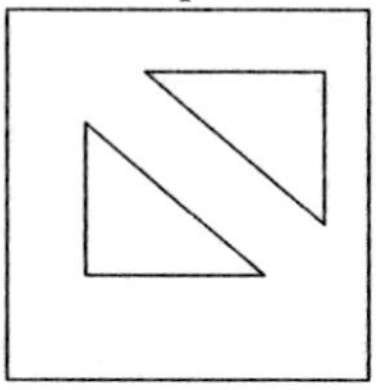

Set A

Set B

Neither

Test Shape 3

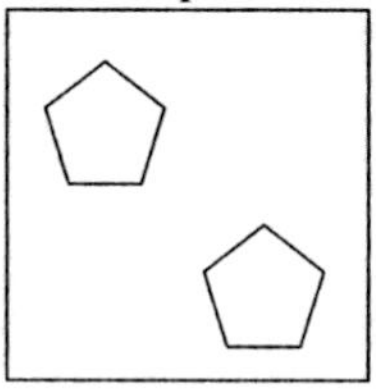

Set A

Set B

Neither

Test Shape 4

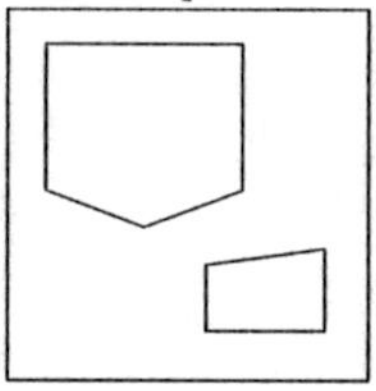

Set A

Set B

Neither

Test Shape 5

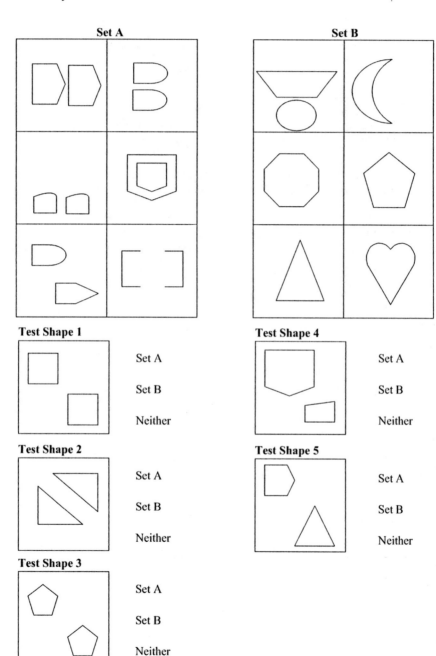

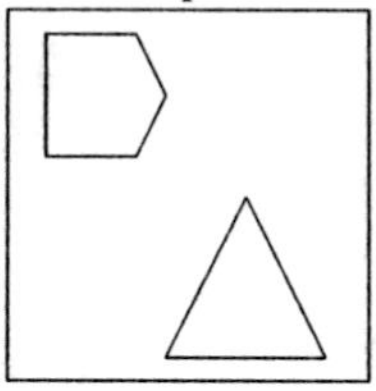

Set A

Set B

Neither

Example 23

Set A

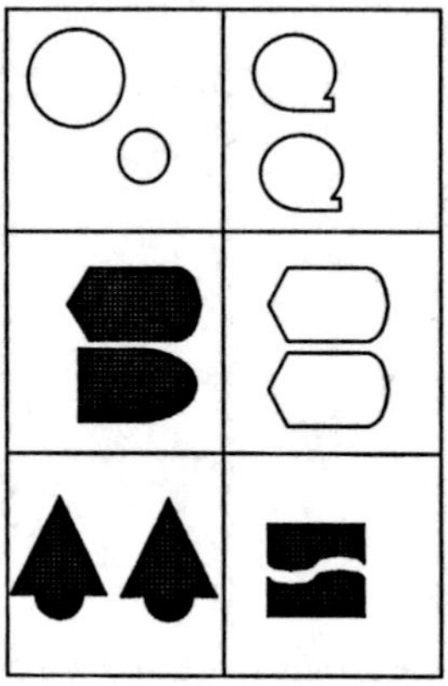

Set B

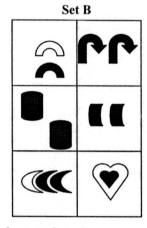

1. Which of the following shapes belong to Set A?

A B C D E

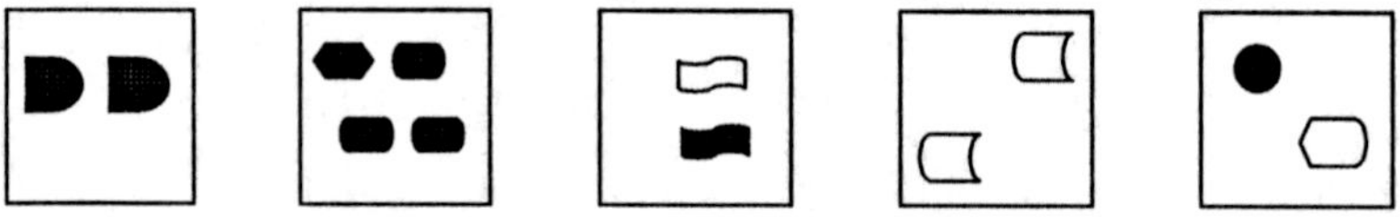

2. Which of the following shapes belong to Set A?

A B C D E

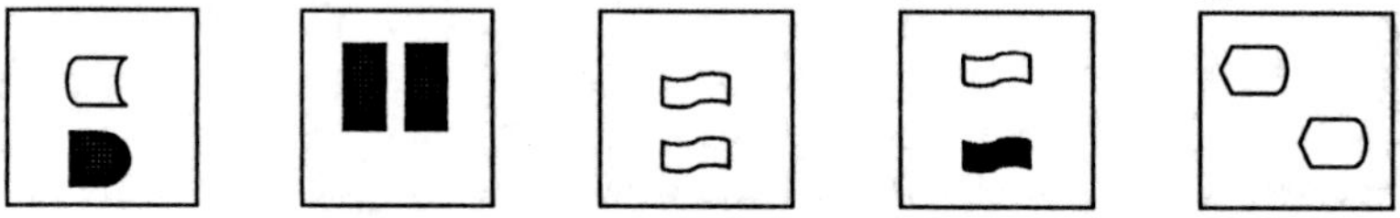

3. Which of the following shapes belong to Set B?

A B C D E

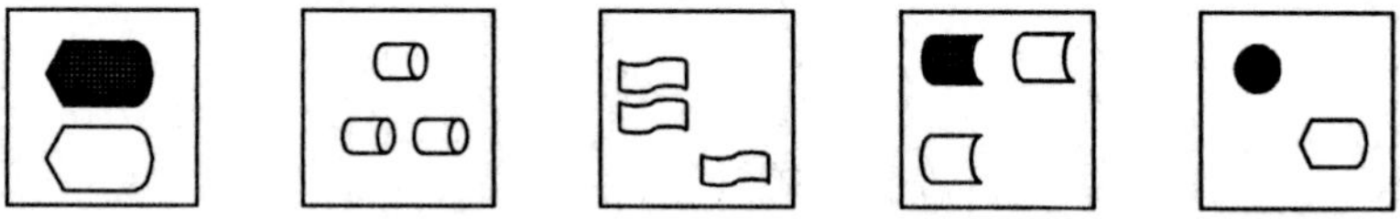

4. Which of the following shapes belong to Set B?

A B C D E

5. Which of the following shapes belong to Set A?

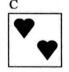

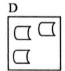

A B C D E

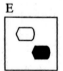

Example 24

Set A

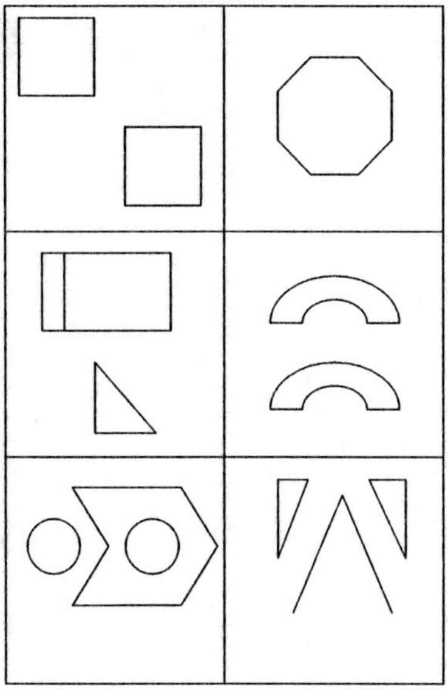

Set B

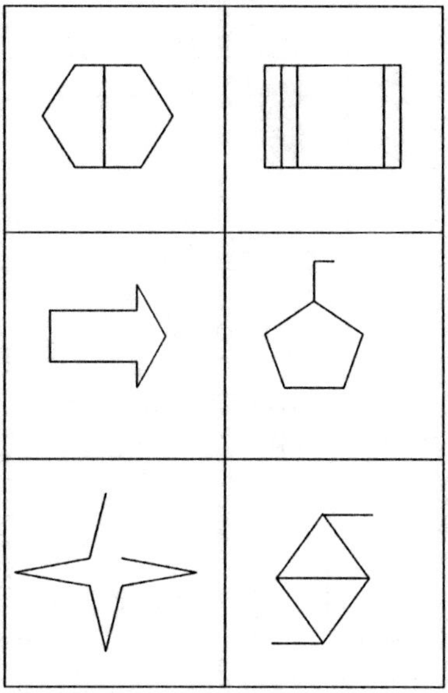

Test Shape 1

Set A

Set B

Neither

Test Shape 2

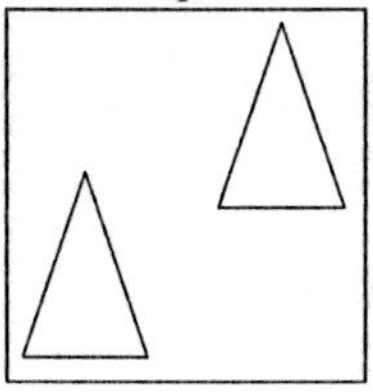

Set A

Set B

Neither

Test Shape 3

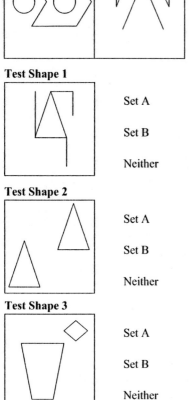

Set A

Set B

Neither

Test Shape 4

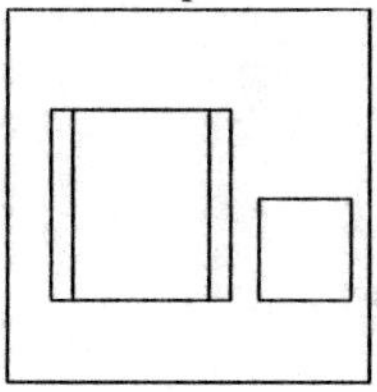

Set A

Set B

Neither

Test Shape 5

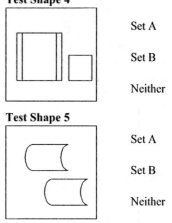

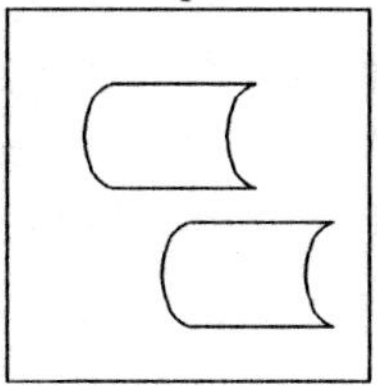

Set A

Set B

Neither

Example 25

Set A **Set B**

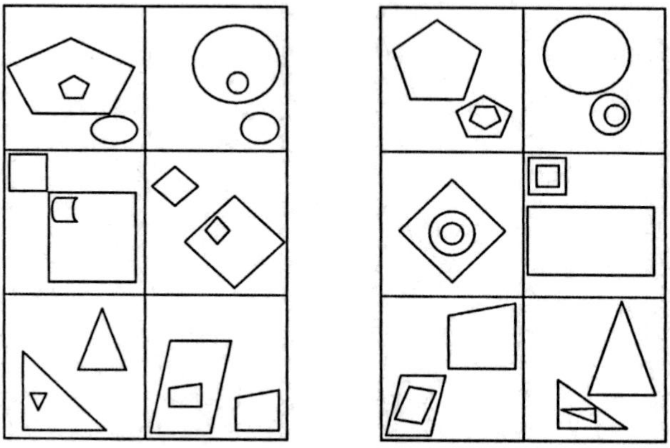

1. Which of the following shapes belong to Set A?

A B C D E

2. Which of the following shapes belong to Set A?

A B C D E

3. Which of the following shapes belong to Set B?

A B C D E

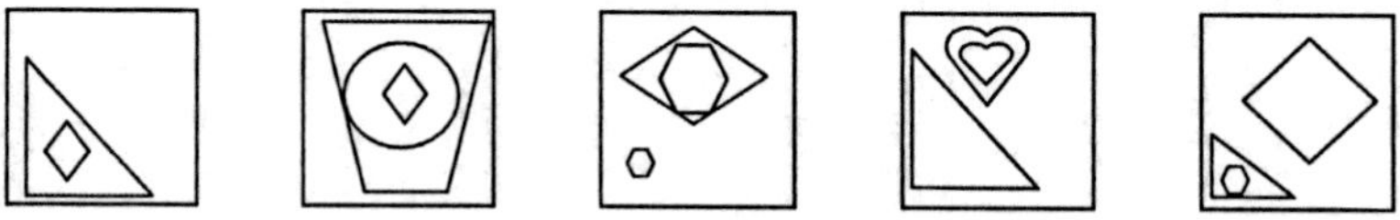

4. Which of the following shapes belong to Set B?

A B C D E

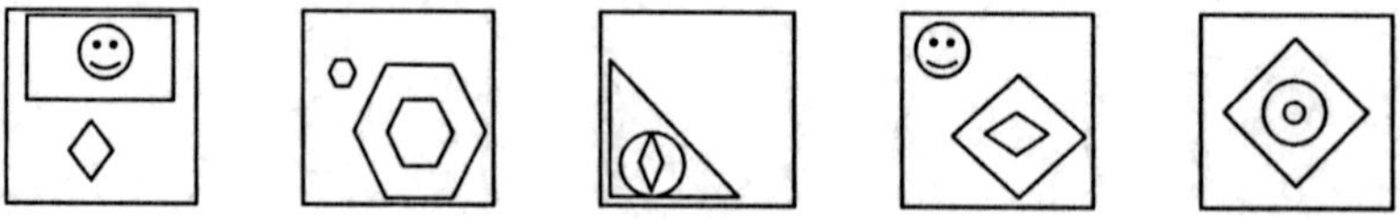

5. Which of the following shapes belong to Set B?

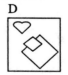

A B C D E

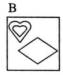

Example 26

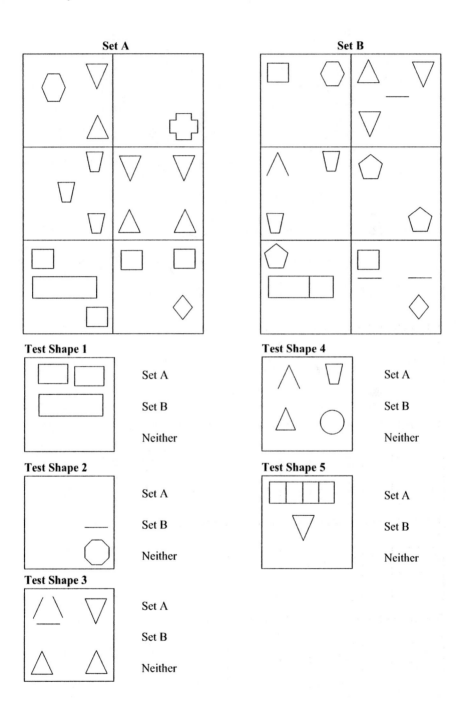

Set A

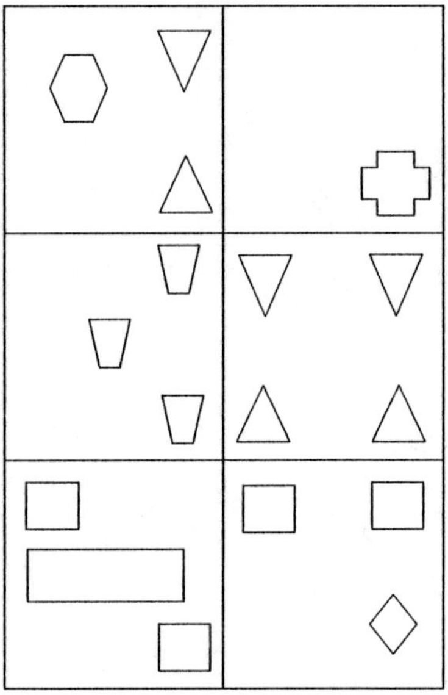

Set B

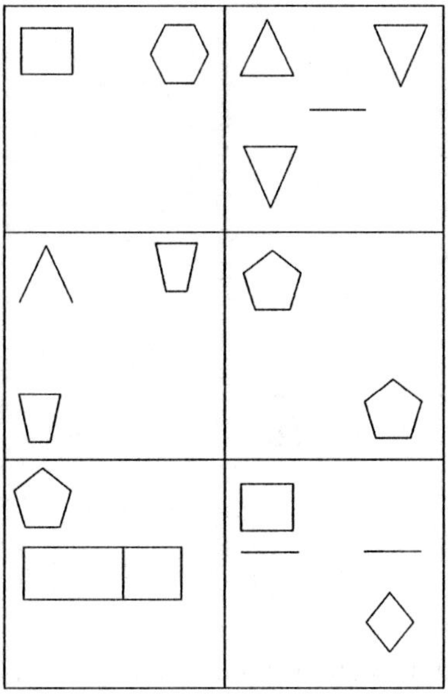

Test Shape 1

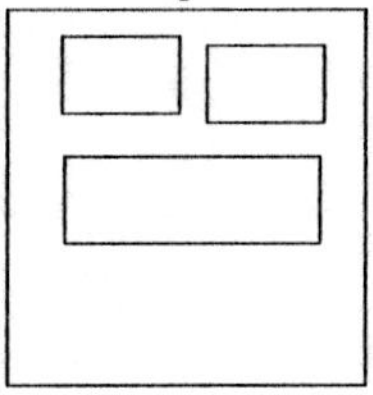

Set A

Set B

Neither

Test Shape 2

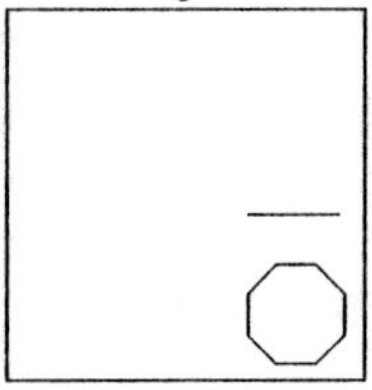

Set A

Set B

Neither

Test Shape 3

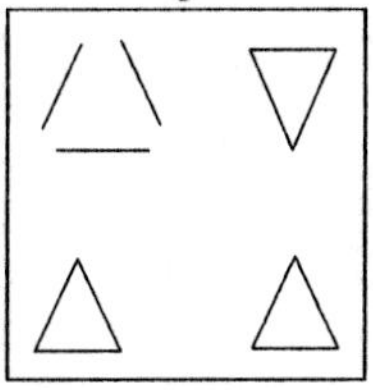

Set A

Set B

Neither

Test Shape 4

Set A

Set B

Neither

Test Shape 5

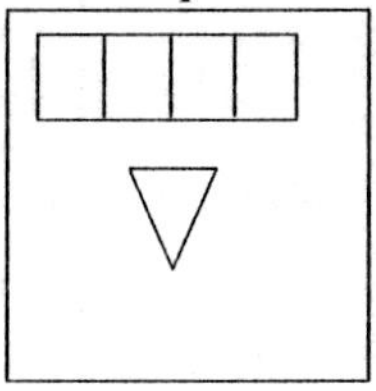

Set A

Set B

Neither

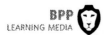

Example 27

Set A **Set B**

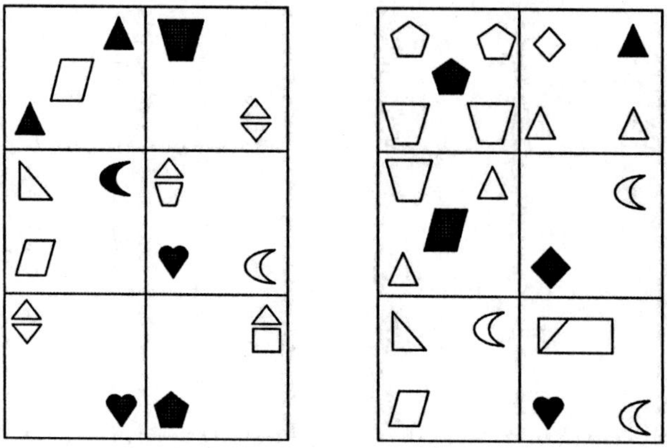

1. Which of the following shapes belong to Set A?

A B C D E

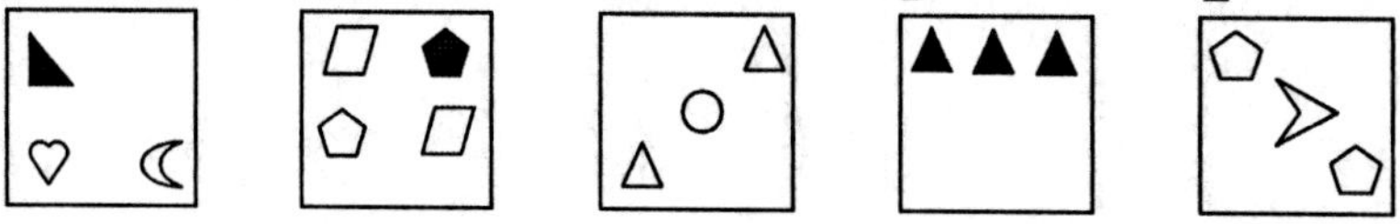

2. Which of the following shapes belong to Set A?

A B C D E

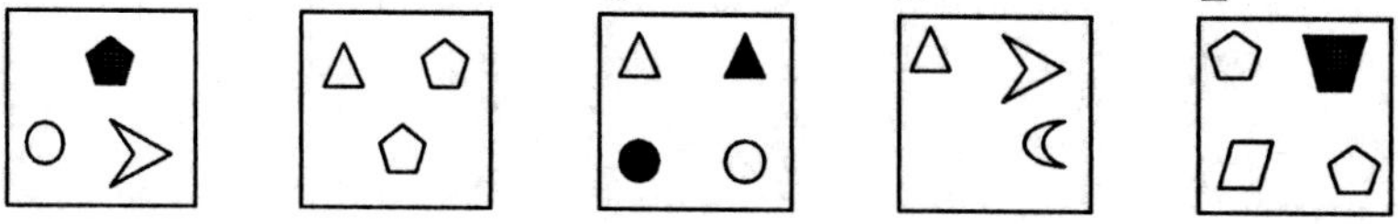

3. Which of the following shapes belong to Set A?

A B C D E

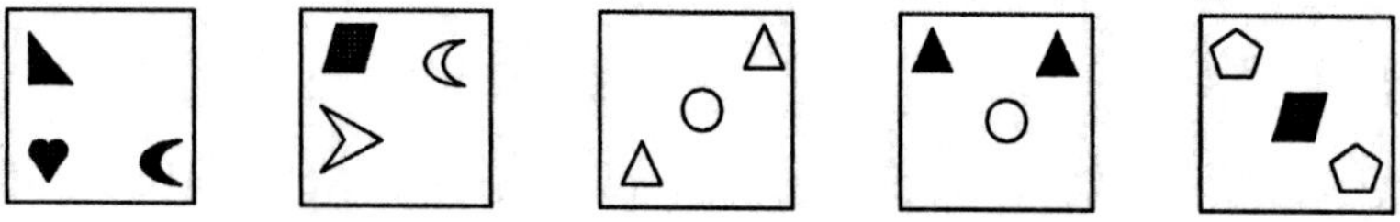

4. Which of the following shapes belong to Set B?

A B C D E

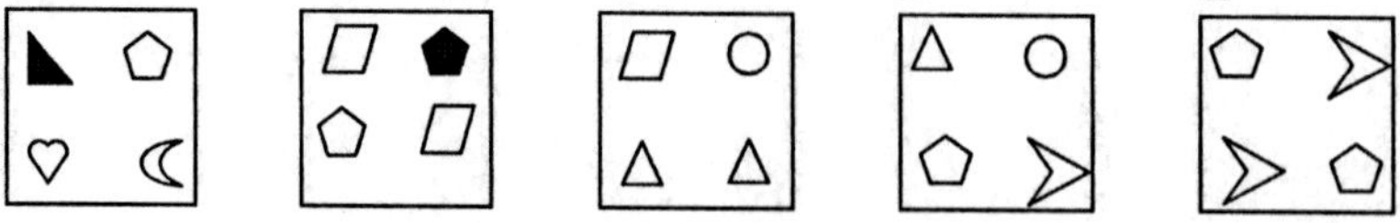

5. Which of the following shapes belong to Set B?

A B C D E

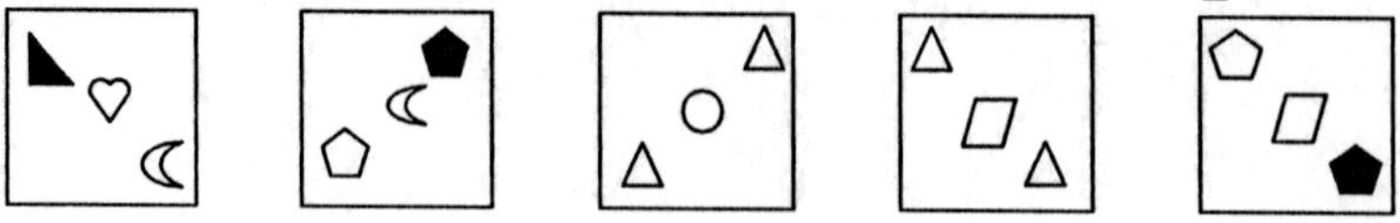

Example 28

Set A

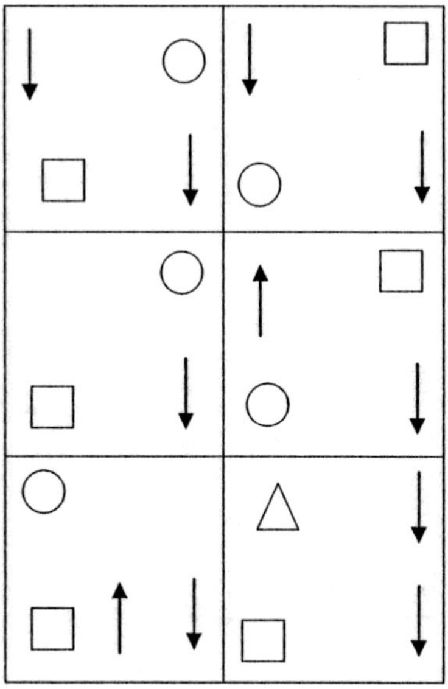

Set B

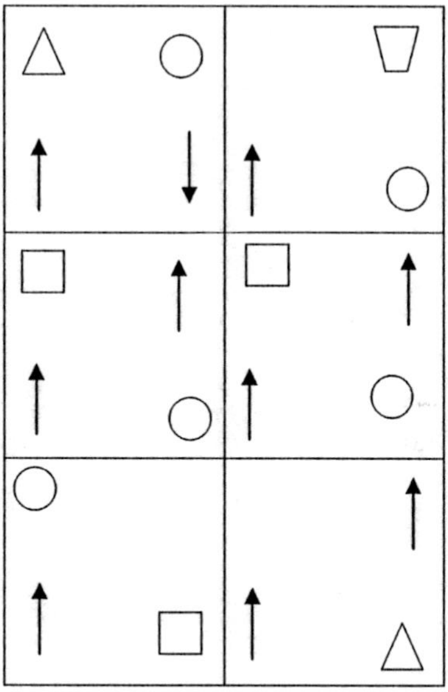

Test Shape 1

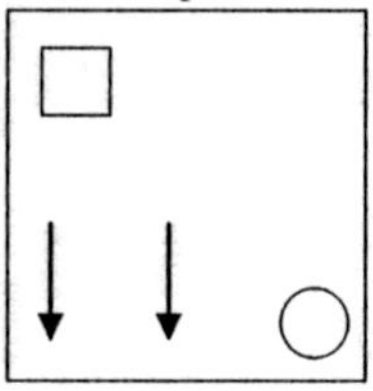

Set A

Set B

Neither

Test Shape 2

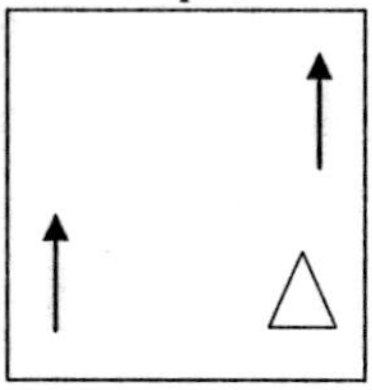

Set A

Set B

Neither

Test Shape 3

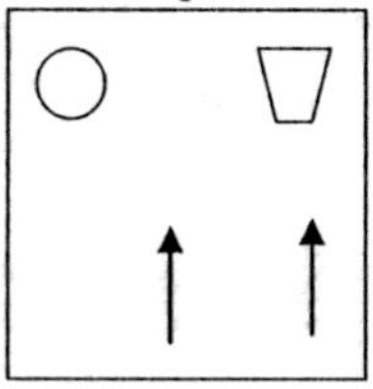

Set A

Set B

Neither

Test Shape 4

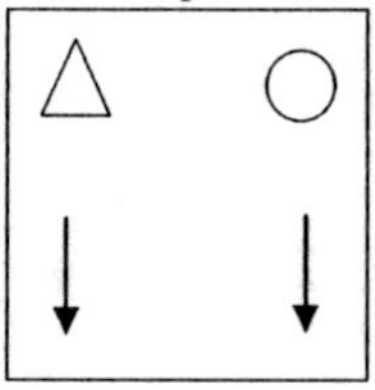

Set A

Set B

Neither

Test Shape 5

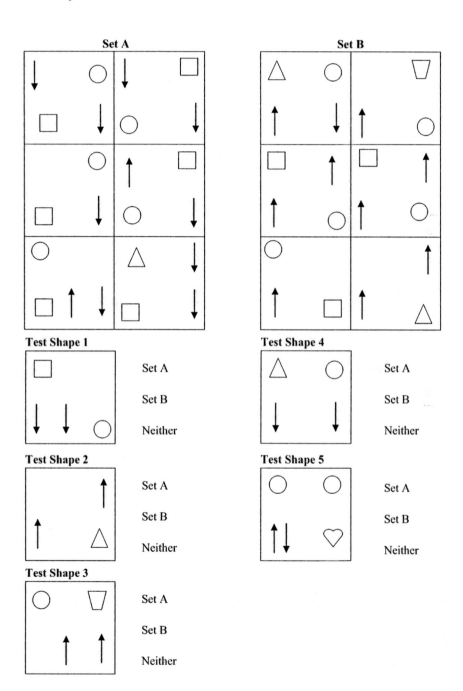

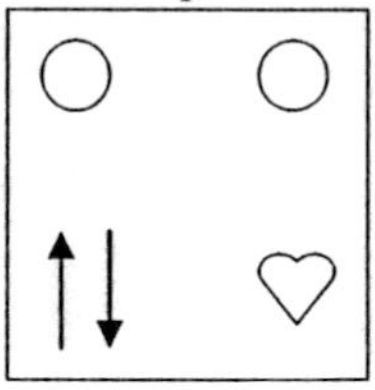

Set A

Set B

Neither

Example 29

Set A

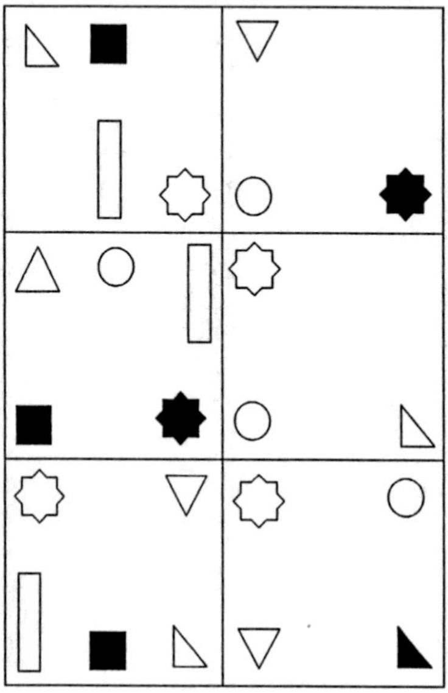

Set B

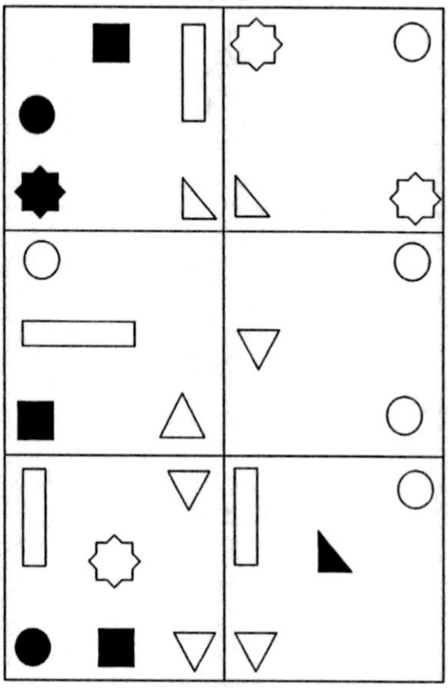

Test Shape 1

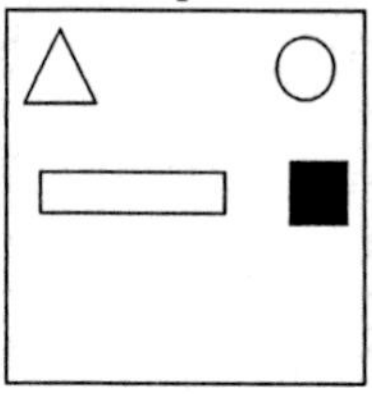

Set A

Set B

Neither

Test Shape 2

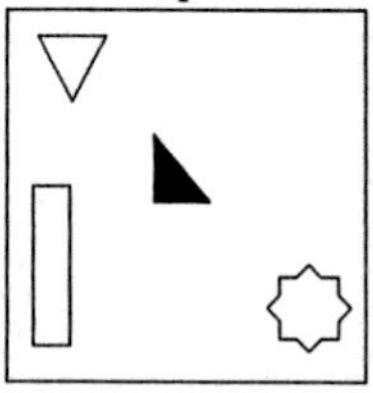

Set A

Set B

Neither

Test Shape 3

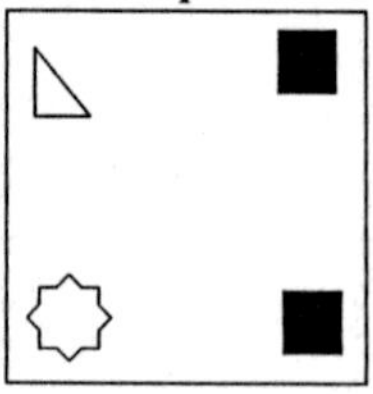

Set A

Set B

Neither

Test Shape 4

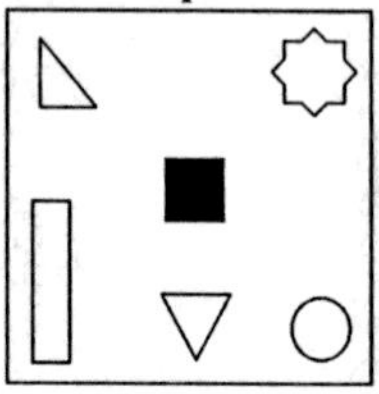

Set A

Set B

Neither

Test Shape 5

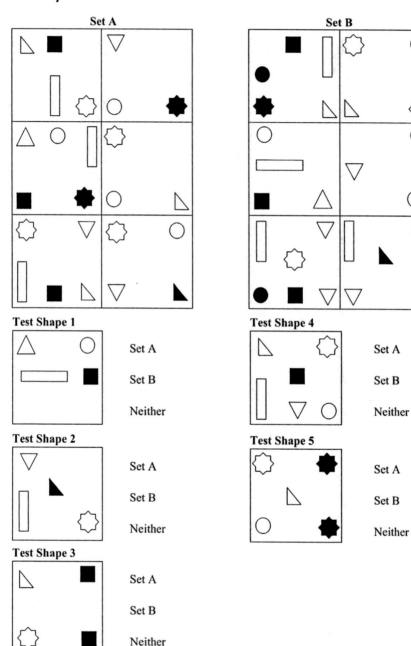

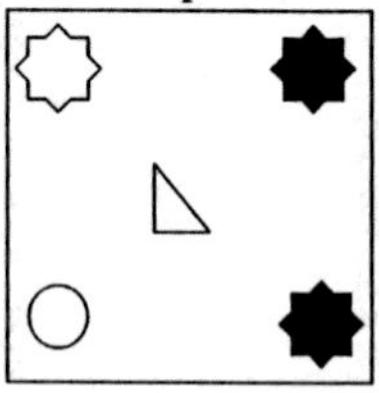

Set A

Set B

Neither

Example 30

Set A **Set B**

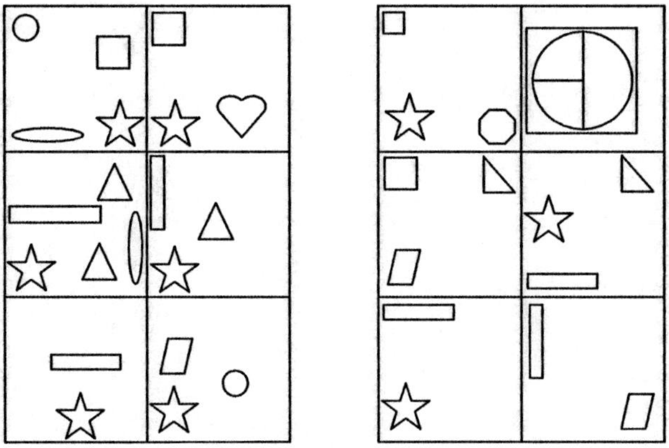

1. Which of the following shapes belong to Set A?

A B C D E

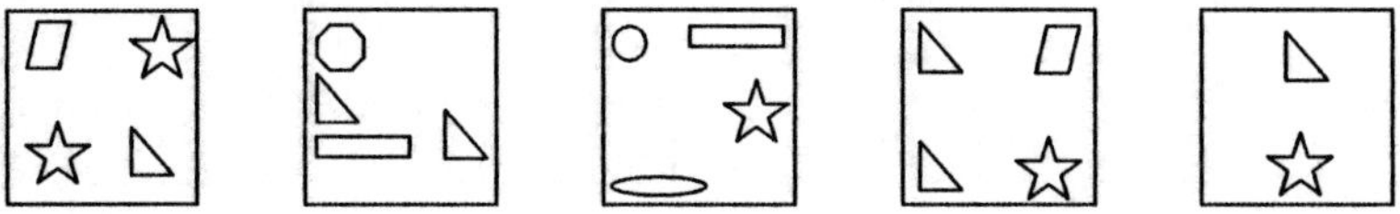

2. Which of the following shapes belong to Set A?

A B C D E

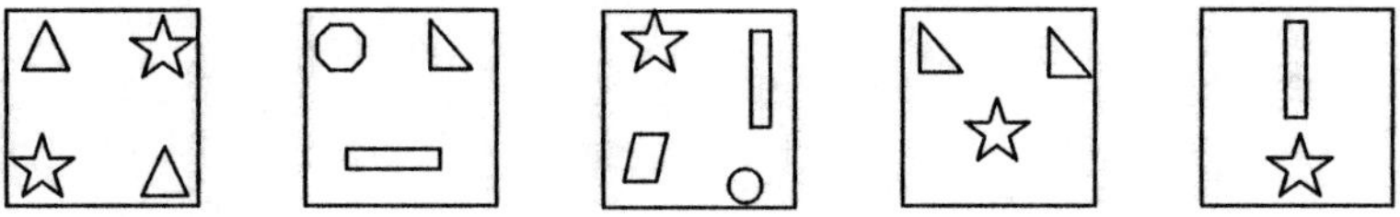

3. Which of the following shapes belong to Set A?

A B C D E

4. Which of the following shapes belong to Set B?

A B C D E

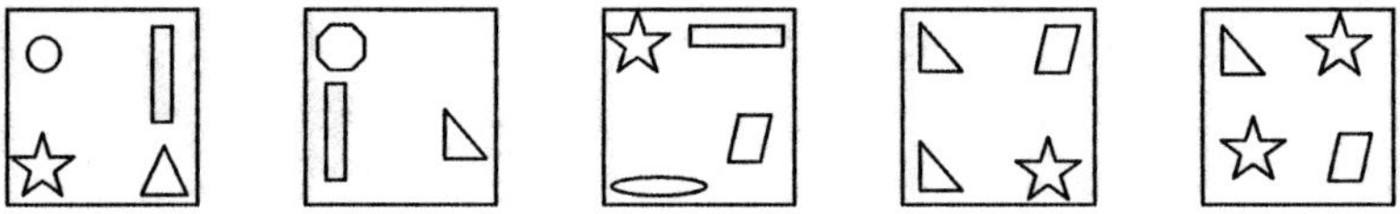

5. Which of the following shapes belong to Set B?

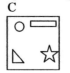

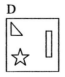

A B C D E

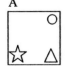

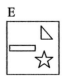

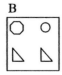

Example 31

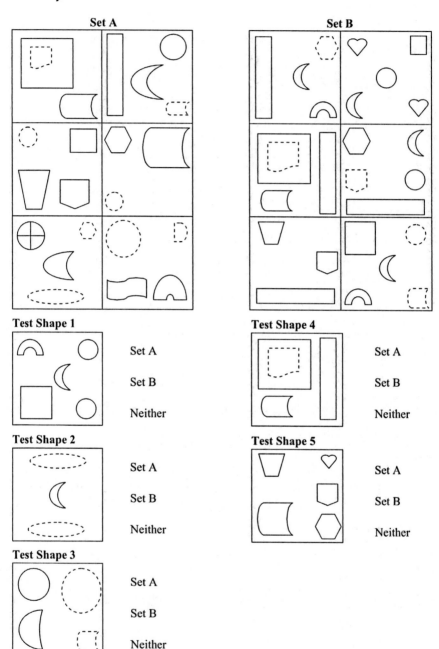

Set A

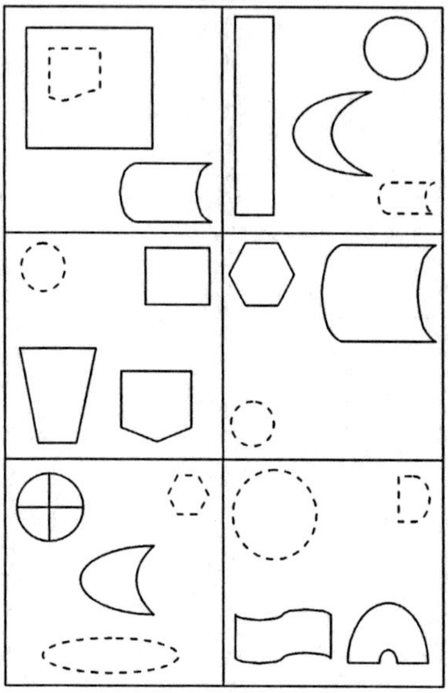

Set B

Test Shape 1

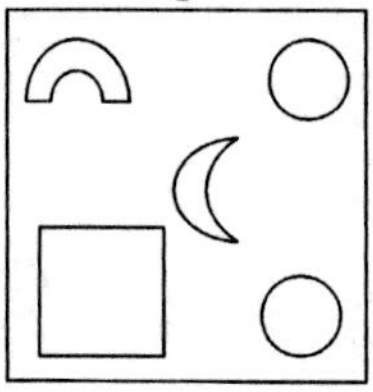

Set A

Set B

Neither

Test Shape 2

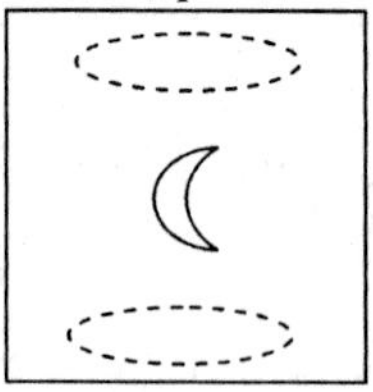

Set A

Set B

Neither

Test Shape 3

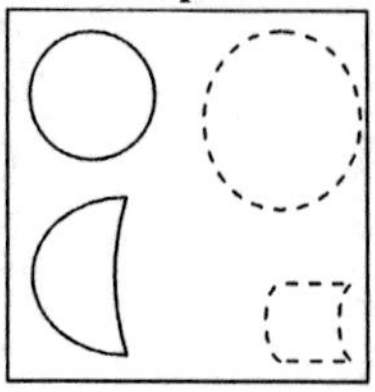

Set A

Set B

Neither

Test Shape 4

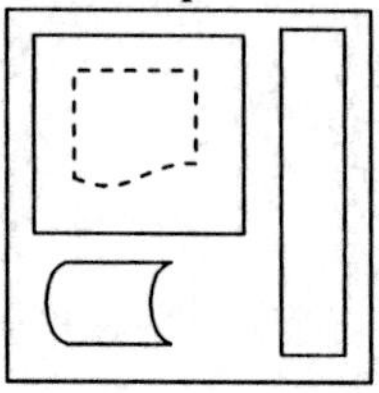

Set A

Set B

Neither

Test Shape 5

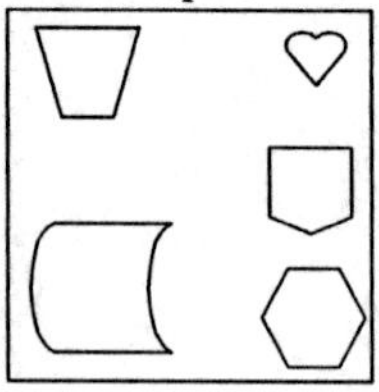

Set A

Set B

Neither

Justifications of Abstract Reasoning practice examples

Example 1

Set A

In this set there is a large shape with at least one corresponding smaller shape, both shapes are made of solid lines.

- The rule here is that the smaller shape must be identical to the larger shape in everything but size
- The smaller shape can be present either inside, or outside the larger shape
- A smaller non identical shape to the larger shape is used as a distracter

Set B

In this set there is a large shape and at least one small shape, both shapes are made of solid lines.

- The smaller shape must be identical to the larger shape except in size and shading
- Also, the smaller shape must be outside the larger shape
- A second smaller shape is used as a distracter

Test Shape 1 Answer: Set B
The smaller shape is shaded whereas the larger shape is unshaded. The smaller shape is also outside the larger shape; therefore it follows the rule of Set B.

Test Shape 2 Answer: Neither
The smaller shape is within the larger shape but it is shaded, whereas the larger shape is unshaded. Therefore it follows neither rule for Set A or B.

Test Shape 3 Answer: Neither
Both shapes are the same size and therefore they can go into neither set.

Test Shape 4 Answer: Set A
The small and large shapes are identical to each other following the rule in Set A.

Test Shape 5 Answer: Neither
The larger shape and smaller shape correspond to each other. However, they consist of dashed lines. Therefore they can go into neither set.

Example 2

Set A

In this set there is a combination of shapes used. The shapes consist of straight lines or curved lines.

- The rule is that the number of lines on the straight line shapes add up to 8
- Circles are used as distracters

Set B

In this set there are various shapes used. The shapes consist of straight lines or curved lines.

- The main rule is that the numbers of lines on the straight line shapes add up to 8
- Also, there are always three small circles in each box
- An oval is a distracter

1. **Correct answer B:** The number of straight lines equals 8, therefore it belongs to set A.
2. **Correct answer A:** The number of straight lines equals 8. therefore it belongs to set A.
3. **Correct answer E:** The number of straight lines equals 8. therefore it belongs to set A.
4. **Correct answer B:** The number of straight lines equals 8, there are 3 small circles present, therefore it belongs to set B.
5. **Correct answer C:** The number of straight lines equals 8, there are 3 small circles present, therefore it belongs to set B.

Example 3

Set A

In this set there is a combination of faces, triangles, and ovals made up of solid lines only. The rules in this set are:

- Where there are three faces, there should be one corresponding triangle
- Where there are three triangles there should be one corresponding face
- The ovals in this set are used as distracters

Set B

As above, in this set there is a combination of faces, triangles and ovals made up of solid lines only. The rules in this set are:

- Where there are three faces, there should be one corresponding oval
- Where there are three ovals there should be one corresponding face
- The triangles are distracters

Test Shape 1 Answer: Set A
This test shape belongs to Set A as there are three faces to one triangle. In this instance the ovals are a distracter.

Test Shape 2 Answer: Set B
This test shape belongs to Set B as there are three faces to one oval; the triangles are used as a distracter.

Test Shape 3 Answer: Neither
This test shape belongs to neither set as there are four faces. There would need to be three faces for this test shape to follow either rule.

Test Shape 4 Answer: Set A
This test shape belongs to Set A as there are three faces to one triangle. The ovals are used as distracters.

Test Shape 5 Answer: Set A
This test shape belongs to Set A as there are three faces to one triangle. The ovals in this case are distracters.

Example 4

Set A

In this set there are various shapes used. Each box has two shapes. The shapes can be shaded or unshaded.

- The rule in this set is that all shapes should have at least one line of symmetry
- Shading is used as a distracter

Set B

In this set various shapes are used. The shapes can be shaded or unshaded. Each box includes two shapes.

- The rules in this set are that only one shape should have symmetry
- Shading is used as a distracter

Test Shape 1 **Answer: Set A**
There are two shapes used, each of which has at least one line of symmetry.

Test Shape 2 **Answer: Set A**
There are two shapes used, each of which has at least one line of symmetry.

Test Shape 3 **Answer: Set B**
This follows Set B as there are two shapes and only one has a line of symmetry.

Test Shape 4 **Answer: Neither**
This follows neither rule as neither shape has one line of symmetry.

Test Shape 5 **Answer: Neither**
Although all shapes have at least one line of symmetry, there are three shapes, therefore the test shape belongs to neither set.

Example 5

Set A

There are various shapes made up of straight and curved lines. There can be up to three shapes in each box. Some of the shapes are shaded, others are not.

- The rule in this set is that the test shape must contain a square
- Shaded and unshaded shapes that are not squares are used as distracters

Set B

There are various shapes made up of straight lines which may be shaded or unshaded.

- The rule in this set is that the test shape must contain at least one right angle

Test Shape 1 **Answer: Neither**
The shape follows neither rule as there is not a square and there are no right angles.

Test Shape 2 **Answer: Neither**
The shape contains four non-right angled triangles and follows the rules of neither set.

Test Shape 3 Answer: Set A
The shapes are squares and therefore follows the rules of Set A.

Test Shape 4 Answer: Set B
Neither shape is a square so it cannot follow Set A. A right angle is present in both of the shapes. It therefore follows Set B.

Test Shape 5 Answer: Neither
As neither shape is a square and there are no right angles present in either shape, it therefore follows neither rule.

Example 6

Set A

In this set there are various shapes made up of straight and curved lines. Dashed and solid lines may be used and shapes may be shaded or unshaded.

- The rule of this set is that there should be at least two right angles
- Other shapes used are distracters

Set B

In this set there are various shapes made up of straight and curved lines.

- The rule of this set is that there should be only one right angle
- Also an oval shape is present

1. **Correct answer A:** There are at least 2 right angles present, therefore it belongs to set A.
2. **Correct answer D:** There are at least 2 right angles present, therefore it belongs to set A.
3. **Correct answer B:** There are at least 2 right angles present, therefore it belongs to set A.
4. **Correct answer E:** There is only 1 right angle present and an oval shape is present, therefore it belongs to set B.
5. **Correct answer E:** There is only 1 right angle present and an oval shape is present, therefore it belongs to set B.

Example 7

Set A

The set contains various shapes made up of straight or curved lines. The lines can be dashed or solid. Within each box there are always three shapes.

- The rule in this set is that one circle needs to be present, regardless of size
- Also, there must never be more than one of the same shape, regardless of size

Set B

The set contains various shapes made up of straight or curved lines. The lines are either dashed or straight.

- The rule in this set is that there should be at least one smaller version of the largest shape, which may be shaded or unshaded

Test Shape 1 Answer: Neither
There are three shapes in this test box with none of them being repeated. It may therefore be thought that the test shape follows Set A. However there is no circle present. It therefore follows neither rule.

Test Shape 2 Answer: Set B
There are three shapes in this test box, so it could belong to Set A. However, two of the three shapes are repeated: a large oval and a small oval. Since there is a smaller version of the large shape, the test shape therefore follows Set B.

Test Shape 3 Answer: Set B
There are four shapes in this set, including three hearts; therefore it cannot belong to Set A. As there is one large heart and at least one small heart the test shape belongs to Set B.

Test Shape 4 Answer: Neither
There are three shapes present. As the two circles are repeated it cannot belong to Set A and as there is no smaller version of the large shape then it cannot belong to Set B.

Test Shape 5 Answer: Set A
There are three shapes present that do not relate to each other. It cannot therefore follow rule B. There is a circle present, therefore it belongs to Set A.

Example 8

Set A

In this set, there are various shapes consisting of triangles, squares, circles and arrows. Some of the shapes are shaded others are not. Each box in the set contains at least one arrow and a triangle of fixed size. The triangle can be pointing either downwards or upwards.

- The rule in this set is that at least one arrow should always be pointing east and situated at the top of the box
- Also a triangle must always be in one of the corners of the box
- The remaining shapes including an additional arrow are randomly placed and are used as distracters

Set B

This set contains the same shapes as Set A. Some of the shapes are shaded others are not.

- The rule in this set is that an arrow should always be present and facing south
- Also a triangle should be present, and should always face upwards and should not be positioned in a corner.

1. **Correct answer A:** One arrow is located at the top of the box and is pointing East and a triangle is present in a corner, therefore it belongs to set A.
2. **Correct answer C:** One arrow is located at the top of the box and is pointing East and a triangle is present in a corner, therefore it belongs to set A.
3. **Correct answer C:** At least one arrow is present and is facing South. A triangle is present and is positioned upwards and is situated in the corner. It therefore belongs to set B.
4. **Correct answer D:** At least one arrow is present and is facing South. A triangle is present and is positioned upwards and is situated in the corner. It therefore belongs to set B.
5. **Correct answer E:** At least one arrow is present and is facing South. A triangle is present and is positioned upwards and is situated in the corner. It therefore belongs to set B.

Example 9

Set A

The set contains various shapes made up of straight, curved, solid and dashed lines. Within each box there are always three shapes. There are no number patterns or rules of symmetry to follow.

- The rule is that there must be three differently sized shapes.
- Also, none of the shapes must be repeated in the box.

Set B

This set contains various shapes made up of straight, curved, solid and dashed lines. Within each box there are three or four shapes. There are no number pattern or rules of symmetry to follow.

- The only rule is that the largest shape must be replicated elsewhere within the test box by a smaller version of itself.
- Other shapes are randomly arranged and are used as distracters

Test Shape 1 Answer: Set B
A heart is repeated three times. It therefore does not follow rule A. The large shape is replicated by a smaller version of itself. Thus it follows Set B.

Test Shape 2 Answer: Set B
The shapes are repeated so it cannot follow Set A. The large shape is replicated elsewhere by a smaller version of itself therefore it follows Set B.

Test Shape 3 Answer: Set A
This test box belongs to Set A as none of the three shapes are repeated and they are in different sizes.

Test Shape 4 Answer: Neither
Of the three shapes two are repeated so it does not belong to Set A. The large shape, an oval, is not replicated. Therefore, it belongs to neither set.

Test Shape 5 Answer: Set B
A shape is replicated, so this test shape cannot belong to Set A and must belong to Set B as it contains a large shape that is replicated by a smaller version of itself.

Example 10

Set A

Within this set there are a number of different sized curved shapes. All curved shapes are made of solid lines. There is always a large and a small curved shape.

- The rule in this set is that the smallest circular shape must always be inside the largest shape

Set B

Within this set there are a number of curved shapes.

- The rule in this set is that the smallest curved shape must always be within one of the middle sized curve shapes

Test Shape 1 Answer: Neither
The test shape belongs to neither set as the smallest shape is not in either the middle or the larger sized shape.

Test Shape 2 Answer: Set A
There are three different sized shapes, ranging from small, medium and large. The smallest shape is inside the largest shape. It therefore follows the rule of Set A.

Test Shape 3 Answer: Set A
The test shape follows the rule of Set A as the smallest shape is present within the largest shape.

Test Shape 4 Answer: Set B
Within one of these medium sized ovals there is a smaller circle within it. Therefore the shapes follow the rule of Set B.

Test Shape 5 Answer: Set B
The smallest shape is within a medium sized shape.

Example 11

Set A

In this set there are various curved and straight shapes.

- The main rule is that there must be two symmetrical shapes present
- Also, a triangle must always be present

Set B

In this set there are various curved and straight symmetrical shapes.

- The main rule is that there must be a large and small symmetrical shape present
- Also, there must be least one small circle present

Test Shape 1 Answer: Set A
The test box contains two symmetrical shapes. Also a triangle is present. This shape follows the rule of Set A.

Test Shape 2 Answer: Set A
This test box follows the rule of Set A as there are two shapes present that are symmetrical, both a large and a smaller one. There is also a triangle present.

Test Shape 3 Answer: Set B
This test box follows Set B, as there is a large shape present that is symmetrical and a small shape that is symmetrical. Also, a small circle is present. There are no triangles present for this test box to follow the rules of Set A.

Test Shape 4 Answer: Neither
This test box follows neither rule as the large shape is not symmetrical.

Test Shape 5 Answer: Set B
Excluding the circles, there is a large shape and a small shape that are symmetrical. There are also two circles present so this must follow the rule of Set B. There are no triangles present for it to follow the rule of Set A.

Example 12

Set A

This set consists of hearts, circles and a large shape divided into four segments.

- The rule is that each large shape must be divided into four segments
- Also, the large divided shape must contain at least one right angle
- Hearts and circles have been used as distracters

Set B

This set consists of hearts, circles and a large shape divided into four segments.

- The rule is that each large shape must be divided into four segments
- Also, the large shape divided must not contain a right angle
- Hearts and circles have been used as distracters

Test Shape 1 Answer: Neither

This test shape follows neither rule as the large shape is not divided into four segements.

Test Shape 2 Answer: Set A

This test shape follows Set A as it is divided into four segments and there is at least one right angle present.

Test Shape 3 Answer: Set A

This test shape follows Set A as it is divided into four segments and there is at least one right angle present.

Test Shape 4 Answer: Set A

Again this test shape follows Set A as it is divided into four segments and there is at least one right angle present.

Test Shape 5 Answer: Set B

This test shape follows Set B as it is divided into four segments and there is no right angle present.

Example 13

Set A

In this set there are various shaded and unshaded shapes.

- The rule is that the large unshaded shape must contain at least one right angle.
- Also, there must be at least one circle present.
- The shaded object is used as a distracter

Set B

In this set there are various shaded and unshaded shapes used.

- The rule is that the large unshaded shape must contain at least one right angle.
- Also, there is always one shaded shape.

Test Shape 1 Answer: Neither
This set follows neither rule as there are no right angles present in the large unshaded shape.

Test Shape 2 Answer: Neither
This set follows neither rule as there are no right angles present in the large unshaded object.

Test Shape 3 Answer: Set A
This test shape follows Set A as there are two right angles present and two circles.

Test Shape 4 Answer: Set B
This test shape follows Set B as there are two right angles present and no circles.

Test Shape 5 Answer: Set A
This test shape follows Set A as the arrow contains two right angles and there is also a circle present.

Example 14

Set A

In this set various straight and curved shapes are used. There are no pattern rules to follow.

- The only rule is that there must be at least one shape present that is symmetrical.

Set B

In this set there are various straight and curved shapes used. There are no number pattern rules to follow.

- The only rule is that there must be no symmetrical shapes present

1. **Correct answer D:** One shape present is symmetrical, therefore it belongs to set A.
2. **Correct answer C:** One shape present is symmetrical, therefore it belongs to set A.
3. **Correct answer B:** There are no symmetrical shapes present, therefore it belongs to set B.

4. **Correct answer E:** There are no symmetrical shapes present, therefore it belongs to set B.
5. **Correct answer B:** There are no symmetrical shapes present, therefore it belongs to set B.

Example 15

Set A

This set contains circles, triangles and arrows pointing north and south.

- The rule in this set is that the triangles are always in a corner.
- Also, where the triangle is in the top corner, an arrow is always pointing down. Where a triangle is in the bottom corner an arrow is always pointing up.
- Circles are always present.

Set B

This set contains circles, triangles and arrows pointing north and south.

- The rule in this set is that triangles are always in the corner.
- There is always a triangle or a circle in the top left corner. Where the triangle is in the top left corner, a circle is always in the bottom right corner; and where a circle is in the top left corner a triangle is in the bottom right corner.
- Arrows are used as distracters.

Test Shape 1 Answer: Neither
This test shape follows neither set as the triangle is in the centre.

Test Shape 2 Answer: Set A
This test shape follows Set A as a triangle is present in the corner and an arrow facing upwards is present. For the shape to follow Set B the triangle should be in either the bottom right or top left corner and a circle in the opposing corner.

Test Shape 3 Answer: Neither
There is no triangle present in this test box so it can follow neither rule.

Test Shape 4 Answer: Neither
This test shape follows neither set as the triangle is not in a corner.

Test Shape 5 Answer: Set B
This test shape follows the rule of Set B as the triangle is in the top left corner and there is a circle in the bottom right corner. The arrow is facing in the wrong way for it to follow Set A.

Example 16

Set A

In this set there are various shapes used.

- The rule is that there is always one shaded non-symmetrical shape.
- Also, at least two unshaded triangles are present.
- The other unshaded shapes are distracters.

Set B

In this set there are various shapes used that are unshaded or shaded.
- The rule is that there is always one non-symmetrical shape.
- Other shapes used are distracters.

Test Shape 1 Answer: Neither
The test shape cannot belong to Set A as the shaded shape is symmetrical. It does not follow the rule of Set B as there are two non-symmetrical shapes.

Test Shape 2 Answer: Set B
This test shape follows Set B as there is one non-symmetrical shape present. It does not follow the rule of Set A as there are no triangles.

Test Shape 3 Answer: Set A
This test shape follows Set A as the non-symmetrical shape is shaded and there are two unshaded triangles present. It does not follow the rule of Set B as there is more than one non-symmetrical shape present.

Test Shape 4 Answer: Neither
This test shape follows neither rule as all the shapes are symmetrical.

Test Shape 5 Answer: Set A
This test shape follows Set A as the non symmetrical shape is shaded and there are two unshaded triangles present. It does not follow the rule of Set B as there is more than one non symmetrical shape present.

Example 17

Set A

In this set there are small circles, faces and triangles. The rules are:

- There must be either five circles and three triangles, or five triangles and three circles.
- The faces are used as distracters.

Set B

In this set there are small circles, faces and triangles. The rules are:

- There must be either five faces and three circles, or five circles and three faces.
- The triangles are used as distracters.

Test Shape 1 Answer: Neither
This test shape belongs to neither set as there are six circles present.
Test Shape 2 Answer: Set B
This test shape follows Set B as there are five circles with three faces.

Test Shape 3 Answer: Set A
This test shape follows Set A as there are five triangles with three circles.

Test Shape 4 Answer: Set A
This test shape follows Set A as there five circles with three triangles.

Test Shape 5 Answer: Neither
This test shape follows neither set as there are four circles with five faces.

Example 18

Set A

This set contains various shapes which can be either shaded or unshaded. All shapes are made from straight lines. There are no curved shapes in this set. Some shapes are on their own, some are mixed with others.

- The rule is that lines making up the shapes must add up to 12.
- Shading is used as a distracter.

Set B

This set contains various shapes which can be either shaded or unshaded. All shapes are made from straight lines.

- The rule is that the lines making up the shapes must add up to 6
- Shading is used as a distracter

1. **Correct answer D:** The number of lines making up the shapes equals 12, therefore it belongs to set A.
2. **Correct answer A:** The number of lines making up the shapes equals 12, therefore it belongs to set A.
3. **Correct answer C:** The number of lines making up the shapes equals 12, therefore it belongs to set A.
4. **Correct answer B:** The number of lines making up the shapes equals 6, therefore it belongs to set B.
5. **Correct answer E:** The number of lines making up the shapes equals 6, therefore it belongs to set B.

Example 19

Set A

In this set there is a combination of curved rectangles, circles, and arrows facing south and north. All shapes are made up of solid lines only. The rules in this set are:

- Where there are three curved rectangles, there should be one corresponding circle.
- Where there are three circles there should be one corresponding curved rectangle.
- The arrows facing south and north are used as distracters.

Set B

In this set there is a combination of curved rectangles, circles, arrows facing south and north. All shapes are made up of solid lines only. The rules in this set are:

- Where there are three south facing arrows, there should be one corresponding circle.
- Where there are three circles there should be one arrow facing south.
- The curved rectangles, and north facing arrows are used as distracters.

Test Shape 1 Answer: Set A
This test shape belongs to Set A as there are three curved rectangles to one circle. It does not belong to Set B as there are not three south facing arrows to the one circle.

Test Shape 2 Answer: Set B
This test shape belongs to Set B as there are three south facing arrows to one circle.

Test Shape 3 Answer: Neither
This test shape belongs to neither as there are four circles.

Test Shape 4 Answer: Neither
This test shape contains three circles to one arrow facing south but the circles included are made of dashed lines which is a feature of neither set.

Test Shape 5 Answer: Neither
This test shape belongs to neither as there are three circles to one curved rectangle.

Example 20

Set A

In this set are various shapes that are either shaded, or unshaded. The shapes are composed of straight and curved lines.

- The rule in this set is that each shape must have at least two lines of symmetry.

Set B

In this set are various shapes which are either closed, or unclosed. The shapes are composed of straight and curved lines.

- The rule in this set is that each shape cannot have any lines of symmetry.
- Also, none of the shapes are shaded.

Test Shape 1 Answer: Neither
The shape has a single line of symmetry and therefore does not belong in Set A or Set B.

Test Shape 2 Answer: Set A
The test shape belongs to Set A as the shape has a horizontal and a vertical line of symmetry.

Test Shape 3 Answer: Neither
Although the curved arrow does not have any lines of symmetry, it cannot belong to Set B because the shape is shaded. Therefore, the shape does not belong to either group.

Test Shape 4 Answer: Set B
The oval shape is not complete and therefore does not have any lines of symmetry. It therefore belongs to Set B.

Test Shape 5 Answer: Neither
The test shape does not have any lines of symmetry. However, the line is not continuous therefore the test shape belongs to neither set.

Example 21

Set A

In this set there are a combination of pentagons, rounded rectangles and quadrilateral shapes. Within each box there are four or five shapes.

- The rule in this set is that each box must contain two pentagons.
- Also, each box must contain at least one quadrilateral shape and at least one rounded rectangle.

Set B

As with Set A, there are a combination of pentagons, rounded rectangles and quadrilateral shapes. Also, within each box there are four or five shapes.

- The rule in this set is that each box must contain at least one rounded rectangle.
- Also, each box must contain at least one quadrilateral shape and only one pentagon. All other shapes are distracters.

Test Shape 1 Answer: Neither
The test shape does not belong to Set A or Set B because there are too many shapes within it.

Test Shape 2 Answer: Set A
As there are two pentagons and at least one quadrilateral shape and at least one rounded rectangle, the test shape belongs to Set A. Since there is one pentagon it cannot belong to Set B.

Test Shape 3 Answer: Set A
As there are two pentagons and at least one quadrilateral shape and at least one rounded rectangle, the test shape belongs to Set A. Since there are two pentagons it cannot belong to Set B.

Test Shape 4 Answer: Set B
As there is one rounded rectangle and at least one quadrilateral shape and one pentagon, the test shape belongs to Set B. It does not fit Set A because there is only one pentagon.

Test Shape 5 Answer: Neither
The text shape does not belong to Set A or Set B because there are too many shapes within it.

Example 22

Set A

In this set there are two shapes in each box. In most cases the shapes are identical. However, this is not always the case.

- The rule in this set is that there are always two shapes.
- Also, each shape must contain two right angles.

Set B

In this set there are either one or two shapes in each box.

- The rule in this set is that each shape in the box must not contain any right angles.

Test Shape 1 Answer: Neither
Although at first sight, the test shape appears to fit into Set A, each square has four right angles. Therefore, it cannot belong to either set.

Test Shape 2 Answer: Neither
The test shape contains two right-angled triangles. Each triangle contains one right angle, therefore, the test shape cannot belong to either set.

Test Shape 3 Answer: Set B
The test shape contains two pentagons. As neither shape contains right angles, it therefore belongs to Set B.

Test Shape 4 Answer: Set A
The test shape contains a pentagon and a rhomboid. Although the shapes are not similar, they both contain two right angles. Therefore the shape belongs to Set A.

Test Shape 5 Answer: Neither
The test shape contains a pentagon and an isosceles triangle. The pentagon contains two right angles, however the triangle does not contain any right angles. Therefore, the test shape does not belong to either set.

Example 23

Set A

In this set there are two shapes in each box. In most cases the shapes are identical.

- The rule in this set is that there are always two shapes in each box.
- Also, each shape must contain a total of one curved line.
- Also, all the shapes must have corresponding shading, that is, they must both be shaded, or both unshaded.

Set B

In this set there are two or three shapes in each box.

- The rule in this set is that each shape must contain two curved lines.
- Also, there must be at least one shaded shape.

1. **Correct answer A:** There are two identical shapes in the box, which both contain one curved side, one shape is shaded, one is not, therefore it belongs to set A.
2. **Correct answer E:** There are two identical shapes in the box, which both contain one curved side, one shape is shaded, one is not, therefore it belongs to set A.
3. **Correct answer D:** There are two or more shapes in the box, each shape contains two curved sides and at least one shape is shaded, therefore it belongs to set B.
4. **Correct answer B:** There are two or more shapes in the box, each shape contains two curved sides and at least one shape is shaded, therefore it belongs to set B.
5. **Correct answer C:** There are two or more shapes in the box, each shape contains two curved sides and at least one shape is shaded, therefore it belongs to set B.

Example 24

Set A

In this set there are between one to three shapes in each box. The shapes are composed of straight and / or curved lines.

- The rule in this set is that within each box there must be exactly eight lines, which can be either curved or straight.

Set B

In this set there is one straight lined shape.

- The rule in this set is that there is always one shape in each box.
- Also, the shape must be composed of seven straight lines.

Test Shape 1 Answer: Set B
The test shape consists of seven straight lines in total. Therefore, the test shape belongs to Set B.

Test Shape 2 Answer: Neither
The test shape contains two triangles, which total six straight lines altogether. Therefore, the test shape does not belong to either set.

Test Shape 3 Answer: Set A
The test shape contains two quadrilateral shapes. In total there are eight straight lines. Therefore, the test shape belongs to Set A.

Test Shape 4 Answer: Neither
The test shape contains two squares, with an additional two vertical lines within the larger square. As there are a total of ten lines, the test shape belongs to neither set.

Test Shape 5 Answer: Set A
The test shape contains two four-sided shapes. Although four of the lines are curved, the total number of lines equals eight. Therefore the test shape belongs to Set A.

Example 25

Set A

In this set there are three unshaded shapes within each box. The shapes are composed of straight and / or curved lines. There is always one shape within another shape.

- The rule in this set is that the smallest shape in the box is always positioned inside the largest shape

Set B

In this set there are three unshaded shapes in each box. The shapes are composed of straight and curved lines. There is always at least one shape within another shape.

- The rule in this set is that the smallest shape in the box is always positioned inside the medium sized shape.
- Also, this shape is always a smaller copy of the medium sized shape.

1. **Correct answer A:** The smallest shape is positioned inside the **largest** shape, therefore it belongs to set A.
2. **Correct answer D:** The smallest shape is positioned inside the largest shape, therefore it belongs to set A.
3. **Correct answer D:** The smallest shape is positioned inside the medium sized shape, both shapes are the same, therefore it belongs to set B.
4. **Correct answer E:** The smallest shape is positioned inside the medium sized shape, both shapes are the same, therefore it belongs to set B.
5. **Correct answer B:** The smallest shape is positioned inside the medium sized shape, both shapes are the same, therefore it belongs to set B.

Example 26

Set A

In this set there are a range of straight lined shapes within each box.

- The rule in this set is that the total number of lines must equal 12.

Set B

In this set, as above, there are a range of straight lined shapes within each box.

- The rule in this set is that the total number of lines must equal ten.

Test Shape 1 Answer: Set A
Each rectangle contains four straight lines, totaling 12 altogether. Therefore, the test shape belongs to Set A.

Test Shape 2 Answer: Neither
The total number of straight lines within the box is nine. Therefore, the shape does not belong to either set.

Test Shape 3 Answer: Set A
There are 12 straight lines in total. Therefore the test shape belongs to Set A.

Test Shape 4 Answer: Neither
There are ten lines altogether, which is the correct number to belong to Set B. However, the circle is composed of a curved line which is not permitted within Set B. Therefore, the test shape belongs to neither set.

Test Shape 5 Answer: Set B
The total number of straight lines is ten. Therefore the test shape belongs to Set B.

Example 27

Set A

In this set there are may be a range of straight and curved shapes.

- The rule in this set is that there must be at least one triangle within each box
- Also, one of the shapes must be shaded and one of the shapes must be unshaded

Set B

In this set, as above, there may be a range of straight and curved shapes within each box.

- The rule in this set is that there must be at least one quadrilateral and one shaded shape within each box

1. **Correct answer A:** There is at least one triangle in the box, there is at least one shaded and one unshaded shape, therefore it belongs to set A.
2. **Correct answer C:** There is at least one triangle in the box, there is at least one shaded and one unshaded shape, therefore it belongs to set A.

3. **Correct answer D:** There is at least one triangle in the box, there is at least one shaded and one unshaded shape, therefore it belongs to set A.

4. **Correct answer B:** There is at least one quadrilateral and one shaded shape present therefore it belongs to set B.

5. **Correct answer E:** There is at least one quadrilateral and one shaded shape present therefore it belongs to set B.

Example 28

Set A

In this set there are three to four shapes in each box consisting of arrows and unshaded shapes.

- The rule in this set is that there must always be a least one downward facing arrow.
- Also, there must be one square.

Set B

In this set, as above, there are three to four shapes in each box consisting of arrows and unshaded shapes.

- The rule in this set is that there must always be an upward facing arrow in the bottom left hand corner.

Test Shape 1 Answer: Set A
As there is a downward facing arrow and a square, the test shape belongs to Set A.

Test Shape 2 Answer: Set B
As there is an upward facing arrow in the bottom left hand corner, the test shape belongs to Set B.

Test Shape 3 Answer: Neither
Although the test shape includes at least one upward facing arrow, it does not belong to Set B because neither arrow is located in the bottom left hand corner.

Test Shape 4 Answer: Neither
Although there is at least one downward facing arrow, there is no square. Therefore, the test shape does not fit into Set A. As there are no upward facing arrows, the test shape also cannot belong to Set B.

Test Shape 5 Answer: Set B
There is an upward facing arrow in the bottom left hand corner. Therefore the test shape belongs to Set B.

Example 29

Set A

In this set there is a mixture of triangles, rectangles, circles and 16-sided shapes, which are called hexadecagons.

- The rule in this set is that there is always a triangle in the top left hand corner and a hexadecagon in the bottom right hand corner, or vice versa.

Set B

As above, there is a mixture of triangles, rectangles, circles and hexadecagons.

- The rule in this set is that there must always be a circle on the left hand side of the box and a triangle on the right hand side of the box, or vice versa

Test Shape 1 Answer: Set B
There is no hexadecagon so the test shape cannot belong to Set A. There is a triangle on the left side and a circle on the right side. Therefore the test shape belongs to Set B.

Test Shape 2 Answer: Set A
There is a triangle in the top left hand corner and a hexadecagon on the bottom right hand corner. Therefore the test shape belongs to Set A.

Test Shape 3 Answer: Neither
The triangle is positioned in the top left hand corner and the hexadecagon in the bottom left hand corner. To belong to Set A, the two shapes have to diagonally face each other, therefore the test shape does not belong to this set. The test shape also cannot belong to Set B because it does not contain a circle.

Test Shape 4 Answer: Set B
Although there is a hexadecagon, it is incorrectly positioned for the test shape to belong to Set A. However, there is a circle on the right hand side of the box and a triangle on the left hand side of the box. Therefore the test shape belongs to Set B.

Test Shape 5 Answer: Neither
Although the triangle is diagonally aligned with all three hexadecagons, it is not positioned in either the top left hand corner or the bottom right hand corner, therefore the test shape cannot belong to Set A. Also, the test shape cannot belong to Set B because the triangle is not positioned on either the left, or right hand side. Therefore, the test shape does not belong to either set.

Example 30

Set A

In this set there is a mixture of straight and curved shapes.

- The rule in this set is that there is always a star positioned along the bottom of the box.
- Also, there is always a quadrilateral shape positioned above the star.

Set B

In this set there is a mixture of straight and curved shapes.

- The rule in this set is that there is always a quadrilateral shape positioned along the left side of the box.

1. **Correct answer D:** The star is positioned along the bottom of the box with a quadrilateral shape above it, therefore it belongs to set A.
2. **Correct answer E:** The star is positioned along the bottom of the box with a quadrilateral shape above it, therefore it belongs to set A.
3. **Correct answer A:** The star is positioned along the bottom of the box with a quadrilateral shape above it, therefore it belongs to set A.
4. **Correct answer B:** There is a quadrilateral shape positioned at the left of the box, therefore it belongs to set B.
5. **Correct answer E:** There is a quadrilateral shape positioned at the left of the box, therefore it belongs to set B.

Example 31

Set A

In this set there is a mixture of continuous and dashed lined shapes of varying size. There are three to four shapes in each box.

- The rule in this set is that the smallest shape, in terms of total area covered, is always dashed.

Set B

In this set there is a mixture of continuous and dashed lined shapes of varying size. There are three to five shapes in each box.

- The rule in this set is that the largest sized shape, in terms of total area covered, is always continuous

Test Shape 1 Answer: Set B
The largest shape within the box is the square. As this is composed of a continuous line, the test shape belongs to Set B.

Test Shape 2 Answer: Neither
The smallest shape is continuous, therefore the test shape cannot belong to Set A. The largest shape is dashed, therefore, the shape cannot belong to Set B. As such, the test shape belongs to neither set.

Test Shape 3 Answer: Set A
The largest shape is composed of a dashed line, therefore the test shape cannot belong to Set B. The smallest shape is composed of a dashed line, therefore, the test shape belongs to Set A.
Test Shape 4 Answer: Set B
The smallest shape is composed of a continuous line, therefore the test shape cannot belong to Set A. The largest shape is composed of a continuous line, therefore the test shape belongs to Set B.

Test Shape 5 Answer: Set B
The smallest shape is continuous, therefore, the test shape cannot belong to Set A. The largest shape is composed of a continuous line, therefore, the test shape belongs to Set B.

Chapter 6

The Decision Analysis subtest

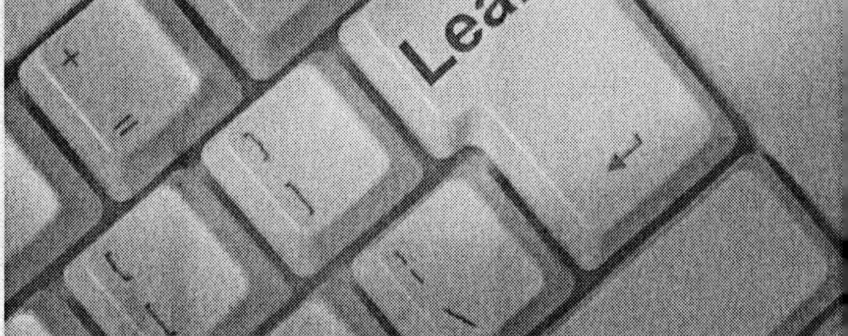

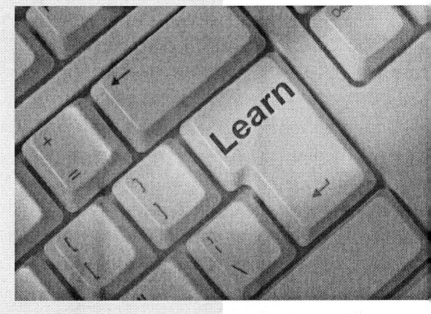

Chapter 6

The Decision Analysis subtest

The Decision Analysis test measures a candidate's ability to translate and make sense of coded information. This type of test measures a candidate's quality of decision-making in terms of accuracy, adequacy and the time taken in which the decision is made. Individuals must possess an exceptional ability to translate and identify related information, separate facts from fiction and consider all issues they are presented with. Achieving a high score in the Decision Analysis subtest reflects a candidate's ability to make decisions in real life situations where the information provided is complex and from various sources.

The UKCAT Decision Analysis subtest consists of one scenario and 28 related items which form the basis of questions asked. The scenario itself may contain a table, text and various other sources of information and codes. You will be requested to interpret information given in the questions using the facts provided in the scenario.

You will find at times that the information which you have is either incomplete or that it does not make sense. You will then need to make your best judgement based on the codes, rather than what you expect to see or what you think is reasonable. **Ensure that you base your decisions solely on the information provided to you.** There will always be a best answer which makes the most sense based on all the information presented. It is important that you understand that this test is based on judgements rather than simply applying rules and logic.

The Decision Analysis subtest differs from the other UKCAT subtests in that there can be either four or five answer options for each question. Another notable difference from the other subtests is that candidates may be asked to give more than one response for a particular question. However, if this is the case then this will always be clearly stated within the question. You will have a time limit of 32 minutes for this section, which includes one minute for administration purposes, to answer 28 questions equating to just under one minute per question.

You may be asked to give a confidence rating in this subtest. You will be asked to rate between 1 and 5 (low to high) how confident you are that you have given the correct answer to each question.

This is something which is being trialled by UKCAT and will NOT contribute to your score or be communicated to the universities. It has been included in an attempt to measure a candidates awareness of their capacity and self monitoring skills. You should therefore answer as honestly as you can.

Summary of Decision Analysis structure

Stem

In this subtest you will be presented with one scenario comprising various facts and information, including codes.

Lead-in question

There will be 28 individual lead-in questions, based on just the one scenario (the stem).

Choices

For each of the lead-in questions you will be given a choice of five or more answers. These will be represented as A, B, C, D or E. In the previous subtests there was always only one correct answer. In this subtest you may be given the option of choosing more than one correct answer. This will always be clearly indicated in the lead-in question.

The time limit is 31 minutes. Therefore you will have 66 seconds per question. When you are working through the UKCAT subtests it can be distracting to monitor exactly how long you spend on answering each question, especially when you have the stems to read. Therefore a more useful time management approach is to divide each subtest into four quarters. So in the case of the Decision Analysis subtest, allowing for one minute's administration at the start, after approximately eight minutes you should be working on the seventh question, at approximately fifteen minutes you should be commencing the fourteenth question, and so on. If you find yourself falling behind at these points you know that you need to pick up the pace.

Example of a Decision Analysis question

A team of explorers have stumbled across an ancient civilisation in the Amazon rainforest. There are many buildings with strange symbols and codes, some of which have been deciphered by the team and are shown below. Your task is to examine particular codes or sentences and then choose the best interpretation of the code from one of five possible choices.

You will find that, at times, the information you have is either incomplete or does not make complete sense. You will then need to make your best judgement based on the codes rather than what you expect to see or what you think is reasonable. There will always be a best answer which makes the most sense based on all the information presented. It is important that you understand that this test is based on judgements rather than simply applying rules and logic.

Operating codes	Basic codes
1 = opposite 2 = increase 3 = merge 4 = weak 5 = positive 6 = past 7 = present 8 = condition 9 = similar 10 = hard 11 = open 12 = plural 13 = attribute	A = cold B = oxygen C = rain D = night E = sun F = today G = tomorrow H = danger I = person J = he K = run L = building M = win N = weapon O = construct P = wind Q = summer R = fight S = fire T = earth

Question

Examine the following coded message: **(1, G), 13(C, E)**

Now examine the following sentences and try to determine the most likely interpretation of the code.

A Today there was a rainbow.
B Yesterday was windy and there was a rainbow.
C Yesterday there was a rainbow.
D Yesterday was sunny and rainy.
E Tomorrow there will be a rainbow.

Decision Analysis hints and tips

The following are common mistakes to look for when interpreting codes in a Decision Analysis subtest:

- **Various interpretations** of the same word can be used, eg 'present', which could refer to time, as in 'the present moment', or otherwise to a gift, as in 'a birthday present'.
- Some of the answer options may include all of the encoded words but may not make logical or grammatical sense.
- Some answer options **may not include all of the interpreted code words.**

- The interpreted words are **not necessarily in a specific order.** Therefore do not make the mistake of necessarily interpreting the codes in the exact order they are presented.
- **Do not spend too long on a difficult question.** Difficult questions are often easily identifiable by the length and complexity of the code – effective time management is key.
- Words within brackets are usually combined to give one meaning and should not be used as separate words within answer options.
- Certain codes require you to give your answer in a specific tense such as 'past', 'present' or 'future'. These answers do not require you to actually state the word unless specified by other codes.

Three simple steps to Decision Analysis

Step 1

Interpret the coded information given in the lead-in question and write the words down on your whiteboard – remember to pay special attention to words in brackets.

Step 2

Translate the meaning of combined codes where applicable.

Step 3

Relate the words to each of the answer options; remember to take the following into account:

- Do the answer options make use of all of the words within the code?
- Which of the answer options are clearly incorrect or contain information not referred to in the scenario, and are therefore easy to eliminate?
- Do the answer options make use of the combined words and words in brackets correctly?
- Which answer options are clearly correct, and of these, which potential correct answer options arrive at the best interpretation of the code?
- An answer can still be correct if it does not contain the exact interpretation but is the best fit of all the answer options provided.
- Base your answer on the information provided – do not make subjective judgements.
- Where you are unable to distinguish between two answer options go with your gut feeling as this is normally correct.
- As you work through each question use your whiteboard to make a note of the code interpretations, to avoid confusion.
- You may be asked a question where you are provided with a line of text that you must convert into the correct code sequence.

Decision Analysis practice examples

Scenario

A team of explorers have stumbled across an ancient civilisation in the Amazon rainforest. There are many buildings with strange symbols and codes, some of which have been deciphered by the team and are shown below. Your task is to examine particular codes or sentences and then choose the best interpretation of the code from one of five possible choices.

You will find that, at times, the information you have is either incomplete or does not make complete sense. You will then need to make your best judgement based on the codes rather than what you expect to see or what you think is reasonable. There will always be a best answer which makes the most sense based on all the information presented. It is important that you understand that this test is based on judgements rather than simply applying rules and logic.

Operating codes	Basic codes
1 = opposite	A = cold
2 = increase	B = oxygen
3 = merge	C = rain
4 = weak	D = night
5 = positive	E = sun
6 = past	F = today
7 = present	G = tomorrow
8 = condition	H = danger
9 = similar	I = person
10 = hard	J = he
11 = open	K = run
12 = plural	L = building
13 = attribute	M = win
	N = weapon
	O = construct
	P = wind
	Q = summer
	R = fight
	S = fire
	T = earth

Example 1

Examine the following coded message: **(1, G), 13(C, E)**

Now examine the following sentences and try to determine the most likely interpretation of the code.

A Today there is a rainbow.
B Yesterday was windy and there was a rainbow.
C Yesterday there was a rainbow.
D Yesterday was sunny and rainy.
E Tomorrow there will be a rainbow.

Example 2

Examine the following coded message: **H, S, (4, L), 7**

Now examine the following sentences and try to determine the most likely interpretation of the code.

A The building is on fire and is at risk of collapsing.
B Danger. The building was on fire and is at risk of collapsing.
C Danger. The building is on fire and is at risk of collapsing.
D Danger. The building is at risk of collapsing.
E Danger. The buildings are on fire and are at risk of collapsing.

Example 3

Examine the following coded message: **(6, Q), (1, A), Q(1, 6), (2, A)**

Now examine the following sentences and try to determine the most likely interpretation of the code.

A Last summer was warm, but next summer should be cooler.
B This summer has been warm, but in the future they will be warmer still.
C This summer was warm, but in the future summers will be cooler.
D Recent summers have been warm, but in the future they will be warmer still.
E Last summer was warm and the winter was very cold.

Example 4

Examine the following coded message: **(J, K), G, 8, 13(P, E, C), 5**
Now examine the following sentences and try to determine the most likely interpretation of the code.

A They run tomorrow if the weather is right.
B He runs tomorrow if the weather is right.
C He runs if the weather is favourable.
D He runs tomorrow if the report is favourable.
E They run tomorrow when the sun rises.

Example 5

Examine the following coded message: **(I, 12), R, T, (9, L)**

Now examine the following sentences and try to determine the most likely interpretation of the code.

A The earth is worth fighting for.
B The land had been fought upon many times.
C If you fight you will conquer them.
D They fought to save the earth.
E They fight for land and shelter.

Example 6

Examine the following coded message: **(J, 4, 2), (1, M), R, 6**

Now examine the following sentences and try to determine the most likely interpretation of the code.

A They had lost all the battles.
B He was weak and so lost the fight.
C He was weak after his illness.
D He was very weak after losing the battle.
E He is stronger despite losing the fight.

Example 7

Examine the following coded message: **(12, J), R, (1, 6), 8, (2, N)**

Now examine the following sentences and try to determine the most likely interpretation of the code.

A The soldiers will fight provided they have weapons.
B The men fought because they had more weapons.
C The men will fight provided they have more weapons and better armour.
D The men are fighting because they have better weapons.
E The men will fight provided they have more swords.

Example 8

Examine the following coded message: **D, (2, A), S(4, 2), 6**

Now examine the following sentences and try to determine the most likely interpretation of the code.

A It became colder that night as the fire began to die out.
B It was cold that night after the fire went out.
C It became colder that day as the fire went out.
D The night became colder as the fire was blown out by the wind.
E It became warmer once the fire was lit.

Example 9

Examine the following coded message: **(6, A, T), (1, O), 13(2, E), 7**

Now examine the following sentences and try to determine the most likely interpretations of the code.

A The temperatures had been freezing but the summer was fast approaching.
B As the sun rose, it is clear the overnight frost has destroyed the crops.
C The earth had been frozen all winter.
D The glaciers are melting because of global warming.
E The ice age helped illuminate our understanding of geology.

Example 10

Examine the following sentence: **'He has sunstroke because the wind makes it seem cooler'.**

Now examine the following codes and try to determine the most likely interpretation of the sentence.

A I, E(1, 4), H, P, A, 7
B J, E, Q, H, P, A, 7
C J, E(1, 4), H, P, A, 7
D J, E(2, 4), H, P, A, 7
E J, E(1, 4), H, P, A, 6

Example 11

Examine the following coded message: **F, (2, H), 12(R, I), (H, N)**

Now examine the following sentences and try to determine the most likely interpretation of the code.

A Soldiers are at increased risk of danger from artillery fire.
B Today some soldiers are at increased risk of danger because of artillery fire.
C Today soldiers are more at risk because of artillery fire.
D Today soldiers are at risk of danger because of friendly fire.
E A soldier is always at risk of danger because of friendly fire.

Example 12

Examine the following coded message: **8, O, (12, I), 13(S, T), (2, H)**

Now examine the following sentences and try to determine the most likely interpretation of the code.

A The lava presents a hazard to the local population if they build near it.
B More people will die if the lava flow worsens.
C Volcanoes are dangerous and large cities should not be near them.
D Many houses are near the volcano and present a hazard.
E Fumes from volcanoes present a hazard providing people live near them.

Example 13

Examine the following coded message: **(12, I), (1, O), L, 6, 8, (2, C)**

Now examine the following sentences and try to determine the **two most likely** interpretations of the code.

A The workers could have carried on and demolished the home had the heavy rain not come.
B The builders may have demolished everything but the heavy rain stopped them.
C The builder nearly destroyed the home but the heavy rain prevented this.
D The builders could have demolished the shelter providing the heavy rain had not come.
E The builders will knock down the home until the heavy rain stops them.

Scenario

The explorers have discovered some additional 'Specialist' codes.

Operating codes	Basic codes	Specialist codes
1 = opposite	A = cold	♋ = happy
2 = increase	B = oxygen	♌ = angry
3 = merge	C = rain	♍ = trusting
4 = weak	D = night	♎ = sociable
5 = positive	E = sun	♐ = scared
6 = past	F = today	♒ = clever
7 = present	G = tomorrow	♓ = strange
8 = condition	H = danger	☺ = intelligent
9 = similar	I = person	
10 = hard	J = he	
11 = open	K = run	
12 = plural	L = building	
13 = attribute	M = win	
	N = weapon	
	O = construct	
	P = wind	
	Q = summer	
	R = fight	
	S = fire	
	T = earth	

Example 14

Examine the following coded message: **(1, 6), (13, ♋), 13(2, A, C)**

Now examine the following sentences and try to determine the most likely interpretation of the code.

A I will enjoy the snow.
B I enjoyed the snow.
C I will enjoy the heavy rain tomorrow.
D I will enjoy the heavy snow and rain tomorrow.
E I will not be happy if it snows tomorrow.

Example 15

Examine the following coded message: **G, (1, H), K, 8, 13(P, A), D, ☺**

Now examine the following sentences and try to determine the most likely interpretation of the code.

A It will be wise and safe to run tomorrow as long as the storm passes in the night.
B He should run tomorrow as long as the storm passes in the night.
C It will be better to run tomorrow if the storm has passed in the night.
D Once the storm has passed he can run tomorrow.
E It is more intelligent and safer to run today if the storm passes tonight.

Example 16

Examine the following coded message: **13(4, L), ♐, 6, (13, C), I**

Now examine the following sentences and try to determine the most likely interpretation of the code.

A I worry that damp may damage my shelter.
B Damp can damage buildings.
C I was worried that my shelter would be damaged by rain.
D I was concerned that my home would be damaged by damp.
E They were worried that damp can damage homes.

Example 17

Examine the following sentence: **'She panicked when the mob was about to fight'.**

Now examine the following codes and try to determine the most likely interpretation of the sentence.

A (1, J), ♐, (12, I, H), R
B 1, J, ♐, (12, I, H), R, 6
C (1, J), ♐, (12, I, H), R, 6
D (1, J), ♐(1, 2), (12, I, H), R, 6
E (1, J), (1, ♋) (12, I, H), R, 6

Example 18

Examine the following sentence: **'They smile at danger'.**

Now examine the following codes and try to determine the most likely interpretation of the sentence:

A (12, I), (13, ♋), (7, 1)
B J, (13, ♋), 7
C (12, I), (13, ♋), H
D 12, (J, 13) (♋, 7)
E (12, I), (1, ♋), 7, H

Example 19

Examine the following coded message: **13{☺(12, I)}, O(L, 12), (I, 12), 6**

Now examine the following sentences and try to determine the most likely interpretation of the code.

A The clever engineers developed a huge office for the workers.
B It took many clever people many years to build the new city.
C The students gathered in the marquee amongst friends and family.
D The scientists are working hard to develop new medicines for the patients.
E The advanced civilisation built vast cities for their people.

Example 20

Examine the following coded message: **2(P, C), (1, O), (L, 12), 6**

Now examine the following sentences and try to determine the most likely interpretation of the code.

A The storm is causing widespread damage to the buildings.
B The storm caused fire and destruction to the village.
C The wind and rain caused damage of the village.
D The storm caused widespread destruction of the village.
E The storm led to the construction of a new village.

Example 21

Examine the following coded message: **(I, 12, ♋), L, 13(♎, D), 7**
Now examine the following sentences and try to determine the most likely interpretation of the code.

A The disco is full of revellers dancing the night away.
B The partygoers had enjoyed the wedding reception by dancing the night away.
C The bride and groom were pleased they had married in a church.
D Many people attended the festival, which lasted for several nights.
E The evening entertainment was attracting quite a crowd.

Example 22

Examine the following coded message: **I, 13(K, 4), 2(12, D, H)**

Now examine the following sentences and try to determine **the two most likely** interpretations of the code.

A The man's injured leg made him more vulnerable to infection.
B The man's limp made him more vulnerable to nocturnal predators.
C The man's shoulder injury made him more vulnerable to nocturnal predators.
D Nocturnal predators are more likely to catch a poor runner.
E The man's limp made him more likely to be caught by predators.

Example 23

Examine the following coded message: **(12, I), ♋, (Q, C), (2, A), 6**

Now examine the following sentences and try to determine the most likely interpretation of the code.

A The people were happy because the shower cooled the air.
B The people were happy because the summer shower warmed the air.
C The people are happy because the summer shower is cooling the air.
D The people were happy because the summer breeze cooled the air.
E The people were happy because the summer shower cooled the air.

Example 24

Examine the following coded message: **(1, J), ♍, J, (O, S), ♐, (H, ♓, 12), 7**
Now examine the following sentences and try to determine the most likely interpretation of the code.

A She's trusting him to put out the fire to protect them from any unknown predators.
B She's trusting him to build them a fire to scare away any ambushers.
C She trusted him to build them a fire to protect them from any unknown predators.
D She trusted him to build them a tent to protect them from any unknown predators.
E She's trusting him to build them a fire to scare away any strangers.

Example 25

Examine the following coded message: **(I, ☺, 4), R, M, ♒**

Now examine the following sentences and try to determine **the two most likely** interpretations of the code.

A By using their intelligence, the weak can win in a contest by being cunning.
B By using all their strength, even the weak can win fights.
C The strong boy won all his fights by being cunning.
D The bright little boy managed to win the fight by using his fists.
E The bright little boy managed to win the fight by using his wit.

Example 26

Examine the following message: **'When it's sunny even the most unsociable people smile.'**

Now examine the following codes and try to determine the most likely interpretation of the sentence.

A E, I (1, ♎), (13, ♋)
B E, (I, 12), (1, ♎), (2, ♋)
C E, (I, 12), (1, ♋), (13, ♋)
D E, (I, 12), (1, ♋), (13, ♋)
E E, (I, 12, 1), ♎, (13, ♋)

Scenario

A group of archaeologists have discovered an ancient crypt in Athens. There are many chambers and passageways with strange symbols and codes, some of which have been deciphered by the team and are shown below. Your task is to examine particular codes or sentences and then choose the best interpretation of the code from one of five possible choices.

You will find that, at times, the information you have is either incomplete or does not make complete sense. You will then need to make your best judgement based on the codes rather than what you expect to see or what you think is reasonable. There will always be a best answer which makes the most sense based on all the information presented. It is important that you understand that this test is based on judgements rather than simply applying rules and logic.

Operating codes	Basic codes
1 = opposite 2 = present 3 = past 4 = future 5 = increase 6 = past 7 = conditional 8 = strong 9 = prefer 10 = hard 11 = close 12 = enjoyable 13 = attribute	A = wind B = season C = food D= secret E = earth F = gift G = speak H = liquid I = day J = sun K = today L = yesterday M = danger N = person O = she P = public Q = building R = cold S = achievement T = watch

Example 27

Examine the following coded message: **L, N, 12, (H, Q, P)**

Now examine the following sentences and try to determine the most likely interpretation of the code.

A Tomorrow, I will go to the public baths.
B Yesterday, I enjoyed the public baths.
C Yesterday, I swam at the public baths.
D Yesterday, I planned to go to the public baths.
E Today, I went to the public baths.

Example 28

Examine the following coded message: **O, 12, 7, (S, G), 8, 4**

Now examine the following sentences and try to determine the most likely interpretation of the code.

A She will be happy if her speech goes well.
B She was happy that her acceptance speech went well.
C She will be happy if she remembers her lines.
D She will be happy if the acceptance speech goes well.
E He will be happy if the acceptance speech goes well.

Example 29

Examine the following coded message: **(8, A), E, N(C, H), 2**

Now examine the following sentences and try to determine the most likely interpretation of the code.

A The gale is blowing dust onto my food and drink.
B The gale blew dust onto my food and drink.
C The breeze is blowing dust onto my food and drink.
D The wind blew over my food and drink.
E The gale is blowing dust onto my food.

Example 30

Examine the following coded message: **O, M, G, O, 12(G, D, P)**

Now examine the following sentences and try to determine the most likely interpretation of the code.

A She's a dangerous person to speak to because she likes to spread news.
B She's a useful person to speak to because she doesn't like to spread gossip.
C She's a pleasant person to speak to because she likes to spread gossip.
D She's a dangerous person to listen to because she likes to spread gossip.
E She's a dangerous person to speak to because she likes to spread gossip.

Example 31

Examine the following coded message: **(Q, P, H), 12, 7, (8, N), 6**

Now examine the following sentences and try to determine the **two most likely** interpretations of the code.

A The library was an enjoyable place so long as you were quiet.
B The pub was a great place to be so long as you could stand up for yourself.
C The brewery was an enjoyable place so long as you were strong.
D The pub was a great place to be so long as you didn't start a fight.
E The pub was a great place to be so long as you could tell a joke.

Example 32

Examine the following coded message: **E(5, D), 7, N(1, G), 10**

Now examine the following sentences and try to determine the most likely interpretation of the code.

A The earth has many secrets that you will hear if you really want to.
B The earth has many secrets which you will hear if you speak with it.
C The earth never gives up its secrets, even if you listen hard.
D I have many secrets to tell you if you want to listen.
E The earth has many secrets that you will hear if you listen hard.

Example 33

Examine the following coded message: **O, 9, (13, C), (13, H), 6**

Now examine the following sentences and try to determine the most likely interpretation of the code.

A She always favoured the smell of food rather than drink.
B He has always favoured the smell of food rather than drink.
C She prefers the smell of food rather than drink.
D She always preferred the taste of drink rather than food.
E She always favoured food rather than drink.

Example 34

Examine the following coded message: **(1, L), (5, 11), 7, (9, S), K**

Now examine the following sentences and try to determine the most likely interpretation of the code.

A The future arrives more quickly if you keep yourself busy today.
B The past goes quicker if you make the most of your achievements today.
C Tomorrow arrives sooner if you enjoy the achievements of yesterday.
D The future arrives quicker if you enjoy the achievements of today.
E Tomorrow comes sooner if you try to succeed today.

Example 35

Examine the following coded message: **(P, Q, T), T, (5, N), M, 3**

Now examine the following sentences and try to determine the most likely interpretation of the code.

A The stadium will witness many killings.
B The stadium had witnessed many slaves be killed before.
C The public stand will witness many more people in danger.
D The crowd had seen many people in danger before.
E The public stand had witnessed many people in danger before.

Example 36

Examine the following coded message: **(N, T), O, D, (5, M, H), H, 3**

Now examine the following sentences and try to determine the most likely interpretation of the code.

A I saw her secretly lacing the drink with poison.
B We saw her drinking the poisoned wine.
C I saw her sipping the poisoned liquid.
D I saw her secretly lacing the food with poison.
E She secretly laced the wine with poison.

Example 37

Examine the following coded message: **K(5, A), H(1, 5), L**

Now examine the following sentences and try to determine the most likely interpretation of the code.

A It will be windier tomorrow, but warmer than today.
B It was windy today, but wetter yesterday.
C It was windy yesterday, but colder today.
D It was windy today but will be rainier tomorrow.
E It was windier today, but less wet yesterday.

Example 38

Examine the following coded message: **7, (5, H), (5, M), Q, 4**

Now examine the following sentences and try to determine the most likely interpretation of the code.

A The house is flooded heavily and may be at risk of collapsing.
B If the water level rises, the house may become unstable.
C The water level is rising causing the building to become more unstable.
D If the water enters into the house, it may be more dangerous.
E If the water recedes, the building may fall down.

Example 39

Examine the following coded message: **O, 9((B, J,)H), C, 3**

Now examine the following sentences and try to determine the **two most likely** interpretations of the code.

A She enjoys summer wine more and food.
B She enjoyed the summer wine more than the food.
C Summer fruit juice is always better than the fruit.
D She preferred summer showers more than anything, including food.
E She enjoyed wine more than any other type of drink or food.

Scenario

The archaeologists have discovered a number of additional 'Specialist' codes.

Operating codes	Basic codes	Specialist codes
1 = opposite	A = wind	♏ = hope
2 = present	B = season	♦ = excited
3 = past	C = food	⍓ = sad
4 = future	D= secret	♓ = agressive
5 = increase	E = earth	☐ = nervous
6 = past	F = gift	● = strange
7 = conditional	G = speak	⌘ = angry
8 = strong	H = liquid	❖ = curious
9 = prefer	I = day	♒ = happy
10 = hard	J = sun	
11 = close	K = today	
12 = enjoyable	L = yesterday	
13 = attribute	M = danger	
	N = person	
	O = she	
	P = public	
	Q = building	
	R = cold	
	S = achievement	
	T = watch	

Example 40

Examine the following coded message: **O, (1, ♒), (1, G), D, 6**

Now examine the following sentences and try to determine the most likely interpretation of the code.

A She felt guilty when she passed on the secret.
B She was glad to finally hear the secret.
C She was not happy to have to pass on the message.
D She was not happy when she heard the secret.
E She was not happy to have to say the secret out loud.

Example 41

Examine the following coded message: **O, (13, □), (1, G), M, (8, A, H), 3**

Now examine the following sentences and try to determine the most likely interpretation of the code.

A She felt herself shaking as she heard the threatening storm.
B She felt herself shaking as she saw the storm ahead.
C She felt herself shaking as she heard the volcano erupt.
D She is shaking as she hears the threatening storm.
E She was nervous as she heard the storm.

Example 42

Examine the following coded message: **(8, J), I, (P, ♓), 7(5, N)**

Now examine the following sentences and try to determine the most likely interpretation of the code.

A A heat wave cannot cause riots, unless the police are ineffective.
B A heat wave can cause fires provided there are sufficient people.
C A heat wave can cause traffic chaos provided there are sufficient people.
D A heat wave can cause riots provided it is hot enough.
E A heat wave can cause riots provided there are sufficient people.

Example 43

Examine the following coded message: **O, ●, (1, G), H, 10, (O, Q), 3**

Now examine the following sentences and try to determine the most likely interpretation of the code.

A She felt strange as she felt the rain on her skin.
B She didn't feel herself as she heard the rain smash on her roof.
C They felt strange as they heard the rain on the roof of her house.
D She feels strange as she hears the water on the roof of her house.
E She felt strange as she heard the rain on the roof of her house.

Example 44

Examine the following coded message: **(5, N), (13, ⍓), 7, H, 13(H, J)**

Now examine the following sentences and try to determine the most likely interpretation of the code.

A The villagers will cry if there is a flood.
B The villagers will cry when the water dries up.
C The villagers will cry if the water dries up.
D The villagers will cry if the water doesn't dry up.
E The villagers will celebrate when the rains come.

Example 45

Examine the following coded message: **P(♦, G), (5, N, S, 8), 4**

Now examine the following sentences and try to determine the most likely interpretation of the code.

A The people will jeer their losing athletes.
B The crowd will cheer for their victorious athletes.
C The men will cheer their victorious athletes.
D The crowd will cheer for their athletes if they win.
E The people cheered their victorious athletes.

Example 46

Examine the following coded message: **N, ♏, (1, L), (5, J), (1, H)**

Now examine the following sentences and try to determine the most likely interpretation of the code.

A Tomorrow, I hope it will be sunny and dry.
B Tomorrow, I hope it will be sunny and very dry.
C Tomorrow, will be sunny and very dry.
D Tomorrow, I predict that it will be dry and sunny.
E Tomorrow, I hope there will be a lot of sun and no rain.

Example 47

Examine the following message: **'The spy will hope the dangerous people can't see him'.**

Now examine the following codes and try to determine the most likely interpretation of the sentence.

A (8, N), ♏, (M, P), 1(13, T), 3
B (D, N), ♏, (M, P), 1(13, T), 4
C (D, N), ♏, (M, P), (13, G), 3
D (D, N), O, ♏, 1(13, T), 3
E (D, N), ♏, (M, P), 1(13, T), 2

Example 48

Examine the following message: **'She felt frightened as the flood approached the school.'**

Now examine the following codes and try to determine the most likely interpretation of the sentence.

A O, □, (M, H), 11, (P, Q), 2
B O, □, (F, M), 11, (P, Q), 3
C O, □, (M, H), 11, P, 2
D (1, O), □, (M, H), 11, (P, Q), 3
E O, □, (M, H), 11, (P, Q), 3

Example 49

Examine the following message: **'I like a drink with my friends on a warm day'.**

Now examine the following codes and try to determine the most likely interpretation of the sentence.

A N, 12, H, (9, 5, N), B(1, R)
B N, 12, C, (9, 5, N), I(1, R)
C N, 12, H, (9, 5, N), I(1, R)
D N, 12, H, (9, 5, N), I(R)
E N, 12, H, (O, 5, N), I(1, R)

Example 50

Examine the following coded message: **(5, M), (N, T), (8, H), K**

Now examine the following sentences and try to determine the **two most likely** interpretations of the code.

A Beware, the water today is extremely cold and choppy today.
B Beware, I've been observing and the current is unexpectedly strong today.
C Beware, I've been watching and the drinks are very strong today.
D Beware, I've been watching and the waters are very strong at the moment.
E Beware, I've heard the drinks are very strong here.

Example 51

Examine the following message: **'He's not curious to see what his present is'**.

Now examine the following codes and try to determine the most likely interpretation of the sentence.

A (1, O), (1, ❖), T, (P, F), 3
B (1, O), ❖, T, (N, F), 2
C (1, O), (1, ❖), G, (N, F), 2
D (1, O), (1, ❖), T, (N, F), 3
E (1, O), (1, ❖), T, (N, F), 2

Example 52

Examine the following message: **'She was annoyed that the food didn't look appetising for her guests'**.

Now examine the following codes and try to determine the most likely interpretation of the sentence.

A O, ⌘, C, G(1, 12), (5, N), 3
B O, ⌘, C, T(1, 12), (5, N), 3
C O, ⌘, C, T(1, 12), N, 3
D O, ⌘, H, T(1, 12), (5, N), 2
E N, ⌘, C, T(1, 12), (5, N), 3

Justifications of Decision Analysis practice examples

Example 1

Answer: C

(1, G), 13(C, E)

The code combines the words: (opposite, tomorrow), attribute (rain, sun).

A Is incorrect as it uses the present tense rather than the past tense.

B Is incorrect as it introduces the word 'windy'.

C Is the correct answer as it uses all the codes and the rules within the brackets. It correctly combines 'opposite' and 'tomorrow' to imply 'yesterday'. An attribute of 'sun' and 'rain' is a 'rainbow'.

D Ignores the combination of the words '(sun, rain)'.

E Ignores combining 'opposite' and 'tomorrow' to make 'today'.

Example 2

Answer: C

H, S, (4, L), 7

The code combines the words: danger, fire, (weak, building), present.

A Is incorrect as it ignores the word 'danger'.

B Is incorrect as it is in the past tense.

C Is the correct answer as it uses all the words within the code and correctly combines '(weak, building)' as 'collapsing'.

D Ignores the word 'fire'.

E Wrongly includes more than one building.

Example 3

Answer: A

(6, Q), (1, A), Q(1, 6), (2, A)

The code combines the words: (past, summer), (opposite, cold), summer (opposite, past), (increase, cold).

A Is the correct answer as it correctly combines 'past' and 'summer' to imply 'last summer' and '(opposite, cold)' as 'warm'. 'Summer' is combined with '(opposite, past)' to mean 'next summer' and '(increase, cold)' to imply 'cooler'.

B Incorrectly combines '(increase, cold)' as 'warmer still'.
C Is incorrect as it ignores '(past, summer)' by stating 'this summer'.
D Introduces the word 'recent'.
E Is incorrect as it introduces the word 'winter'.

Example 4

Answer: B

(J, K), G, 8, 13(P, E, C), 5

The code combines the words: (he, run), tomorrow, condition, attribute (wind, sun, rain), positive.

A Is incorrect as it states the word 'they' when no plural code is provided.
B **Is correct as it uses all the words and correctly combines 'he' and 'run' to imply 'he runs', while an attribute of 'wind', 'sun' and 'rain' is the 'weather'. The use of 'right' is substituted for 'positive'.**
C Ignores the word 'tomorrow'.
D Is incorrect as it introduces the word 'report'.
E Incorrectly uses the plural of 'they'. Also, 'when the sun rises' is not an attribute of '(wind, sun, rain)'.

Example 5

Answer: E

(I, 12), R, T, (9, L)

The code combines the words: (person, plural), fight, earth, (similar, building).

A Is incorrect as it ignores '(person, plural)'.
B Is incorrect as it ignores '(similar, building)'.
C Introduces the word 'conquer'.
D Is incorrect as it introduces the word 'save' and ignores '(similar, building)'.
E **Is the correct answer as it combines 'person' and 'plural' to mean 'they'. The word 'land' has been substituted for 'earth' while 'similar' and 'building' are combined to imply 'shelter'.**

Example 6

Answer: D

(J, 4, 2), (1, M), R, 6

The code combines the words: (he, weak, increase), (opposite, win), fight, past.

- A Is incorrect as 'they' is in the plural.
- B Is incorrect as it ignores combining 'weak, increase' to imply becoming weaker or very weak.
- C Introduces the word 'illness'.
- D **Is the most correct as it is set in the past tense and combines 'he', 'weak' and 'increase' to give 'he was very weak' and combines 'opposite' and 'win' to give 'losing'. 'Battle' is substituted for 'fight'.**
- E Is incorrect as it ignores the word 'past' and is phrased in the present tense.

Example 7

Answer: E

(12, J), R, (1, 6), 8, (2, N)

The code combines the words: (plural, he), fight, (opposite, past), condition, (increase, weapon).

- A Is incorrect as it ignores the word 'increase'.
- B Incorrect as it is in the past tense.
- C Incorrect as it introduces the words 'better armour'.
- D Incorrect as it is in the present tense.
- E **Is the correct answer as it uses all the codes and the rules within the brackets. It correctly combines 'opposite' and 'past' to imply the future tense. It also correctly infers 'increase' and 'weapon' to mean 'more swords'.**

Example 8

Answer: A

D, (2, A), S(4, 2), 6

The code combines the words: night, (increase, cold), fire (weak, increase), past.

A **Is the correct answer as it uses all the codes and the rules within the brackets. It correctly combines 'increase' and 'cold' to imply 'colder'. It also correctly combines 'fire', 'weak' and 'increase' to mean 'the fire began to die'.**
B Is incorrect as it does not combine 'increase' and 'cold'.
C Incorrect as it refers to day rather than night.
D Incorrect as it refers to the wind blowing out the fire.
E Incorrect as it replaces 'colder' with 'warmer'.

Example 9

Answer: D

(6, A, T), (1, O), 13(2, E), 7

The code combines the words: (past, cold, earth), (opposite, construct), attribute (increase, sun), present.

A Is incorrect as it ignores the words '(opposite, construct)'.
B Is incorrect because it introduces 'crops'.
C Is incorrect as it is set in the past tense and ignores '(opposite, construct)' and 'attribute (increase, sun)'.
D **Is correct as it combines 'attribute (past, cold, earth)' to mean 'glaciers', '(opposite, construct)' as 'are melting', and 'attribute (increase, sun)' as 'because of global warming'. The sentence is correctly phrased in the present tense.**
E Is incorrect as the sentence is in the past tense.

Example 10

Answer: C

J, E(1, 4), H, P, A, 7

The code combines the words: he, sun (opposite, weak), danger, wind, cold, present.

A Is incorrect as it introduces the word 'person'.
B Is incorrect as it introduces the word 'summer' and the word 'strong' is missing.
C **Is correct as 'He has sunstroke' is implied by 'sun (opposite, weak)' and 'danger'. 'Wind' and 'cold' are used to imply 'wind makes it seem cooler'. The sentence is set in the present tense.**
D Is incorrect because it introduces a code for 'increase' suggesting the sun became weaker.
E Is incorrect as it is set in the past tense.

Example 11

Answer: C

F, (2, H), 12(R, I), (H, N)

The code combines the words: today, (increased, danger), plural (fight, person), (danger, weapon).

A Is incorrect as it ignores the use of the word 'today'.
B Is incorrect as it introduces the word 'some'.
C **Is correct as it uses all the words within the code. It correctly combines 'increased, danger' as 'more at risk'. It also correctly combines 'plural', 'fight' and 'person' as 'soldiers' and 'danger' and 'weapon' as 'artillery fire'. It also correctly uses 'today'.**
D Is incorrect as it introduces the concept of 'friendly fire' which is not part of the coding.
E Is incorrect as it does not use 'today', incorrectly combines 'increased' and 'risk' to mean 'always at risk' and introduces the concept of 'friendly fire'.

Example 12

Answer: A

8, O, (12, I), 13(S, T), (2, H)

The code combines the words: condition, construct, (plural, person), attribute (fire, earth), (increase, danger).

A **Is correct as it uses all the words in the code and combines 'plural' and 'person' to mean 'population'. It also combines 'fire' and 'earth' as 'volcano', of which an attribute is 'lava'. It also combines 'increase' and 'danger' as 'hazard' and correctly uses 'condition' to imply 'if'.**
B Is incorrect as it ignores 'construct'. It also adds the words 'more' and 'die'.
C Is incorrect as 'volcanoes' and 'large' are added. It also ignores 'condition'.
D Is incorrect as it ignores 'construct', does not combine 'plural' and 'person' and introduces 'volcano'.
E Is incorrect as it adds 'fumes' and uses 'live' rather than 'construct'.

Example 13

Answers: A & D

(12, I), (1, O), L, 6, 8, (2, C)

The code combines the words: (plural, person), (opposite, construct), building, past, condition, (increase, rain)

A **Is the correct answer as it uses all the words in the code: 'plural' and 'person' are combined to mean 'workers'. Also 'opposite' and 'construct' are combined to mean 'demolished' and 'increase' and 'rain' mean 'heavy rain'.**

B Is incorrect as 'building' is not used and the condition is not used correctly to imply 'if the rain had not come'.

C Is incorrect as 'builder' is singular and it does not use 'condition'.

D **Is also the correct answer as it uses all the words in the code and correctly combines 'plural' and 'person' as 'builders', 'opposite' and 'construct' as 'demolish', and 'increase' and 'rain' as 'heavy rain'. 'Building' is replaced with 'shelter' and 'condition' is used. The statement is also set in the past.**

E Is incorrect as it is not set in the past.

Example 14

Answer: A

(1, 6), (13, ♋), 13(2, A, C)

The code combines the words: (opposite, past), (attribute, happy), attribute (increase, cold, rain).

A **Is correct as it uses all the words within the code and combines 'attribute' and 'happy' as 'enjoy', and 'attribute (increase, cold, rain)' as 'snow'. It also correctly sets the statement in the future tense.**

B Is incorrect as the statement is set in the past.

C Is incorrect as it ignores 'cold'.

D Is incorrect as it does not interpret the attribute of 'increase, cold and rain' as 'snow'.

E Is incorrect as it introduces the negative 'not'.

Example 15

Answer: A

G, (1, H), K, 8, 13(P, A), D, ☺

The code combines the words: tomorrow, (opposite, danger), run, condition, attribute (wind, cold), night, intelligent.

A **Is the best answer, even though there is no code for 'passes', as it uses all the words in the code and combines them correctly. 'Opposite' and 'danger' are combined as 'safe', and an attribute of 'wind' and 'rain' is 'storm'. Also, 'tomorrow' and 'night' are used, and 'wise' replaces the word 'intelligent'.**

B Is incorrect as it introduces the word 'he' and does not include 'intelligent' or combine 'opposite' and 'danger'.

C Is incorrect as it does not use 'intelligent' or combine 'opposite' and 'danger'.

D Is incorrect as it does not use 'intelligent', 'night' or 'conditional', and does not combine 'opposite' and 'danger'.

E Is incorrect as it introduces 'today' instead of 'tomorrow'.

Example 16

Answer: D

13(4, L), ⤯, 6, (13, C), I

The code combines the words: attribute (weak, building), scared, past, (attribute, rain), person.

A Is incorrect as it is not set in the past.

B Is incorrect as it does not mention a person and is not set in the past.

C Is incorrect as it does not combine 'attribute' and 'rain'.

D **Is the best answer as it combines 'attribute, weak, building' as 'damaged home'. It correctly uses 'scared' as 'concerned' and combines 'attribute, rain' as 'damp'. The statement is also set in the past. 'Person' is interpreted as 'I'.**

E Is incorrect as it uses the plural 'they', and also the plural 'homes'.

Example 17

Answer: C

(1, J),⤯, (12, I, H), R, 6

The code combines the words: (opposite, he), scared, (plural, person, danger), fight, past.

A Is incorrect as it does not include the past.

B Does not correctly use brackets to combine 'opposite' and 'he' to denote 'she'.

C **Is correct as it provides the most accurate interpretation of the sentence. She ('opposite, he') panicked ('scared') when the mob ('plural, person, danger') was about to fight. Note the sentence is set in the past.**

D Combines 'opposite' with 'increased' and 'panic'. This would suggest her panic did not get worse.
E Adds 'opposite, happy' which would imply unhappiness rather than panic.

Example 18

Answer: C

(12, I), (13, ♋), H

The code combines the words: (plural, person), (attribute, happy), danger.

A Is incorrect as it omits 'danger'.
B Implies that 'he' smiles, not 'they'.
C **Is correct as it provides the most accurate interpretation of the sentence. They ('plural, person') smile '(attribute, happy)' at 'danger'.**
D Incorrectly combines the brackets.
E Adds 'opposite' to 'happy', which would imply being unhappy at danger.

Example 19

Answer: E

13 {☺(12, I)}, O(L, 12), (I, 12), 6

The code combines the words: attribute {intelligent (plural, person)}, construct (building, plural), (person, plural), past.

A Ignores the combination of 'construct (building, plural)' to imply many buildings.
B Introduces 'many years', which cannot be implied from the code.
C Is incorrect as it ignores the word 'construct'.
D Is incorrect as it is set in the present tense and ignores the words 'construct (building, plural)' and introduces the concept of medicine, which is not part of the code.
E **Is the best fit and is constructed in the past tense. The key to the double brackets is to decode 'intelligent (plural, person)' as a 'group of intelligent' people and combine this with 'attribute' to give 'advanced civilisation'. 'Construct (building, plural)' implies 'vast cities' and (person, plural) is substituted for 'their people'.**

Example 20

Answer: D

2(P, C), (1, O), (L, 12), 6

The code combines the words: increase (wind, rain), (opposite, construct), (building, plural), past

A Is incorrect as it is in the present tense.

B Is incorrect as it introduces the word 'fire'.

C Is incorrect as it ignores the word 'increase', denoting a storm.

D Is the correct answer as it uses all the codes and the rules within the brackets. It correctly combines 'increase', 'wind' and 'rain' to imply a 'storm'. It also correctly combines 'opposite' and 'construct' to indicate 'destruction', and 'plural' and 'building' to suggest a village.

E Is incorrect as it ignores the word 'opposite'.

Example 21

Answer: A

(I, 12, ♋), L, 13(♎, D), 7

The code combines the words: (person, plural, happy), building, attribute (sociable, night), present.

A Is the best fit as it combines the words '(person, plural happy)' as 'revellers', 'building' is substituted for 'disco', while an attribute of '(sociable, night)' is 'dancing'. The sentence is in the present tense.

B Is incorrect as it is set in the past tense rather than the present tense.

C Is incorrect as it is set in the past tense and ignores '(sociable, night)'.

D Is incorrect as the sentence is set in the past tense.

E Ignores the word building.

Example 22

Answers: B & D

I, 13(K, 4), 2(12, D, H)

The code combines the words: person, attribute (run, weak), increase (plural, night, danger).

A Is incorrect because it introduces the concept of infection.

B Is the correct answer as it uses all the codes and the rules within the brackets. It correctly combines 'attribute (run, weak) to indicate 'a limp'. It also correctly combines 'increase' with 'plural, night, danger' to mean 'more vulnerable to nocturnal predators'.

C Is incorrect because it does not refer to 'running'.

D Is also correct. It correctly combines 'attribute (run, weak)' to indicate 'a poor runner'.

E Is incorrect because it does not refer to 'night'.

Example 23

Answer: E

(12, I), ♋, (Q, C), (2, A), 6

The code combines the words: (plural, person), happy, (summer, rain), (increase, cold), past.

A Is incorrect because it ignores the word 'summer'.

B Is incorrect as it wrongly combines the words 'increase' and 'cold' to mean 'warmed'.

C Incorrect as the present tense is used.

D Incorrect as 'summer, rain' is interpreted as 'summer breeze'.

E Is correct as it uses all the words and correctly combines 'person, plural' to imply 'people', while 'summer' and 'rain' are combined to imply 'summer shower'. 'Increase, cold' are combined to imply 'cooled'. The sentence is set in the 'past' tense.

Example 24

Answer: B

(1, J), ♍, J, (O, S), ♐, (H, ♓, 12), 7

The code combines the words: (opposite, he), trusting, he, (construct, fire), scared, (danger, strange, plural), present.

A Is incorrect as it introduces 'put out the fire'.

B Is correct as it is the best interpretation of the code. 'Construct' and 'fire' are combined to imply 'build a fire'. In addition, 'danger, strange, plural' are all combined to imply 'ambushers'.

C Is incorrect as it is in the past tense.

D Is incorrect as it omits mention of 'fire' and introduces the word 'tent'.

E Is incorrect as it ignores 'danger'.

Example 25

Answers: A & E

(I, ☺, 4), R, M, ♒

The code combines the words: (person, intelligent, weak), fight, win, clever.

A **Is correct as it uses all the codes and the rules within the brackets. 'People', 'intelligent' and 'weak' are combined to mean 'by using their intelligence, the weak'. Also 'clever' is interpreted as 'cunning'.**
B Is incorrect as it ignores 'clever'.
C Is incorrect as it ignores 'weak'.
D Is incorrect as it ignores 'clever' and introduces 'fists'.
E **Is also correct. 'Person, intelligent, weak' is combined to imply 'bright little boy'. In addition, 'clever' is interpreted as 'wit'.**

Example 26

Answer: D

E, (I, 12), (1, ♎), (13, ♋)

The code combines the words: sun, (person, plural), (opposite, sociable), (attribute, happy).

A Is incorrect as only one person is referred to, whereas the sentence states 'people'.
B Is incorrect as it implies increasing happiness, rather than an attribute of happiness (a smile).
C Is incorrect as 'opposite' is combined with 'happy', which suggests unhappiness rather than unsociability.
D **Is the correct answer as it provides the most accurate interpretation of the sentence. 'Person' and 'plural' are combined to mean 'people', while 'opposite' and 'sociable' are combined to mean 'unsociable'. Also 'attribute' and 'happy' are combined to mean 'smile'.**
E Is incorrect as the brackets are misplaced, which means 'person' and 'plural' are combined with 'opposite'.

Example 27

Answer: B

L, N, 12, (H, Q, P)

The code combines the words: yesterday, person, enjoyable, (liquid, building, public).

A Incorrect as yesterday is replaced with 'tomorrow'.

B Is the correct answer as it uses all the codes and the rules within the brackets. It correctly combines the words '(liquid, building, public)' to infer 'public baths'.

C Incorrect as it introduces the word 'swam'.

D Incorrect as it introduces the word 'planned'.

E Incorrect as yesterday is replaced with 'today'.

Example 28

Answer: D

O, 12, 7, (S, G), 8, 4

The code combines the words: she, enjoyable, conditional, (achievement, speak), strong, future.

A Incorrect as it ignores the term achievement.

B Incorrect as it uses the past tense.

C Incorrect as it ignores the term achievement and introduces the word 'remembers'.

D Is the correct answer as it uses all the codes and the rules within the brackets. It correctly combines 'speech' and 'achievement' to imply 'acceptance speech' and 'strong' to imply 'well'.

E Incorrect as 'she' is replaced with 'he'.

Example 29

Answer: A

(8, A), E, N(C, H), 2

The code combines the words: (strong, wind), earth, person (food, liquid), present.

A Is the correct answer as it uses all the codes and the rules within the brackets. It correctly combines 'strong' and 'wind' to make 'gale' and also correctly combines 'person' with 'food' and 'liquid' to mean 'my food and drink'.

B Incorrect as it is in the past tense.

C Incorrect as a breeze is not a 'strong wind'.

D Incorrect as there is no reference in the code to the food and drink being blown over. The sentence is also set in the past and not the present tense.

E Incorrect as there is no reference to liquid.

Example 30

Answer: E

O, M, G, O, 12(G, D, P)

The code combines the words: she, danger, speak, she, enjoyable (speak, secret, public).

A Incorrect as 'speak', 'secret' and 'public' are wrongly interpreted to mean 'spread news'.
B Incorrect as 'dangerous' is replaced with 'useful'.
C Incorrect as 'dangerous' is replaced with 'pleasant'.
D Incorrect as 'speak' is replaced with 'listen'.
E **Is the correct answer as it uses all the codes and the rules within the brackets. It correctly combines 'speak', 'public' and 'secret' to mean 'spread gossip'.**

Example 31

Answers: B & C

(Q, P, H), 12, 7, (8, N), 6

The code combines the words: (building, public, liquid), enjoyable, conditional, (strong, person), past.

A Incorrect as 'building', 'public' and 'liquid' are wrongly combined to mean 'library'.
B Is the correct answer as it uses all the codes and the rules within the brackets. It correctly combines 'building, public, liquid' to mean 'pub'. Also, 'strong' and 'person' are combined to imply 'stand up for yourself'.
C Is also the correct answer as it uses all the codes and the rules within the brackets. It correctly combines 'building, public, liquid' to mean 'brewery'. Also, 'strong' and 'person' are combined to imply 'you were strong'.
D Incorrect as the term 'fight' is introduced.
E Incorrect as the term 'joke' is introduced.

Example 32

Answer: E

E(5, D), 7, N(1, G), 10

The code combines the words: earth (increase, secret), conditional, person (opposite, speak), hard.

A Incorrect as it introduces 'if you really want to', which is not part of the coding.
B Incorrect as it introduces 'if you speak with it'.
C Incorrect as it introduces the term 'never'.
D Incorrect as it introduces 'I' and makes no reference to the earth.
E **Is the correct answer as it uses all the codes and the rules within the brackets. It correctly combines 'earth' with 'increase' and 'secrets' to mean 'the earth has many secrets', as well as combining 'person' with 'opposite' and 'speak' to imply 'listen'.**

Example 33

Answer: A

O, 9, (13, C), (13, H), 6

The code combines the words: she, prefer, (attribute, food), (attribute, liquid), past.

A **Is the correct answer as it uses all the codes and the rules within the brackets. 'Prefer' is synonymous with 'favoured' and 'liquid' with 'drink'. An attribute of food and drink is 'smell'.**
B Incorrect as 'she' is replaced with 'he'.
C Incorrect as the present tense is employed.
D Incorrect as the smell of food should be preferred over that of drink.
E Incorrect as no attribute of food and drink is mentioned.

Example 34

Answer: E

(1, L), (5, 11), 7, (9, S), K

The code combines the words: (opposite, yesterday), (increase, close), conditional, (prefer, achievement), today.

A Incorrect as 'prefer' and 'achievement' are wrongly combined to mean 'keep yourself busy'.
B Incorrect as 'opposite, yesterday' is interpreted as 'past' rather than 'tomorrow'.
C Incorrect as 'today' is replaced with 'yesterday'.
D Incorrect as 'tomorrow' is replaced with 'the future'.
E **Is the best answer as it uses all the codes and the rules within the brackets. It correctly combines 'opposite' and 'yesterday' to imply 'tomorrow'. Also, 'increase' and 'close' are combined to mean 'sooner', while 'prefer' and 'achievements' are combined to make 'try to succeed'.**

Example 35

Answer: E

(P, Q, T), T, (5, N), M, 3

The code combines the words: (public, building, watch), watch, (increase, person), danger, past.

A Incorrect as the future tense is used.
B Incorrect as it introduces the word 'slaves'.
C Incorrect as the future tense is employed.
D Incorrect as the terms '(public, building, watch)' are wrongly combined to mean 'crowd'.
E **Is the correct answer as it uses all the codes and the rules within the brackets. It correctly combines '(public, building, watch)' to imply 'public stand'.**

Example 36

Answer: A

(N, T), O, D, (5, M, H), H, 3

The code combines the words: (person, watch), she, secret, (increase, danger, liquid), liquid, past.

A **Is the correct answer. Although the code does not make explicit mention of lacing the drink, the sentence is the best interpretation of the code. It correctly combines '(person, watch)' to mean 'I saw her'. Also, the code '(increase, danger, liquid)' is correctly combined to infer 'poison'.**
B Incorrect as it is stated in the code that there is only one person who watches the woman.
C Incorrect as there is no reference to 'secret' in the sentence. Also the term 'sipping' is incorrectly introduced.
D Incorrect as there is no reference to liquid in the sentence.
E Incorrect as there is no reference to a person watching the event.

Example 37

Answer: E

K(5, A), H(1, 5), L

The code combines the words: today (wind, increase), liquid (opposite, increase), yesterday.

A Incorrect as refers to tomorrow's weather and introduces the term 'warmer'.

B Incorrect as it does not combine '(wind, increase)' appropriately.

C Incorrect as it does not refer to today's winds and makes no reference to the previous day's rain.

D Incorrect as it introduces a reference to tomorrow's weather.

E **Is the correct answer as it uses all the codes and the rules within the brackets. It correctly combines 'today (increase, wind)' to make 'it was windier today'. It also correctly combines 'liquid (opposite, increase)' to make 'less wet'.**

Example 38

Answer: B

7, (5, H), (5, M), Q, 4

The code combines the words: conditional, (increase, liquid), (increase, danger), building, future.

A Incorrect as there is no conditional element within the statement.

B **Is the correct answer as it uses all the codes and the rules within the brackets. It correctly combines '(increase, liquid)' to infer 'water level rises'. It also correctly combines '(increase, danger)' to infer 'unstable'.**

C Incorrect as there is no conditional element within the statement.

D Incorrect as the sentence does not make reference to the water entering the building.

E Incorrect as the code ignores reference to an increase in water. Also, 'recedes' is introduced.

Example 39

Answers: B & D

O, 9((B, J,)H), C, 3

The code combines the words: she, prefer ((season, sun) liquid), food, past.

A Incorrect as the present tense is used.

B **Is the correct answer as it uses all the codes and the rules within the brackets. It correctly combines '((season, sun) liquid)' to infer 'summer wine'.**

C Incorrect as no reference is made to a female.

D **Is also the correct answer as it uses all the codes and the rules within the brackets. It correctly combines 'prefer ((season, sun) liquid)' to infer 'preferred summer showers'.**

E Incorrect as no reference is made to '(sun, season)'.

Example 40

Answer: D

O, (1, ♒), (1, G), D, 6

The code combines the words: she, (opposite, happy), (opposite, speak), secret, past.

A Incorrect as the sentence introduces the word 'guilty'.

B Incorrect as ignores the code '(opposite, happy)' and introduces the word 'glad'.

C Incorrect as the sentence makes no reference to secret. Also, '(opposite, speak)' are not combined.

D **Is the correct answer as it uses all the codes and the rules within the brackets. It correctly combines '(opposite, happy)' to imply 'not happy'. Also, '(opposite, speak)' have been combined to imply 'heard'.**

E Incorrect as '(opposite, speak)' have not been combined.

Example 41

Answer: A

O, (13, □), (1, G), M, (8, A, H), 3

The code combines the words: she, (attribute, nervous), (opposite, speak), danger, (strong, wind, liquid), past.

A **Is the correct answer as it uses all the codes and the rules within the brackets. It correctly combines '(attribute, nervous)' to imply 'shaking'. Also, '(opposite, speak)' are combined to imply 'heard'. Finally, 'danger' and '(strong, wind, liquid)' are combined to imply 'threatening storm'.**

B Incorrect as it introduces the word 'saw' and ignores the code '(opposite, speak)'.

C Incorrect as '(strong, wind, liquid)' are incorrectly combined to mean 'volcano'.

D Incorrect as the present tense is used.

E Incorrect as it ignores combining '(attribute, nervous)'. Also, there is no reference to danger.

Example 42

Answer: E

(8, J), I, (P, ♓), 7(5, N)

The code combines the words: (strong, sun), day, (public, aggressive), conditional (increase, person).

- A Incorrect as it introduces information on the police: 'unless the police are ineffective', which cannot be deduced from the code.
- B Incorrect as it introduces 'fires', and there is no reference to '(public, aggression)'.
- C Incorrect as it introduces 'traffic chaos'.
- D Incorrect as it ignores combining 'increase' and 'person'.
- E **Is the correct answer as it uses all the codes and the rules within the brackets. It correctly combines '(strong, sun)' to give 'heat wave', and 'conditional (increase, person)' to give 'provided there are sufficient people'.**

Example 43

Answer: B

O, ●, (1, G), H, 10, (O, Q), 3

The code combines the words: she, strange, (opposite, speak), liquid, hard, (she, building), past.

- A Incorrect as 'felt the rain on her skin' is introduced and '(opposite, hear)' is ignored.
- B **Is the correct answer. The statement is set in the past tense and uses all of the code. '(opposite, speak)' is interpreted as 'heard'. 'Strange' is interpreted as 'didn't feel herself'. Also, '(she, building)' is combined to imply 'her roof'. 'Hard' indicates that the rain 'smashed' onto the roof.**
- C Incorrect as 'she' is replaced with 'they'.
- D Incorrect as the present tense is used.
- E Incorrect as there is no reference to 'hard' in the sentence.

Example 44

Answer: C

(5, N), (13, ⍓), 7, H, 13(H, J)

The code combines the words: (increase, person), (attribute, sad), conditional, liquid, attribute (liquid, sun).

- A Incorrect as 'flood' is introduced. Also, 'attribute (liquid, sun)' have not been combined.
- B Incorrect as there is no conditional element within the statement.

C **Is the correct answer as it uses all the codes and the rules within the brackets. It correctly combines '(increase, person)' to imply 'villagers' and also correctly combines '(attribute, sad)' to imply 'cry'. Finally, 'attribute (liquid, sun)' have been combined to mean 'dry'.**

D Incorrect as the sentence wrongly states the opposite reason for the cause of the villagers crying.

E Incorrect as 'celebrate' is wrongly introduced. Also, the sentence ignores the combining of '(attribute, sad)'.

Example 45

Answer: B

P (♦, G), (5, N, S, 8), 4

The code combines the words: public (excited, speak), (increase, person, achievement, strong), future.

A Incorrect as there is no reference to 'losing' in the code.

B Is the correct answer as it uses all the codes and the rules within the brackets. It correctly combines 'public (excited, speak)' to imply 'will cheer', which is in the future tense. Also the code '(increase, person, achievement, strong)' is combined to imply 'victorious athletes'.

C Incorrect as the sentence wrongly infers 'men' from the word public.

D Incorrect as the sentence introduces a conditional element.

E Incorrect as the past tense is employed.

Example 46

Answer: E

N, ♏, (1, L), (5, J), (1, H)

The code combines the words: person, hope, (opposite, yesterday), (increase, sun), (opposite, liquid).

A Incorrect as '(increase, sun)' have not been combined.

B Incorrect as '(increase, sun)' have not been combined. Also, the code does not imply that it will be 'very dry'.

C Incorrect as the word 'hope' has been ignored. Also, the code does not imply that it will be 'very dry'.

D Incorrect as the word 'hope' has been replaced with 'predict'.

E Is the correct answer as it uses all the codes and the rules within the brackets. It correctly infers 'person, hope' as 'I hope'. Also, '(increase, sun)' are combined to mean 'a lot of sun'. Also, '(opposite, liquid)' are combined to imply 'no rain'.

Example 47

Answer: B

(D, N), ♏, (M, P), 1(13, T), 4

The code combines the words: (secret, person), hope, (danger, public), opposite (attribute, watch), future.

- A Incorrect as '(strong, person)' is a poor interpretation of 'spy'. Also, the past tense is employed.
- **B Is the correct answer. It correctly combines '(secret, person)' to mean 'spy'. Also, '(danger, public)' is combined to imply 'dangerous people'. Finally, 'opposite (attribute, watch)' are combined to imply 'can't see'.**
- C Incorrect as the past tense is employed. Also, the code introduces reference to an attribute of 'speak', which is not relevant in the sentence.
- D Incorrect as 'she' is introduced. Also, the past tense is used and there is no reference to 'enemy'.
- E Incorrect as the present tense use is employed.

Example 48

Answer: E

O, □, (M, H), 11, (P, Q), 3

The code combines the words: she, nervous, (danger, liquid), close, (public, building), past.

- A Incorrect as uses the code for the present tense.
- B Incorrect as it does not include a code which would imply a flood. Also, the code for 'gift' is used.
- C Incorrect as the present tense is used and the code does not make reference to a '(public, building)'.
- D Incorrect as uses the code '(opposite, she)', which would imply 'he'.
- **E Is the most accurate interpretation as: 'nervous' is substituted for 'frightened' while '(danger, liquid)' can be interpreted as 'flood'. Also, '(public, building)' can be interpreted to mean 'school'.**

Example 49

Answer: C

N, 12, H, (9, 5, N), I(1, R)

The code combines the words: person, enjoyable, liquid, (prefer, increase, person), day (opposite, cold).

A Incorrect as there is reference to a 'warm season', but not a 'warm day'.

B Incorrect as there is reference to 'food', but not 'drink'.

C **Is the correct answer as it uses all the codes and the rules within the brackets: '(prefer, increase, person)' is combined to mean 'friends'. Also 'day (opposite, cold)' means 'warm day'.**

D Incorrect as the day is said to be cold.

E Incorrect as there is no reference to 'friends'. Combining '(she, increase, person)' implies a group of females, rather than friends.

Example 50

Answers: B & C

(5, M), (N, T), (8, H), K

The code combines the words: (increase, danger), (person, watch), (strong, liquid), today.

A Incorrect as there is no reference to the water being cold in the code.

B **Is the correct answer as it uses all the codes and the rules within the brackets. It combines '(increase, danger)' to mean 'beware' while '(person, watch)' are combined to mean 'I've been observing'. Also, '(strong, liquid)' are combined to mean 'strong current'.**

C **Is also the correct answer as it uses all the codes and the rules within the brackets. It combines '(increase, danger)' to mean 'beware', while '(person, watch)' is combined to mean 'I've been watching'. Also, '(strong, liquid)' are combined to mean 'the drinks are strong'.**

D Incorrect as the code explicitly states 'today', rather than 'at the moment'.

E Incorrect as 'heard' is wrongly introduced. Also, there is no reference to 'today'.

Example 51

Answer: E

(1, O), (1, ❖), T, (N, F), 2

The code combines the words: (opposite, she), (opposite, curious), watch, (person, gift), present.

A Incorrect as the past tense is used. Also, 'gift' is combined with 'public', rather than a person, which does not make sense in the context.

B Incorrect as the code refers to being curious, rather than not curious.
C Incorrect as 'speak' is introduced and there is no reference to 'see'.
D Incorrect as the past tense is used.
E **Is the correct answer. It correctly combines '(opposite, she)' to imply 'he' and '(opposite, curious)' to imply 'not curious'. Finally, '(person, gift)' are combined to mean 'his present'.**

Example 52

Answer: B

O, ⌘, C, T(1, 12), (5, N), 3

The code combines the words: she, angry, food, watch (opposite, enjoyable), (increase person), past.

A Incorrect as 'speak' is introduced and there is no reference to 'look'.
B **Is the correct answer. It correctly combines 'watch (opposite, enjoyable)' to imply 'didn't look appetising'. Also, '(increase, person)' are combined to mean 'guests'.**
C Incorrect as there is no reference to 'guests'
D Incorrect as 'food' is replaced by 'liquid' and the present tense is used.
E Incorrect as 'she' is replaced with 'person'.

Chapter 7

The Situational Judgement subtest

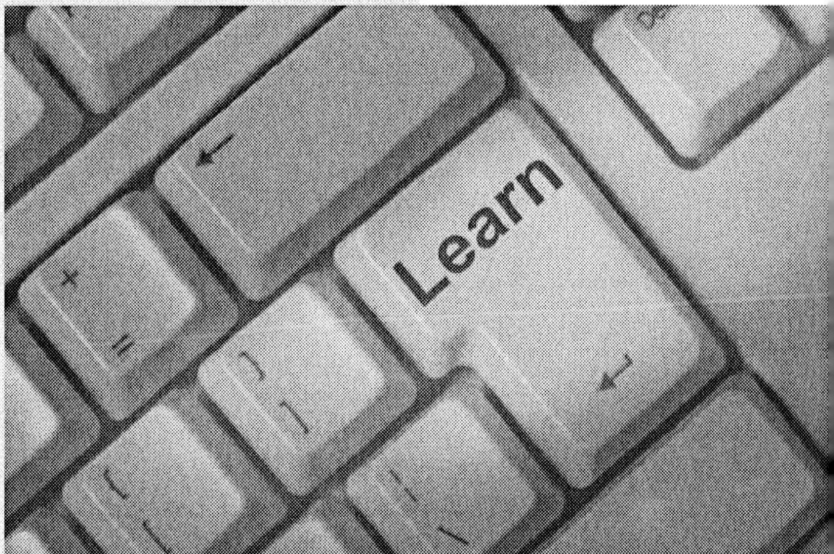

The Situational Judgement subtest

The role of the UKCAT Situational Judgement subtest is to assess a candidate's ability to evaluate information relating to real life scenarios and to select important factors and appropriate responses. The Situational Judgement subtest format is used commonly as part of selection processes to assess a qualified doctor's suitability for progression at various points of their career.

Situational Judgement Tests (SJTs), which are sometimes referred to as Professional Dilemmas, are psychological tests that essentially present the candidate with a real life situation and asks what he/she would do in that particular scenario based on the options available.

The first SJT was used in 1926 before being used extensively by psychologists in the US military during World War II. SJTs are now used by many organisations to identify suitable candidates for particular jobs, assessing whether their responses suit the particular role they are applying for.

The Situational Judgement subtest in the UKCAT comprises of 19 separate scenario stems with a total of 68 action/response items associated with the scenarios. Each of the 19 scenarios comprise a separate passage of information about a hypothetical real life scenario followed by a series of questions relating to an action or response.

The action/response questions associated with each scenario can range from 2 to as many as 5.

For each multiple choice action/response option there will be 4 options centred around two different responses, namely how appropriate a given action/response is or how important a given action/response is.

You will be allocated 27 minutes to complete the Situational Judgement subtest which includes one minute of administration time. This approximately equates to 24 seconds available to answer each of the 68 lead in questions or looking at it another way approximately 85 seconds to spend on each scenario.

For each scenario you will be presented with a passage describing a scenario that assesses your ability to deal with factors including:

- **Empathy and Sensitivity:** Your competency and enthusiasm to take in the perspectives of others and whether you treat others with understanding. This involves handling situations sensitively and treating others as individuals as well as respecting patients' rights to confidentiality.
- **Communication Skills:** The capacity to adjust your behaviour and language to the needs of differing situations. Your ability to deal with individuals of all levels.

- **Conceptual Thinking and Problem Solving:** Your capability to think beyond the obvious, to analyse particular situations and to be flexible in forming an appropriate plan of action.
- **Coping with Pressure:** Your ability to recognise your own limitations and develop appropriate coping mechanisms for stressful and pressured situations.
- **Organisation and Planning:** Your capability to organise all resources (e.g. time/information/people) effectively in a planned manner. The ability to delegate effectively where appropriate.
- **Managing Others and Team Involvement:** Your capacity to work effectively in partnership with others.
- **Professional Integrity:** Your ability to be accountable for your own decisions and to act without delay if you have good reason to believe that you or a colleague may be putting patients at risk.
- **Learning and Personal Development:** Your eagerness to keep your knowledge and skills up to date and to learn from experience.

A significant number of the scenarios will relate to a medical student responding to a given scenario. We would therefore urge you to familiarise yourself with the GMC guidance booklet 'Medical students: professional values and fitness to practise' which is available to on the GMC website (www.gmc-uk.org.uk).

Key factors that should influence your decision as to what priority you place on each of your action/response answers are:

- Placing the needs of the patient first
- Doing no harm – patient safety
- Working within your competency
- The urgency of a situation

Your response is proportionate to the potential severity of the situation.

In terms of scoring for each answer full marks will be awarded for a correct answer and partial marks will be awarded if your response is close to the correct answer. This is because although there will definitely be inappropriate action/response options a number of options may be a reasonable but not fully correct action/response. A candidate's score will then be illustrated through one of four bands rather than a numerical score:

Band 1: Excellent level performance
Band 2: Good level performance
Band 3: Average level performance
Band 4: Low level performance

The Situational Judgement subtest measures non-cognitive abilities and therefore each university will consider this element of candidate's UKCAT results in a slightly different manner.

Summary of Situational Judgement structure

Stem

The stem will consist of a scenario that may be healthcare related or a completely unrelated scenario. The Situational Judgement subtest consists of 19 such stems.

Lead in question

Each of the scenario stems will contain between two and five action/ response item questions. There will be a total of 68 action/response item questions.

Choices

There will be two distinct options for the responses that will be split equally in the UKCAT:

Appropriateness

- **A very appropriate thing to do** – this answer will apply to an action/ response that addresses a key aspect of the situation but does not have to address all aspects of dealing with the scenario.
- **Appropriate, but not ideal** – this answer will apply to an action/ response that could be done but does significantly address the situation.
- **Inappropriate but not awful** – this answer will apply to an action/ response that should not really be done but would not be bad if it was.
- **A very inappropriate thing to do** – this will apply to an action/ response that should definitely not be done and will contribute to making the situation worse.

Importance

- **Very important** – this answer will apply to an action/response that is paramount and must absolutely be considered.
- **Important** – this answer will apply to an action/response that is important but not paramount to be considered.
- **Of minor importance** – this answer will apply to an action/response that could be considered but will not have an impact if it is not considered.
- **Not important at all** – this answer will apply to an action/response that should most certainly not be taken into account/

Example of a Situational Judgement Test

Scenario 1

Upon joining a hospital ward team for a 2-week placement under the supervision of a registrar, a medical student called Jack on his second day suspects that a senior nurse within the team is stealing prescription drugs. On closer observation Jack actually observes the nurse remove drugs from the drug cabinet and place them in her personal bag.

How appropriate are each of the following responses by **Jack** in this situation:

1 **Ignore what they have seen and continue as is.**
   A. A very appropriate thing to do
   B. Appropriate but not ideal
   C. Inappropriate but not awful
   D. A very inappropriate thing to do

Situational Judgement hints and tips

- When reviewing the scenario identify in your mind what the scenario relates to e.g. is it a patient safety issue? A poorly performing colleague? Requires better communication?
- Your number one priority must be the safety and welfare of a patient if applicable to a particular scenario.
- Ensure that the answer you give for each action/response item is based purely on the appropriateness/importance for that particular action/response. The degree of appropriateness/importance should not be influenced by previous answers to a scenario.

- It is important to note that for a particular scenario the same appropriateness/importance answer can be given more than once.
- Understand which individual in a given scenario the question stem is asking you to give the most appropriate/important response.
- When reviewing the response options consider them irrelevant of timeframe. So a response may still be appropriate/important even if is something that can actioned for example weeks after a patient safety incident that also requires immediate action.
- Do not dwell too long on a particular question – remember time management is key throughout and for the Situational Judgement subtest you have less than thirty seconds for each response. You do have the option to flag a question to return to later.
- Attempt all questions and provide a response for each as you will not be penalised for getting a question wrong but you will if you leave a response blank you will stand no chance of scoring full or partial marks.

Simple Steps to Situational Judgement

Step 1

Identify what the issue(s) the scenario relates to.

Step 2

Identify for which individual's action/responses the question relates to.

Step 3

Formulate in your mind what the ideal response to the scenario would be.

Step 4

Read the question and clarify exactly what you are being asked.

Step 5

Re read the scenario if needed.

Step 6

Provide a response based purely on the question that is being asked and that best reflects its appropriateness/importance.

Step 7

If you are unsure enter your best guess at an answer (rather than leaving it blank), flag the question and return to it later.

Situational Judgement practice examples

The following part of this chapter will enable you to work through various examples of Situational Judgement questions together with evaluating your answers with explanations.

Example Scenario 1

Upon joining a hospital ward team for a 2-week placement under the supervision of a registrar, a medical student called Jack on his second day suspects that a senior nurse within the team is stealing prescription drugs. On closer observation Jack actually observes the nurse remove drugs from the drug cabinet and place them in her personal bag.

How **appropriate** is each of the following responses by Jack in this situation:

1. **Ignore what he has seen and continue as is.**
   A. A very appropriate thing to do
   B. Appropriate but not ideal
   C. Inappropriate but not awful
   D. A very inappropriate thing to do

2. **Ask to discuss with the nurse immediately his concerns away from the ward.**
   A. A very appropriate thing to do
   B. Appropriate but not ideal
   C. Inappropriate but not awful
   D. A very inappropriate thing to do

3. **Attempt immediately to seek the opinion of his Registrar who he is assigned under.**
   A. A very appropriate thing to do
   B. Appropriate but not ideal
   C. Inappropriate but not awful
   D. A very inappropriate thing to do

4. **Raise the issue at his review with his educational supervisor next month following the completion of the placement.**
   A. A very appropriate thing to do
   B. Appropriate but not ideal
   C. Inappropriate but not awful
   D. A very inappropriate thing to do

Example Scenario 2

Anthony, a 21-year old dental student on a practice placement, is nearing the end of a busy day. Whilst popping out of his supervisor's examination room to speak to reception, a family member of a patient who is being treated by another dentist confronts Anthony in the middle of the reception. In a very aggressive manner the family member is complaining regarding the time it is taking to treat their Mother and that they need to get home.

How **appropriate** is each of the following responses by **Anthony** in this situation:

1. **Calm the relative down and assure them that you are going to personally look into their concerns.**
   A. A very appropriate thing to do
   B. Appropriate but not ideal
   C. Inappropriate but not awful
   D. A very inappropriate thing to do

2. **Advise the relative that they have nothing to worry about.**
   A. A very appropriate thing to do
   B. Appropriate but not ideal
   C. Inappropriate but not awful
   D. A very inappropriate thing to do

3. **Apologise to the family member and seek the assistance of a senior member of staff who has been involved in the treatment.**
   A. A very appropriate thing to do
   B. Appropriate but not ideal
   C. Inappropriate but not awful
   D. A very inappropriate thing to do

4. **Tell the relative that you have had nothing to do with the patient and that they should raise their concerns with reception.**
   A. A very appropriate thing to do
   B. Appropriate but not ideal
   C. Inappropriate but not awful
   D. A very inappropriate thing to do

Example Scenario 3

A first year medical student is on a placement in a Hospital Trust's maternity unit working alongside a senior midwife in observing a young couple with the birth of their third child in a private delivery room. Whilst the senior midwife has left the room to address a rota issue, the mother to be complains of serious chest pains, to which the father to be responds that she is always complaining and to ignore her.

How **appropriate** is each of the following responses by the **medical student** in this situation:

1. **Reassure the mother that everything is going to be fine.**
   A. A very appropriate thing to do
   B. Appropriate but not ideal
   C. Inappropriate but not awful
   D. A very inappropriate thing to do

2. **Immediately call for the assistance of the senior midwife.**
   A. A very appropriate thing to do
   B. Appropriate but not ideal
   C. Inappropriate but not awful
   D. A very inappropriate thing to do

3. **Agree with the Father to be that there is nothing to worry about and do nothing.**
   A. A very appropriate thing to do
   B. Appropriate but not ideal
   C. Inappropriate but not awful
   D. A very inappropriate thing to do

4. **Ask to examine the mother to be with their stethoscope.**
   A. A very appropriate thing to do
   B. Appropriate but not ideal
   C. Inappropriate but not awful
   D. A very inappropriate thing to do

Example Scenario 4

Kiaria is a member of the university netball team. She enjoys playing in regular matches but is unhappy because of the behaviour of some of the more senior players whilst representing the university in local competitions. This is especially around using bad language in front of children watching the matches.

How **appropriate** is each of the following responses by <u>**Kiaria**</u> in this situation:

1. **Confront the senior players and express her disapproval at their behaviour.**
   A. A very appropriate thing to do
   B. Appropriate but not ideal
   C. Inappropriate but not awful
   D. A very inappropriate thing to do

2. **Write a letter to the University's President of Sport to express her dissatisfaction.**
   A. A very appropriate thing to do
   B. Appropriate but not ideal
   C. Inappropriate but not awful
   D. A very inappropriate thing to do

Example Scenario 5

A final year medical student called Lindsey feels that the Registrar who is supervising her is continually dumping tasks on her at the last minute and is not behaving like this with any other final year medical students.

How **appropriate** is each of the following responses by <u>**Lindsey**</u> in this situation:

1. **Continue as is and not say anything.**
   A. A very appropriate thing to do
   B. Appropriate but not ideal
   C. Inappropriate but not awful
   D. A very inappropriate thing to do

2. **Contact the Medical Director of the hospital to air her concerns.**
   A. A very appropriate thing to do
   B. Appropriate but not ideal
   C. Inappropriate but not awful
   D. A very inappropriate thing to do

3. **Speak to her fellow medical students for advice.**
   A. A very appropriate thing to do
   B. Appropriate but not ideal
   C. Inappropriate but not awful
   D. A very inappropriate thing to do

4. **Confide in one of the patients she has become friendly with on the ward.**
   A. A very appropriate thing to do
   B. Appropriate but not ideal
   C. Inappropriate but not awful
   D. A very inappropriate thing to do

5. **Write a letter to the Clinical Lead complaining about the Registrar.**
   A. A very appropriate thing to do
   B. Appropriate but not ideal
   C. Inappropriate but not awful
   D. A very inappropriate thing to do

Example Scenario 6

A patient on the ward complains to a medical student that their laptop, which is worth a considerable amount of money, and wallet are missing. This is not the first time the medical student has heard of possessions going missing.

How **important** to take into account are the following factors for the medical student when considering how to respond to the situation?

1. **The value of the possessions that have gone missing.**
   A. Very important
   B. Important
   C. Of minor importance
   D. Not important at all

2. **That possessions have gone missing in the past.**
   A. Very important
   B. Important
   C. Of minor importance
   D. Not important at all

3. **The effect of this on other patients staying on the ward.**
   A. Very important
   B. Important
   C. Of minor importance
   D. Not important at all

4. **That the patient whose possessions have gone missing is suffering from moderate dementia.**
   A. Very important
   B. Important
   C. Of minor importance
   D. Not important at all

Example Scenario 7

James is a medical student on a general practice placing. The GP he is observing has just given a child their immunisations and asked him to confirm the details of the batch number and expiry date so they can be recorded in the notes. While doing so James realises that the injection that has been given is one month out of date.

How **important** to take into account are the following factors for **James** when considering how to respond to the situation?

1. **The child appears fine after receiving the injection.**
   A. Very important
   B. Important
   C. Of minor importance
   D. Not important at all

2. **The mother is oblivious to what has happened.**
   A. Very important
   B. Important
   C. Of minor importance
   D. Not important at all

3. **Whether the rest of the batch of the vaccinations in the fridge are within date.**
   A. Very important
   B. Important
   C. Of minor importance
   D. Not important at all

Example Scenario 8

Porick is a final year dental student and is struggling with some of the practical elements that will form the basis of assessment. He is feeling quite disheartened about whether he will complete his course and is considering quitting the course. Janice is one of Porick's close friends on the course and is very worried about Porick's mental health.

How **important** to take into account are the following factors for **Janice** when considering how to respond to the situation?

1. **That Porick refuses to go and see a GP about his mental health.**
   A. Very important
   B. Important
   C. Of minor importance
   D. Not important at all

2. **That Porick has mentioned to Janice that he is feeling suicidal.**
   A. Very important
   B. Important
   C. Of minor importance
   D. Not important at all

3. **The Dental School is holding a final year party next weekend.**
   A. Very important
   B. Important
   C. Of minor importance
   D. Not important at all

4. **Porick's tutor is away at a conference and not due to return until next week.**
   A. Very important
   B. Important
   C. Of minor importance
   D. Not important at all

Example Scenario 9

Debbie is a 3rd year medical student currently working as part of a group of three other students on a project relating to service improvement. Part of the project involves interviewing patients and it has become apparent to Debbie that another member of the group, Francis, is posting confidential patient information in relation to their care on social media.

How **important** to take into account are the following factors for **Debbie** when considering how to respond to the situation?

1. **That the information being shared relates to an elderly patient who is unlikely to see the information posted on the social media site.**
   A. Very important
   B. Important
   C. Of minor importance
   D. Not important at all

2. **That Francis is very popular in the medical school and can be very unpleasant to fellow students he does not like.**
   A. Very important
   B. Important
   C. Of minor importance
   D. Not important at all

Example Scenario 10

It has become apparent to John that one of his fellow students Alan is plagiarising passages from the internet to include in his latest essay.

How **important** to take into account are the following factors for **John** when considering how to respond to the situation?

1. **That the essay will not contribute to the final year mark for the year.**
   A. Very important
   B. Important
   C. Of minor importance
   D. Not important at all

2. **Last month Alan confided in John that he is worried he may have dyslexia.**
   A. Very important
   B. Important
   C. Of minor importance
   D. Not important at all

3. **John's tutor has made it clear to him that if he suspects any of his fellow students plagiarising work he should report it immediately.**
   A. Very important
   B. Important
   C. Of minor importance
   D. Not important at all

Justifications of Situational Judgement practice examples

Example Scenario 1

1. **A very inappropriate thing to do** – ignoring the fact that a colleague is potentially stealing prescription medication and doing nothing would be a very inappropriate thing to do. Also although it may not appear that there is any risk to patients if the nurse is taking the medication whilst on duty there could be a significant risk to patient safety.
2. **Inappropriate but not awful** – although this would be inappropriate it would not put patients at risk. As Jack is new to the ward he may have misinterpreted the nurse's behaviour and there may be an innocent explanation. The nurse may become defensive or aggressive so it would be better to raise it with Registrar in the first instance.
3. **A very appropriate thing to do** – given the Registrar is who Jack has been assigned under this would be an entirely appropriate course of action to take and challenging the nurse should be left to a person in a position of authority.
4. **A very appropriate thing to do** – although in terms of timeframe this is some time after the event the experience is a good case for reflection and discussion with Jack's educational supervisor to aid in his development as a future doctor.

Example Scenario 2

1. **Appropriate but not ideal** – this would be an appropriate course of action although it would be ideal to seek the assistance of a senior who has been involved in the treatment at the earliest opportunity.
2. **A very inappropriate thing to do** – acting within your competency as a student is key. Anthony has no idea what the situation is and no basis to confirm that everything is going to be ok.
3. **A very appropriate thing to do** – demonstrating empathy for the concerns of patients and their families is a key skill and seeking the immediate assistance of senior colleague involved in the treatment is the right course of action here.
4. **Inappropriate, but not awful** – although this is not treating the patient's family with respect and compassion it is not going to cause a serious incident by recommending the family member speaks to reception.

Example Scenario 3

1. **Appropriate but not ideal** – reassuring the patient that everything is going to be ok is not inappropriate however the priority here must be seeking assistance from a senior member of staff especially given the chest pains could be indicative of something serious.
2. **A very appropriate thing to do** – recognising that a given situation is outside of a person's competency is a key component to ensuring the high quality and safe delivery of patient care. In this instance seeking senior assistance as soon as possible is a very appropriate thing to do.
3. **A very inappropriate thing to do** – this would be a very inappropriate course of action especially as the patient is complaining of chest pain and needs addressing immediately.
4. **A very inappropriate thing to do** – the medical student is present in an observational capacity and proceeding to physically examine the mother to be without supervision and more importantly without seeking assistance would be a very inappropriate course of action.

Example Scenario 4

1. **Appropriate but not ideal** – although this is not inappropriate a better course of action may be to speak to the team captain who would be better placed to deal with this in the first instance.
2. **Inappropriate but not awful** – this is an inappropriate course of action as no measures have been taken to address the situation first before escalating it.

Example Scenario 5

1. **Inappropriate but not awful** – although continuing as is will not result in a severe situation nonetheless it is counterproductive to Lindsey's development and wellbeing if the Registrar continues to dump tasks on her at the last minute.
2. **Inappropriate but not awful** – again although this will not have a detrimental effect this is not an appropriate course of action without first attempting to resolve the situation with the Registrar.
3. **Appropriate but not ideal** – this would be an appropriate course of action and help to inform possible ways of solving the situation but it is not directly the addressing the problem by approaching the supervising Registrar.

4. **A very inappropriate thing to do** – professional integrity is key to delivering high quality care. Discussing any grievances that one might have with a patient is not professional.
5. **Inappropriate but not awful** – again this would be an inappropriate course of action without first attempting to speak to the Registrar first.

Example Scenario 6

1. **Not important at all** – regardless of the value of the possessions the fact that possessions have potentially gone missing is very serious.
2. **Of minor importance** – although possessions have gone missing in the past it is important not to jump to conclusions.
3. **Important** – the effect that possessions going missing could have on causing worry to other patients is something that should be considered of importance and taking steps to allay any fears they may have.
4. **Of minor importance** – although this should be considered it is important not to jump to conclusions that the patient may have accidentally misplaced or lost their possessions. All patients' concerns should be considered regardless.

Example Scenario 7

1. **Of minor importance** – although of some importance the condition of the child should not influence the decision on how to respond.
2. **Not important at all** – Regardless of whether the Mother is aware or not of what has happened should not influence the decision to address the situation.
3. **Important** – Although this does not address the matter in question it would still be important to check the rest of the batch to guard against this occurring again.

Example Scenario 8

1. **Very important** – maintaining health and wellbeing is very important in ensuring a student is fit to practice. The fact that Porick seemingly refuses to seek medical help is a very important factor to take into account.
2. **Very important** – this is obviously very serious and should be considered with high importance when determining what to do.

3. **Not important at all** – this has no relevance in informing Janice on what she should take into consideration when helping Porick.
4. **Important** – although this is of importance there are other individuals that could be approached for support.

Example Scenario 9

1. **Not important at all** – regardless of whether a patient can see where their confidential information has been shared, breaching confidentiality is a very serious matter.
2. **Of minor importance** – this is of minor importance as although the primary concern should be addressing the breach of confidentiality Debbie should also be mindful that she should address any fall out aimed at her as a result of reporting the fact that confidentiality has been breached.

Example Scenario 10

1. **Not important at all** – regardless of whether the essay counts towards the final mark or not, plagiarism is very serious and not the behaviour expected of a professional.
2. **Important** – supporting fellow students is an important component of teamwork and the fact that Alan may have dyslexia should be taken into account and help on this matter must be sought.
3. **Very important** – the fact that is has been made clear to John of what steps to take in reporting plagiarism is of high importance.

Chapter 8

Entire mock UKCAT exam 1 questions

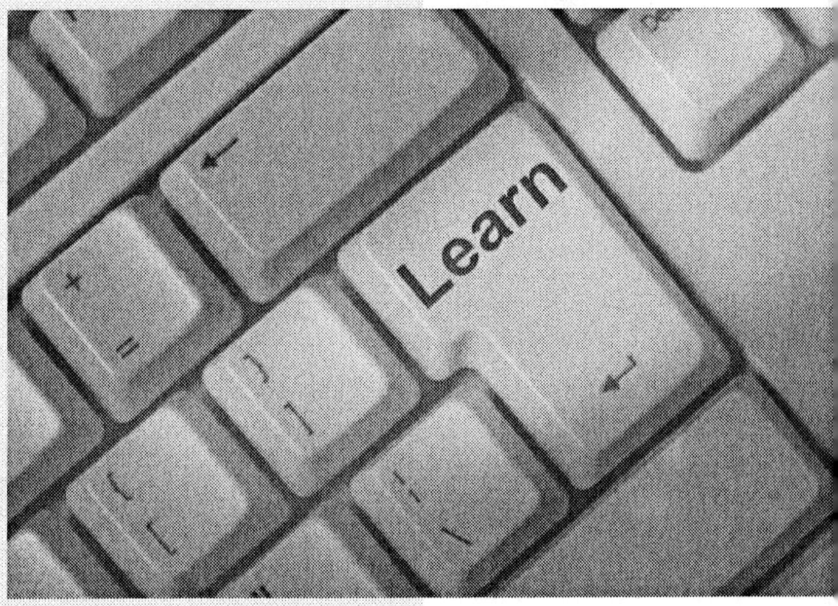

Entire mock UKCAT exam 1 questions

We would recommend that you complete the mock test under timed conditions and that you do not look at the answers until you have completed the test. The mock test should be completed in just over 90 minutes. You will need to print the Answer Sheet which is available to download for free from www.bpp.com/freehealthresources

Verbal Reasoning – 22 minutes

Question 1

Examples of such questions may include a situation where a colleague is viewing child pornography or there is a theft from the ward. As a rule, when answering any of these questions you must always have your facts completely straight before addressing the situation, especially if it may involve incriminating another colleague or patient. Thus it is sensible to prioritise answers that involve establishing the facts about what has happened first before confronting anyone or involving anyone else.

You should also prioritise any actions that involve immediately dealing with the situation, and leave actions such as incident forms and preventative measures until later. You must also be able to use your common sense to assess the severity of the crime and use your judgement in when to involve more senior authorities. For example, although all theft is illegal it may not be necessary to involve the police for a minor theft, and thus you must show that you are able to apply common sense to individual situations.

However, if the criminal issue compromises patient safety or if it involves the work ethic of a colleague, it is necessary to involve someone more senior and escalate the matter to a higher level. This is the case in a scenario where a colleague is stealing prescription drugs or viewing child pornography, as obviously patients may be at risk in these cases. Here you may need to involve your Consultant or even the Clinical Director or GMC if the matter is not dealt with. The ethical principles behind this approach involve the same ethics previously discussed with regard to patient safety and poorly performing colleagues ie you must always safeguard your patients.

Finally you must also use your common sense in deciphering which senior authority to inform first. Although there may be a criminal issue at hand and the police may need to be involved at some point, you are only a foundation doctor, and thus it may be sensible to go to your Registrar or Consultant first before contacting the police yourself. As previously stated, it is common courtesy when dealing with conduct issues in colleagues to deal with the matter locally first. Thus it is perfectly acceptable to discuss the matter with your Registrar or Consultant who can then call the police if necessary. In general, when answering these types of questions, contacting the police should be prioritised after involving someone senior within the hospital to deal with the matter.

From *Succeeding In Your GP ST Stage 2.*

1. **An individual should involve seniors if they suspect a colleague is viewing child pornography.**
   A. True
   B. False
   C. Can't Tell

2. **The passage is solely aimed at medical students.**
   A. True
   B. False
   C. Can't Tell

3. **Ideally the police should be informed only for more serious crimes.**
   A. True
   B. False
   C. Can't Tell

4. **It is considered courteous when dealing with a complaint regarding a colleague to request the views of the colleague in writing within 48 hours of the incident.**
   A. True
   B. False
   C. Can't Tell

Question 2

The game of Arimaa
Arimaa is a two-player board game invented by Omar Syed, a computer engineer trained in artificial intelligence. Inspired by Garry Kasparov's defeat at the hands of the chess computer Deep Blue, Syed wanted to design a new game which would be difficult for computers to play well, but would have rules simple enough for his four-year-old son Aamir to understand. In fact, 'Arimaa' is 'Aamir' spelled backwards plus an initial 'a.' In 2002 Syed published the rules to Arimaa and announced a $10,000 prize, available through 2020, for the first computer program to win matches against top-ranked human players. David Wu's bot Sharp accomplished this in 2015.
Arimaa was specifically designed so that it could be played using a chess set—an 8×8 board is used, and each player has sixteen pieces, in a 1-1-2-2-2-8 distribution. It can also be played on-line at the arimaa.com gameroom. In 2009, Z-Man Games began producing a commercial Arimaa set. Only one face-to-face tournament has taken place, but about 900 games are played on-line every week.
United States Patent number 6,981,700 for Arimaa was filed on the 3rd of October 2003, and granted on the 3rd of January 2006. Omar Syed also holds a trademark on the name 'Arimaa'. Syed has released an experimental license called 'The Arimaa Public License', with the declared intent to 'make Arimaa as much of a public domain game as possible while still protecting its commercial usage'. Items covered by the license are the patent and the trademark.

http://en.wikibooks.org/wiki/Arimaa

1. **Arimaa is best described as:**
   A. A 2-player board game that is popular online
   B. A computer game based on the game of draughts
   C. A game designed for teenagers
   D. Unbeatable by computer programmes

2. **Which of these statements based on the passage is False**
   A. Gary Kasperov has been beaten in the past by a chess computer
   B. The rights of the game is protected by both a patent and a trademark
   C. A physical chessboard is required to play Arimaa
   D. Each player has a sixteen pieces

3. **Upon announcing the competition for a computer to beat a top ranked human Arimaa player it took at least how long for someone to achieve this?**
   A. 15 years
   B. 11 years
   C. 13 years
   D. 10 years

4. **Which of the below statements is not inferred by the passage**
   A. In developing the game it was intended it would be harder for computer's to beat human players than the game of chess
   B. Arimaa is not exploited commercially
   C. People are allowed to use and play Arimaa in a non-commercial manner under a public licence
   D. The inventor of the game derived the name from his child's name

Question 3

Although this may seem obvious, many doctors report that they do not receive much, if any, praise and yet it is a great motivator when given sincerely. When you are developing someone's skills by delegating unfamiliar tasks to them, demonstrating your support is critical. Giving praise and being prepared to listen to concerns and give advice are all powerful ways of building confidence. Confidence is key to all performance issues and once you have instilled it in your colleagues you will be able to delegate to them on a regular basis. If you are asking a colleague to help you with work it will be important to acknowledge their support and assistance and thank them accordingly.

It is unfair to delegate only the jobs you do not like or which are unpleasant. You must delegate any task which is not your priority and that may well include the simple jobs you enjoy. When you delegate it is important during your briefing meeting that you make it clear that the responsibility and authority for completing the task is delegated also. However, what you should not delegate is accountability for the task. Accountability is a similar term to responsibility, so how may accountability be accurately defined?

US President Harry S Truman made famous a slogan which he had on his desk bearing the words, 'The buck stops here'. The meaning of this statement indicated that responsibility was not passed on beyond that point. It meant that Truman never 'passed the buck' to anyone else but always held ultimate responsibility for the way the country was governed.

In delegation terms, accountability is the acknowledgement of responsibility even when the actions may be undertaken by other people. If you delegate a task, it is still you who must answer to someone senior and report on progress. Although many doctors feel this justifies the pointlessness of delegating, all it really means is that you must ensure you are kept fully informed of progress, problems and the ultimate outcome of the task. Do not delegate and walk away, never again to enquire about how the task is progressing. You must review the situation regularly and be able to update senior staff with facts. You must also be prepared to deal with the consequences of problems which may arise. If deadlines are missed it is you who must provide explanations, so delegate properly and be clear about what you expect from your colleagues in return.

From *Effective Time Management Skills for Doctors.*

1. **The slogan made famous by Harry Truman was adopted by all subsequent American presidents.**
   A. True
   B. False
   C. Can't Tell

2. **Accountability and responsibility have the same meaning.**
   A. True
   B. False
   C. Can't Tell

3. **When delegating a task an individual must be prepared to address the consequences of any issues that occur.**
   A. True
   B. False
   C. Can't Tell

4. **Instilling confidence in an individual's colleagues plays a minor role in effective delegation.**
   A. True
   B. False
   C. Can't Tell

Question 4

Polynesian settlement of New Zealand rules

Around 1300 AD, it is believed Polynesian settlers used subtropical weather systems to find their way from their native islands, in Polynesia to New Zealand. As the settlers colonised the country, they developed their distinctive Maori culture.

According to Maori, the first Polynesian explorer to reach New Zealand was Kupe, who travelled across the Pacific in a Polynesian-style voyaging canoe. It is thought Kupe reached New Zealand at Hokianga Harbour, in Northland.

Although there has been much debate about when and how Polynesians actually started settling New Zealand, the current understanding is that they migrated from East Polynesia, the Southern Cook and Society islands region. They migrated deliberately, at different times, in different canoes, first arriving in New Zealand in the late 13th Century.

For a long time during the nineteenth and twentieth centuries, it was believed that the Maori's were descended from the indigenous Morioris people, who hunted giant birds called moas. It has since been established very recently that the population that now form the Maori people in New Zealand originated from Polynesia in a Great Fleet and took New Zealand from the Morioris's, establishing an agricultural society.

http://en.wikibooks.org/wiki/New_Zealand_History/Polynesian_Settlement

1. **Which of the following statement is true according to the passage:**
   A. The Maori people migrated to New Zealand in the 19th century
   B. The Maori people hunted giant birds called Moas
   C. The Maori people are believed to be descended from Polynesian settlers
   D. The Maori people are descended from the Morioris people

2. **According to the passage legend has it that:**
   A. Kupe was the first Polynesian explorer to discover New Zealand
   B. Kupe discovered New Zealand in a Maori style sailing raft
   C. Upon discovering New Zealand Kupe made landfall at Westland
   D. The main Maori God is called Kupe

3. **According to the passage which of the following is inferred:**
   A. The discovery of New Zealand was an accident
   B. Polynesians from East Polynesia, the Southern Cook and Society islands discovered New Zealand over a period of time
   C. The Maori culture was fully developed before discovering New Zealand
   D. Cold weather systems were used to aid the Polynesians discovery of New Zealand.

4. **Although it is unclear exactly when the Polynesians discovered New Zealand according to the passage it is generally accepted that this happened:**
   A. Approximately 500 years ago
   B. Over 2000 years ago
   C. Over 800 years ago
   D. In the 18th Century

Question 5

When organising a meeting establish who needs to attend. If you are chairing the meeting and decide that all the team should be present, consider the advice given previously and think about beginning with non-clinical items and allowing administrative staff the option of leaving after those items have been discussed and actioned. Start the meeting on time and make it clear to everyone that if they are late they will miss what has been discussed. If you are in the position of Chair use your assertiveness skills and ensure that everyone follows the agenda and does not introduce other topics. If they do, question the relevance of the question or debate and remind everyone of the agenda item they are meant to be discussing. Ensure that any actions arising are allocated clearly and that the individuals concerned understand the action they have been given. Agree deadlines for all actions and follow them up after the meeting so that all team members take their tasks seriously.

Circulate the minutes of the meeting in a timely fashion, preferably the same day. This will provide useful information for anyone not in attendance or latecomers who may have missed the beginning. If appropriate, help the minute-taker by advising him or her which items to record. When long discussions ensue it can be difficult for someone to judge accurately. As Chair, you should decide which points are pertinent to capture. This will include all actions.

When attending meetings review all the meetings you currently attend and decide whether you really do need to be there. Could you obtain all the information you need from reading a copy of the minutes? If the answer is yes then consider removing the meeting from your diary. If you need agreement from your senior then discuss it with them. Give your reasons and explain that you can keep up-to-date via the minutes. An alternative to this approach would be to delegate your attendance. Perhaps a colleague in the team, or if you are senior, one of your junior team members, could attend in your place? You can save useful time by having a shorter summary meeting with that individual afterwards. Negotiate with the Chairman your requirement to leave after certain agenda topics have been discussed. This approach works well for many doctors.

From *Effective Time Management Skills for Doctors*.

1. **An effective approach to saving an individual's valuable time regarding attendance at meetings is to request the meeting be recorded onto video and reviewed at a later stage.**
   A. True
   B. False
   C. Can't Tell

2. **Longer discussions within a meeting make it far easier to record the minutes of a meeting.**
   A. True
   B. False
   C. Can't Tell

3. **It is acceptable to introduce additional items that are not on the agenda for discussion as part of an Any Other Business item at the end of the meeting.**
   A. True
   B. False
   C. Can't Tell

4. **Non-attendance at a meeting can be justified by the fact that an individual can potentially glean the salient points discussed at the meeting by reading the minutes.**
   A. True
   B. False
   C. Can't Tell

Question 6

Article 27 of the declaration of Human Rights
According to Article 27 of the Universal Declaration of Human Rights, 'everyone has the right to the protection of the moral and material interests resulting from any scientific, literary or artistic production of which he is the author'. Although the relationship between intellectual property and human rights is a complex one, there are moral arguments for intellectual property.
Various moral justifications for private property can also be used to argue in favour of the morality of intellectual property, such as:
1. Natural Rights/Justice Argument: this argument is based on Locke's idea that a person has a natural right over the labour and/or products which is produced by his/her body. Appropriating these products is viewed as unjust. Although Locke had never explicitly stated that natural right applied to products of the mind, it is possible to apply his argument to intellectual property rights, in which it would be unjust for people to misuse another's ideas.
2. Utilitarian-Pragmatic Argument: according to this rationale, a society that protects private property is more effective and prosperous than societies that do not. Innovation and invention in 19th century America has been said to be attributed to the development of the patent system. By providing innovators with 'durable and tangible return on their investment of time, labour, and other resources', intellectual property rights seek to maximize social utility. The presumption is that they promote public welfare by encouraging the 'creation, production, and distribution of intellectual works'.
3. 'Personality' Argument: this argument is based on a quote from Hegel: 'Every man has the right to turn his will upon a thing or make the thing an object of his will, that is to say, to set aside the mere thing and recreate it as his own'. European intellectual property law is shaped by this notion that ideas are an 'extension of oneself and of one's personality'.

http://en.wikibooks.org/wiki/ Intellectual_Property_and_the_Internet/Intellectual_property

1. **According to the passage the patent system in America was developed as a result of:**
   A. Of the 'Personality Argument' proposed by Hegel
   B. Incentivising innovation and invention
   C. Competition with other countries
   D. To safeguard inventions

2. **It can be inferred from the passage that the aim of Article 27 of the Humans Rights Act is to:**
   A. To protect the rights of individuals to live in a safe environment
   B. To enable individuals to be rewarded for their innovative creations
   C. The relationship between intellectual property and moral rights is a simple one
   D. European intellectual property law was based on the concept of the Natural Rights/Justice argument

3. **A person has a natural right over their creations according to:**
   A. Natural Rights/Justice Argument
   B. Hegel
   C. Utilitarian-Pragmatic Argument
   D. European intellectual property law

4. **Which of the following statements can be inferred from the passage:**
   A. Intellectual property rights reduce social utility
   B. Article 27 is yet to be enshrined in law
   C. The moral component of intellectual property does not play a key part
   D. The morality of intellectual property can be argued by three key arguments

YOU ARE NOW OVER THE HALFWAY STAGE OF THIS SECTION. IDEALLY YOU SHOULD HAVE APPROXIMATELY 10 MINUTES LEFT.
(Please note that this prompt will not be given in your actual test.)

Question 7

Most of these dedicated courses are accelerated and take four years in total. Typically, the pre-clinical part of the course is separate from the undergraduate course of five years. For the clinical years, graduate entry courses and undergraduate courses are often the same.
Graduate entry courses are intense, with shorter holidays, and require a high degree of motivation and self-directed learning. They frequently use problem-based learning (PBL) and interactive styles, and are usually integrated to give early clinical experience. Both science and non-science graduates may be accepted, but this varies according to the institution. Usually a BSc (Hons) science degree is required. Most expect a minimum of a 2:1, although some schools accept a 2:2, particularly if you have a post-graduate qualification (PhD or MSc). The Open University has a specific course to upgrade a 2:2 degree to a 2:1. A health related degree or extenuating circumstances for your 2:2 may be accepted by some medical schools. Be aware that some medical schools stating a 2:1 as minimum are so oversubscribed that they may only select those with 1st class degrees. In practice, an average cohort is a third with 1sts and two-thirds with 2:1s. Some GEPs specify A level requirements too, but the main factor that determines whether or not you get an interview is your score on the GAMSAT or other entrance exam.

GAMSAT is short for the Graduate Australian Medical School Admissions Test. It is required at medical schools such as St. George's, Nottingham / Derby, Swansea and Peninsula (five-year course). It comprises an arduous set of three exams over five hours. Each exam tests a different attribute that you need to have to become a good doctor:

- *Reasoning – social sciences and humanities (75 MCQs).*
- *Communicative ability (two essays).*
- *Scientific reasoning. The exam is 40% chemistry, 40% biology and 20% physics at or above an A level standard (110 MCQs).*

From *Becoming a Doctor*.

1. **An individual with any type of undergraduate degree can apply to a graduate entry programme.**
   A. True
   B. False
   C. Can't Tell

2. **3.5 hours of the GAMSAT is allocated to individuals to complete the total number of MCQs.**
   A. True
   B. False
   C. Can't Tell

3. **A key element for an individual to succeed in their application to graduate entry medicine is scoring in the upper percentile in the GAMSAT.**
   A. True
   B. False
   C. Can't Tell

4. **The clinical component of a graduate entry medicine degree is predominantly the same as an undergraduate course.**
   A. True
   B. False
   C. Can't Tell

Question 8

With the best will in the world a CV guide cannot give you the actual material and content to put on your CV; this is down to the hard work and commitment you have shown since medical school. Early planning of how to improve and develop your CV for a given post is well advised and a friendly Consultant is invaluable in this quest. Approach your Consultant, particularly your educational supervisor, with a copy of your CV and ask if they will go through it with you to see where there are areas you could improve. Most consultants will be happy to do this, as they will remember their own anguish when trying to secure a particular position. If there are gaps in your CV after your previous positions, then take steps to remedy this as quickly as possible. These steps can be relatively easy (eg expand outside interests, book on to relevant courses, involve yourself in an audit) or may require more commitment (volunteer to teach anatomy / physiology at the university, book a college exam and start revising, register for a distance learning qualification). Some of these steps take more time than others to complete, and it depends on how committed you are to following that specialty, and how much time you have before the application deadline, as to what you can achieve. However, do not despair! Print out a copy of your CV. Look at it critically and honestly. Compare yourself with your peers and their achievements, as unfortunately these are the people you are competing with. If there are large gaps in your CV, think practically with the resources you have and the time left that you have to prepare.

From *Preparing the Perfect Medical CV.*

1. **One way an individual can strengthen their CV is through gaining involvement in extra-curricular activities.**
   A. True
   B. False
   C. Can't Tell

2. **Talking to your colleagues about their experience to date in their career can be a helpful exercise for an individual to help them improve their CV.**
   A. True
   B. False
   C. Can't Tell

3. **It is easy and quick for an individual to fill gaps in their CV.**
   A. True
   B. False
   C. Can't Tell

4. **A helpful Registrar can provide invaluable help to individuals wishing to improve their CV.**
   A. True
   B. False
   C. Can't Tell

Question 9

Plato
Plato is regarded by many to be one of the West's greatest ancient philosophers. The student of Socrates and teacher of Aristotle, he wrote many books in his life time. Plato was born into an Athenian

aristocratic family around 427/428 BC. His father Ariston was said to be an ancestor of the last king of Athens, Crodus and his mother Perictione was a relation of the Greek politician Solon.
There is not much external information about Plato's early life and most of what we know has come from his own writings. His father died when Plato was young and his mother was remarried to her uncle Pyrilampes. It is very likely that Plato knew Socrates from early childhood. Perictione's cousin Critias and her brother Charmides are known to have been friends with Socrates and they themselves were part of the oligarchic leadership of 404 BC. These connections should have led to a political career for Plato but at some stage for reasons unknown he made a decision not to enter political life. The oligarchic leadership collapsed and democracy was restored and considering that Plato's family members had been part of the oligarchic terror must have meant that his position in Athenian society was under scrutiny. The condemning to death of Socrates by the democracy seems to have been the final political act of the state that forced Plato into exile at Megara. Plato is known to have taken refuge with Eucleides, founder of the Megarian school of philosophy and it is stated by later historians that during this period in his life he travelled extensively through Greece, Italy and Egypt. Whether these journeys took place is disputed but it is known that Plato did travel to Sicily where he met Dion, brother-in-law of the ruler of Syracuse, Dionysius I.

http://en.wikibooks.org/wiki/Plato

1. **According to the passage what best describes the reason why Plato did not follow a career in politics?**
   A. He was also destined to become a philosopher
   B. He was far to intelligent
   C. It was unsafe for him
   D. For some unknown reason he chose not to

2. **According to the passage which of the following statements is true:**
   A. Plato met Socrates when he was 21
   B. Eucleides was Plato's uncle
   C. Charmides was part of the Oligarchic leadership
   D. Socrates was murdered by poisoning

3. **According to the passage Plato was regarded by many as one of the West's greatest philosophers because:**
   A. He wrote many books in his life time
   B. He was the teacher of Socrates
   C. He travelled extensively in England
   D. He was not able to follow a political career

4. **Which of the following is true:**
   A. Critias is the sister of Perictione
   B. When Crodusdied Plato's mother remarried Eucleides
   C. Critias and Charmides were related
   D. Perictione and Critias were brothers

Question 10

Think about all the things you need to accomplish as a doctor. At some point in your career you will need to create business cases to purchase equipment or hire extra resources. You will often find yourself in situations that require you to negotiate with others to achieve your outcomes. You may need to persuade and convince other people that your plan is the best one. You will definitely need to develop a strategy for the future and to make it inspiring enough that others are motivated to follow. The more senior you become the more you will be expected to manage a team of people, directing their actions in the most productive way for your service. You will be actively involved in the mentoring of junior staff. You will devise training plans and be expected to communicate frequently with your team. Above all you will be expected to defend them from unwarranted criticism and to support and praise them when they are performing well. You will attend senior level meetings and be involved with agreeing major contracts and service level agreements. As you can see, the more senior you become, the more you are drawn away from clinical responsibilities. You do not have to exclude them altogether but it is important that you understand what is expected of you when you hold a senior role. A lot of self-preparation is required and the earlier in your career that you can start, the better it will be for you. You need to be effective in your healthcare organisation as you will have many things to get done. There is a compelling argument for being able to organise yourself and your working day so that you do not become overwhelmed with all that you need to achieve.

From *Effective Time Management Skills for Doctors.*

1. **As a doctor progresses through their career their role and responsibilities will change to involve more management tasks.**
   A. True
   B. False
   C. Can't Tell

2. **Influencing others is a skill required of a doctor.**
   A. True
   B. False
   C. Can't Tell

3. **Mentoring junior staff involves conducting their appraisals.**
   A. True
   B. False
   C. Can't Tell

4. **It can be inferred from the passage that management responsibilities reduce a doctor's clinical responsibilities.**
   A. True
   B. False
   C. Can't Tell

Question 11

Nurses are the most important people to you in the hospital, they make the difference between things going smoothly, and things completely falling apart. It is absolutely essential to work to have them on your side. Find out who is in charge of the ward (Senior Sister / Charge Nurse) and make a special effort to introduce yourself. This person will be incredibly useful to you both practically and educationally. They can solve problems that you might be having trouble with. Remember: you work on their ward, and they will know the systems and the other staff better than you do. Ensure you know who the other nurses and healthcare assistants are, and what skills they have. This may take some time, but it means you can ask the right favour from the right person. Knowing the people you work with on a day to day basis will also make for a much easier start to your job. You must get nurses to complete your Mini-Peer Assessment Tool (Mini-PAT), and they can also observe you completing DOPS assessments. However, they cannot perform Mini-CEX or CbD assessments. Specialist nurses are highly trained in a single field, eg cardiac, endoscopy, diabetes, cancer (MacMillan nurses). They work with consultant doctors in the same field. Use their experience in their specialist field as much as you can, and learn from them. The ward pharmacist knows the dosages and indications for drugs, and they can also tell you if a drug you want to prescribe is in the hospital formulary. Ask them if you are unsure. Pharmacists can also work directly with the hospital pharmacy, to get medications for your patients quickly, especially in emergency situations and prior to discharges. Look out for their green ink on your drug charts. Physiotherapists use physical therapies such as breathing exercises, muscular training and motivational strategies to improve your patient's stability, strength, stamina and confidence. They often use frames and walking aids to get patients moving, especially after operations. They work in rehabilitation, and are an essential part of your discharge planning. They will also help in cases of acute pneumonia, and other respiratory illnesses.

From *The Essential Clinical Handbook for the Foundation Programme.*

1. **Specialist nurses are highly trained in more than one field.**
   A. True
   B. False
   C. Can't Tell

2. **A requirement of the Mini-Peer Assessment Tool (Mini-PAT) is that it must be completed by a pharmacist.**
   A. True
   B. False
   C. Can't Tell

3. **Pharmacists can help doctors with budgeting drugs.**
   A. True
   B. False
   C. Can't Tell

4. **Green ink on a chart suggests the involvement of a physiotherapist.**
   A. True
   B. False
   C. Can't Tell

Quantitative Reasoning – 25 minutes

Below you will find a menu for a café:

Ciabatta with cheese and onion	£3.20
Jacket potato	£1.20
Fries	£1.00
Pizza slice	£2.00
Onion rings	£1.00
Sausage and mashed potato	£2.39

1. What is the mean average of the prices?

A £1.78
B £1.82
C £1.80
D £2.80
E £1.86

2. What is the median of the prices?

A £1.89
B £1.90
C £1.60
D £2.00
E £1.20

3. What is the range of the price list?

A £3.20
B £2.89
C £2.20
D £1.00
E £2.30

4. What is the total of the mean, the median and the range?

A £4.60
B £3.76
C £1.98
D £5.60
E £5.20

Book	Total readership (Millions)		% of total readership reading each book in 1998	
	1981	1998	Male adults	Female adults
A Warm Day	2.2	8.9	22	18
My Best Friend	2.9	6.6	4	3
The Darkness in the Mind	3.5	2.1	24	6
Alive in the Past	6.9	4.8	10	13

5. Which book was read by more females than males in 1998?

A A Warm Day
B My Best Friend
C The Darkness in the Mind
D Alive in the Past
E A Warm Day and My Best Friend

6. What was the combined readership of 'Alive in the Past', 'A Warm Day' and 'My Best Friend' in 1981?

A 11 million
B 12 million
C 13 million
D 11.2 million
E 12.5 million

7. What was the percentage decrease in readership of 'Alive in the Past' from 1981 to 1998?

A 30.43 %
B 30.23 %
C 2.1 %
D 32.9 %
E 32.1%

8. **How many male adult readers read a 'A Warm Day' in 1998?**
   A 89,000,000
   B 1,958,000
   C 1.958
   D 8,900
   E 4,895,000

	B1	B2	B3	B4	B5	B6	B7	B8
A1	23	98	44	9	28	43	3	65
A2	34	87	27	21	78	17	1,123	44
A3	21	54	33	554	45	234	34	68
A4	23	333	46	312	345	22	2	88
A5	56	125	44	455	223	3,354	3	955
A6	54	86	87	321	334	23	4	43
A7	45	36	62	335	264	444	54	234
A8	126	432	145	405	22	707	335	77

The table above is a cipher matrix (Matrix A) used as part of covert operations to communicate commercial information back to Blenheim Park. In the event of being compromised operatives can convert the information in the above matrix by multiplying all values by 20 to produce Matrix B or dividing all values by 15 to produce Matrix C.

9. **Calculate the following: (B1, A6) × (B3, A1) + B8, A8**
   A 4,324
   B 2,354
   C 2,345
   D 2,543
   E 2,453

10. **Calculate the following (B4, A4 × B6, A4) ÷ (B5, A1 + B3, A2) (to 3 significant figures)**
   A 116
   B 120
   C 124
   D 125
   E 124.8

11. What is the ratio of (B2, A8) to (B3, A7) to the nearest whole number?

A 1:6
B 5:1
C 6.96:1
D 1:7
E 7:1

12. What is the mean average of the B1 column (to 1 decimal place)?

A 47.75
B 48
C 47
D 47.8
E 480

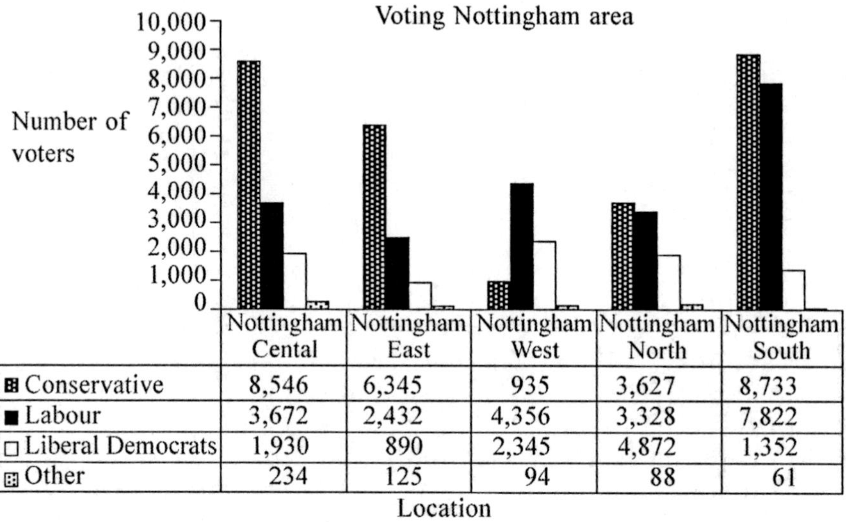

	Nottingham Cental	Nottingham East	Nottingham West	Nottingham North	Nottingham South
Conservative	8,546	6,345	935	3,627	8,733
Labour	3,672	2,432	4,356	3,328	7,822
Liberal Democrats	1,930	890	2,345	4,872	1,352
Other	234	125	94	88	61

Location

The data above show the voter turnout for various areas in Nottingham. The voter turnout was 43% in Nottingham Central, 37% in Nottingham East, 49% in Nottingham West, 61% in Nottingham North and 32% in Nottingham South.

13. What percentage of the vote did Labour win in Nottingham West (to 2 decimal places)?

A 56%
B 1:2
C 56.35%
D 53.65%
E 56.4%

14. **What is the total population of Nottingham East and Nottingham South combined?**
   A 92,340
   B 84,543
   C 82,615
   D 53,546
   E 79,345

15. **What was the total number of Conservative and Labour voters in all five areas?**
   A 52,327
   B 49,796
   C 56,345
   D 48,796
   E 67,345

16. **Who won the vote in Nottingham West?**
   A Conservative
   B Labour
   C Liberal Democrats
   D Other
   E Tied

Height of garage door (metres)	5–5.9	6–6.9	7–7.9	8–8.9	9–9.9
Number of garage doors	4	12	16	24	36

17. **How many garage doors are ≤ 6.9 metres?**
   A 15
   B. 4
   C 12
   D 18
   E 16

18. **Out of the total number of garage doors measured, how many are ≤ 7.9 metres? (Give your answer as the simplest fraction of the total number.)**
   A 32/92
   B 19/23
   C 23/72
   D 8/23
   E 4/23

THIS IS THE HALFWAY STAGE OF THIS SECTION. IDEALLY YOU SHOULD HAVE APPROXIMATELY 12 MINUTES LEFT. (Please note this prompt will not be given in your actual test.)

19. What is the ratio of garage doors which are 6–6.9 metres to those which are 8–8.9 metres?

A 12:36
B 36:12
C 1:2
D 6:2
E 12:24

20. If 5 garage doors are each 12.9 metres high, what is their total height in centimetres (cm)?

A 64.5 cm
B 645 cm
C 6,450 cm
D 6.450 cm
E 6,525 cm

	Calibre	Velocity	Range	Accuracy
Rifle A	0.38	500	100	3
Rifle B	0.45	435	150	4
Rifle C	0.576	650	300	6
Rifle D	0.762	900	500	7
Rifle E	0.9	760	300	4
Rifle F	1.5	567	600	2

The data provided in the table above relates to various rifles and their performance levels. The data provided includes Calibre (centimetres), Velocity (metres/second), Range (metres) and an Accuracy Rating out of ten (the lower the value the higher the accuracy).

21. What is the difference in size between the largest and second smallest calibre?

A 115 mm
B 1.15 cm
C 0.0000015 m
D 1.10 cm
E 1.05 cm

22. The overall effectiveness of a rifle can be calculated using the following formula where the higher the score the better:

Calibre × Velocity × Range × Accuracy = Effectiveness Quotient

What is the difference in Effectiveness Quotient between Rifle F and Rifle B (to 4 significant figures)?

A 903,200
B 903,150
C 903,100
D 90,320
E 93,251

23. What is the mean average velocity of the six rifles (to the nearest whole number)?

A 635 m/s
B 653 m/s
C 365 m/s
D 83 m/s
E 540 m/s

24. Which rifle is the most accurate?

A Rifle B
B Rifle C
C Rifle D
D Rifle E
E Rifle F

Here are two equations. Ian needs help solving them:

C = 4B + 2D (equation 1)

A = C – 4B (equation 2).

25. What is A with relation to D?

A B
B 2D
C D
D 1/2 D
E 4D

26. Make B the subject of equation 1.

A B = (A – 3D)/4
B D = (C – 4B)/2
C B = (C – 2D)/4
D B = 18
E B = (C – D)/2

27. If B = 1.25 and D = 3, what is the value of C?

A 10
B 12.25
C 12
D 8.5
E 11

28. If C = 8 and D = 2, what is the value of B?

A 3
B 5.3
C 1
D 2
E 4.5

Below is a pie chart showing the % market control held by four businesses. The value of the market grew from £15bn in 1990 to £23bn in 2010.

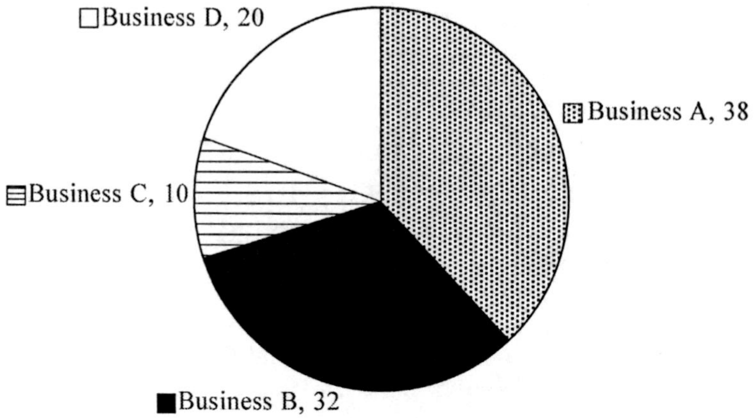

29. If Business A were bought out equally by Business C and D, what market percentage would Business D now have?

A 20%
B 51%
C 36%
D 39%
E 58%

30. If Business B were to go bankrupt and liquidate, and only the other three businesses remained, what would be the new market percentage controlled by Business A?

A 29.41%
B 14.71%
C 47.06%
D 55.88%
E 39.31%

31. What is the difference in the value of Business C from 1990 to 2010?

A £3.10bn
B £2.56bn
C £1.60bn
D £0.80bn
E £2.65bn

32. What is the increase in value of 1% of the market share from 1990 to 2010?

A £0.15bn
B £0.30bn
C £1.00bn
D £0.08bn
E £0.23bn

Below is a bar chart showing the yearly income from the different sectors of Bubble inc. The yearly costs of Bubble inc. are £100 million.

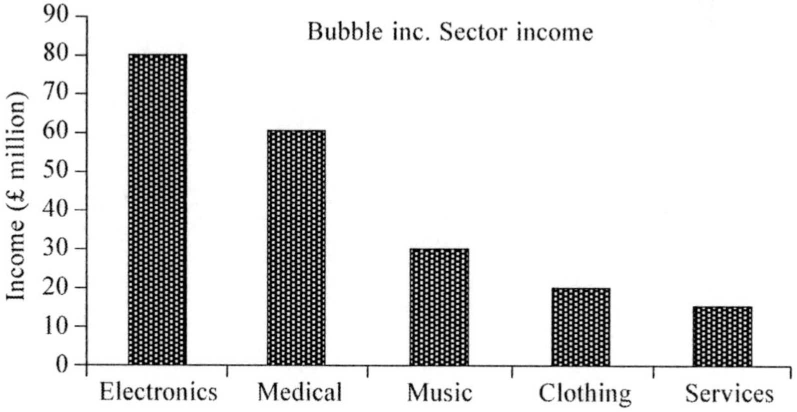

33. What percentage of Bubble inc. income comes from the Electronics sector (to the nearest whole number)?

A 62%
B 45%
C 80%
D 26%
E 39%

34. To expand the Medical sector it will cost £300 million. It will give the Medical sector a boost of 20% of yearly income. How long will it take for it to earn back its investment?

A 25 years
B 14 years
C 32 years
D 30 years
E 43 years

35. What are the total yearly profits of Bubble inc.?

A £108 million
B £85 million
C £90 million
D £105 million
E £95 million

36. The Services sector costs 125% of its income to run. What would be the total yearly profits of Bubble inc. if they were to shut down the Services sector?

A £105.00 million
B £108.75 million
C £123.50 million
D £133.25 million
E £ 98.75 million

Abstract Reasoning – 14 minutes

Question 1

Set A

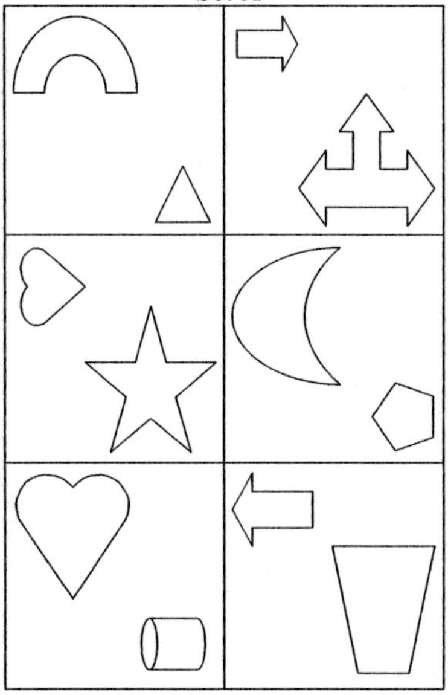

Set B

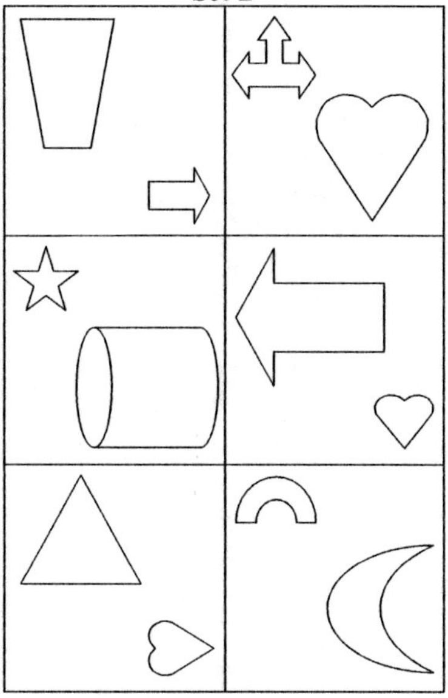

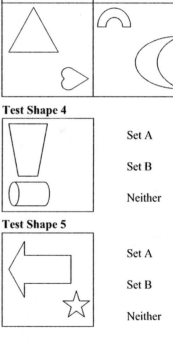

Test Shape 1

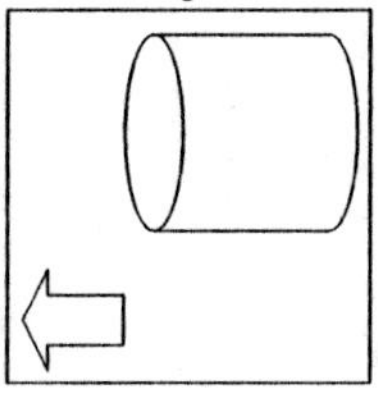

Set A

Set B

Neither

Test Shape 2

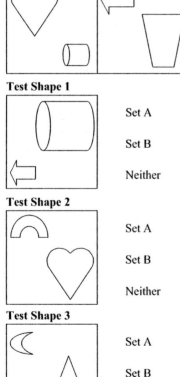

Set A

Set B

Neither

Test Shape 3

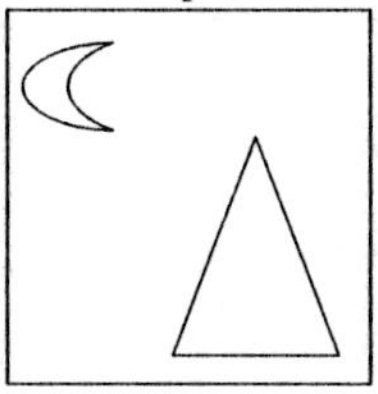

Set A

Set B

Neither

Test Shape 4

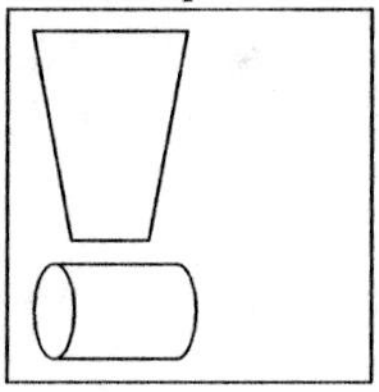

Set A

Set B

Neither

Test Shape 5

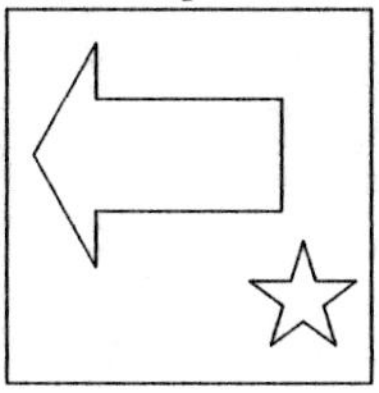

Set A

Set B

Neither

Question 2

Set A

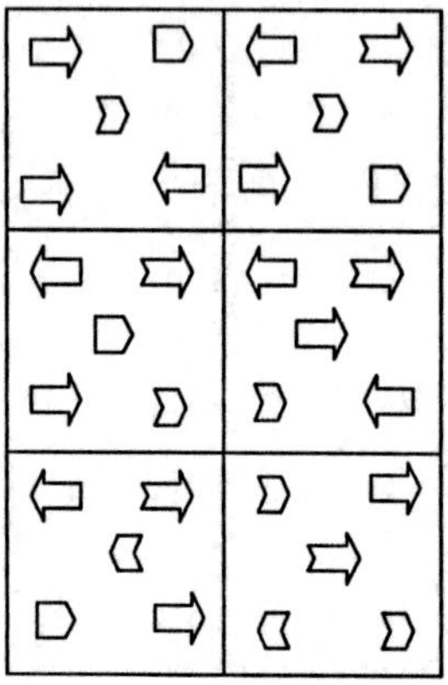

Set B

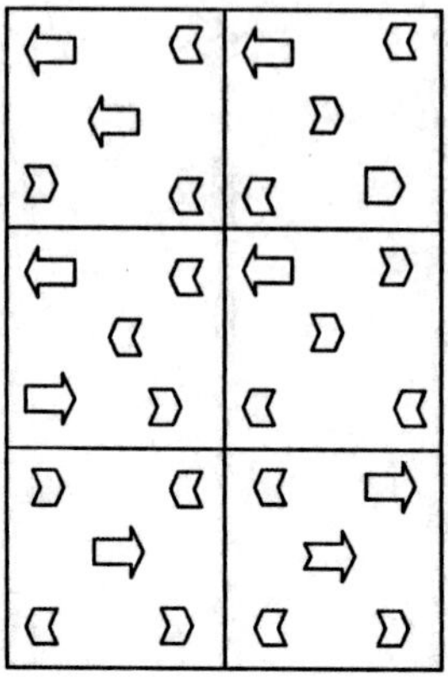

1. Which of the following belong to Set A?

A

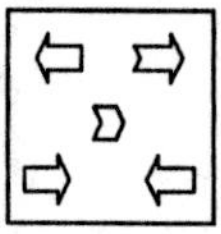

B

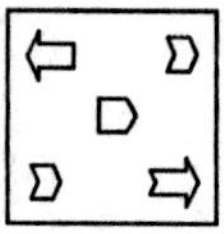

C

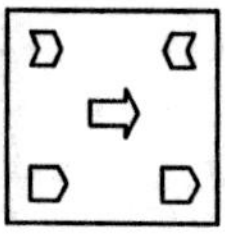

D

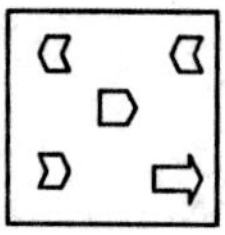

2. Which of the following belong to Set A?

A

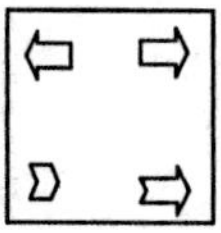

B

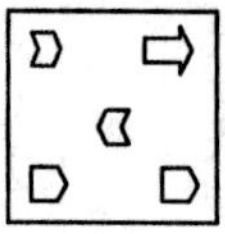

C

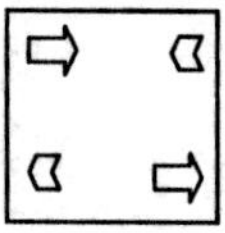

D

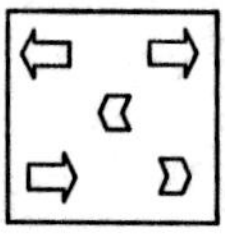

3. Which of the following belong to Set A?

A

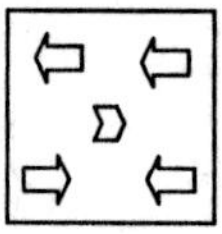

B

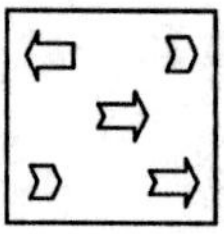

C

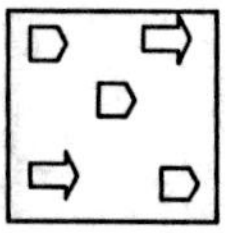

D

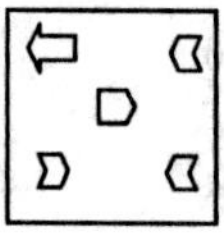

4. Which of the following belong to Set B?

A

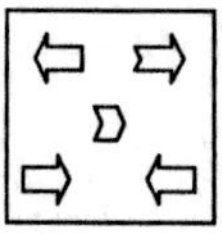

B

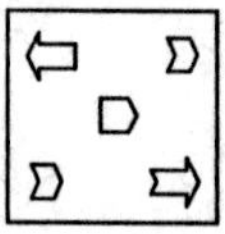

C

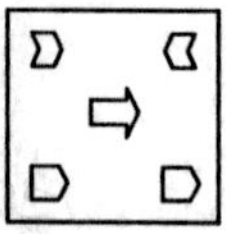

D

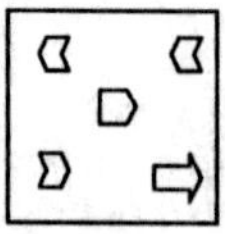

5. Which of the following belong to Set A?

A

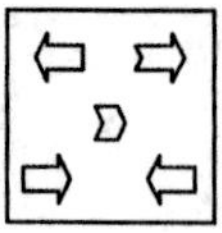

B

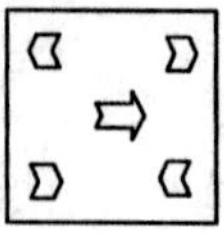

C

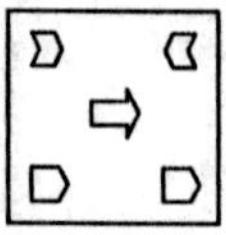

D

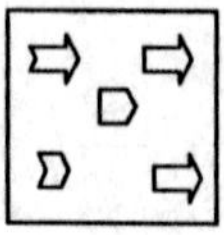

Question 3

Set A

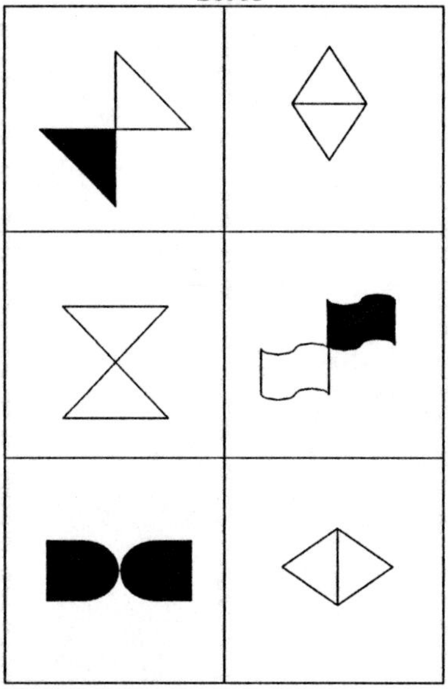

Set B

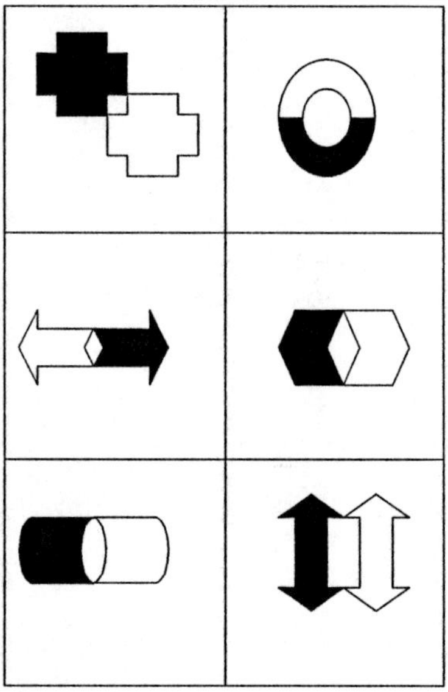

Test Shape 1

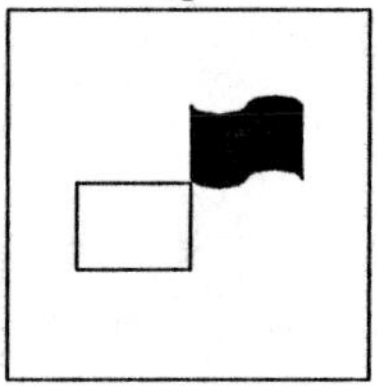

Set A

Set B

Neither

Test Shape 2

Set A

Set B

Neither

Test Shape 3

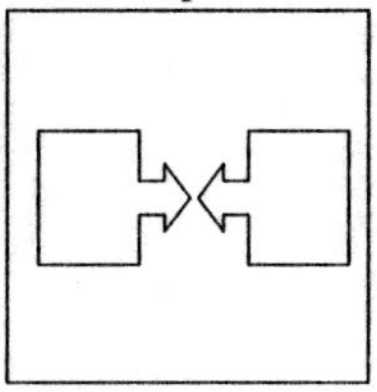

Set A

Set B

Neither

Test Shape 4

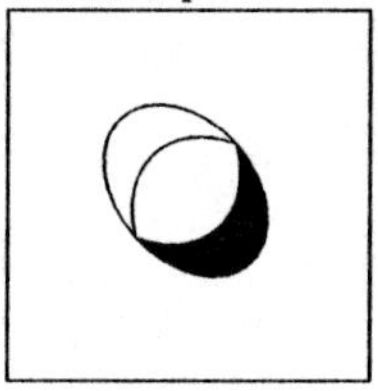

Set A

Set B

Neither

Test Shape 5

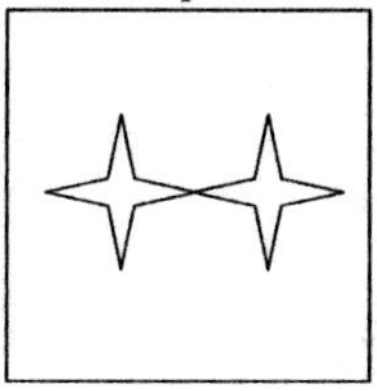

Set A

Set B

Neither

Question 4

Set A

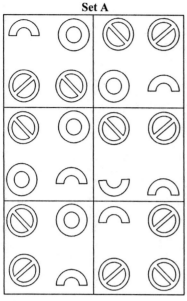

Set B

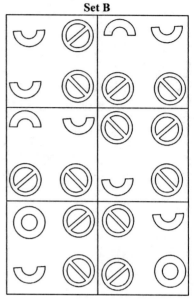

Test Shape 1

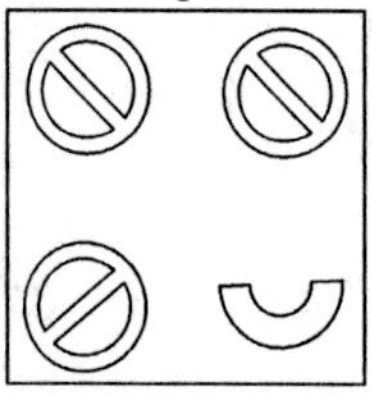

Set A

Set B

Neither

Test Shape 2

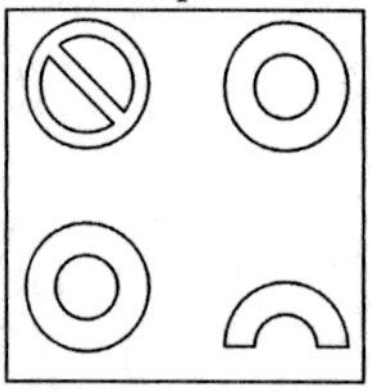

Set A

Set B

Neither

Test Shape 3

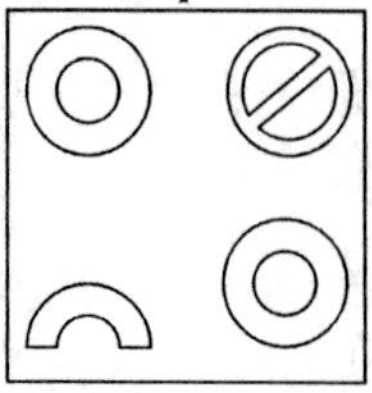

Set A

Set B

Neither

Test Shape 4

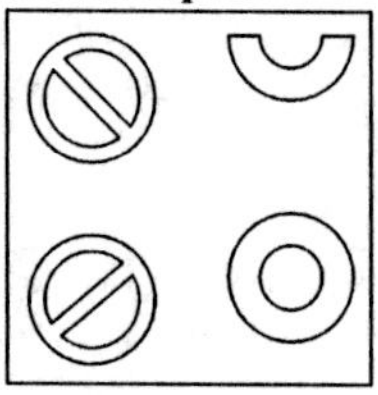

Set A

Set B

Neither

Test Shape 5

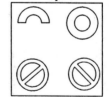

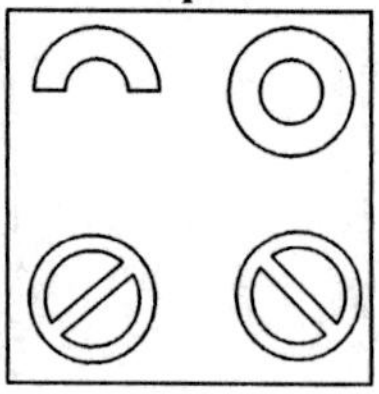

Set A

Set B

Neither

Question 5

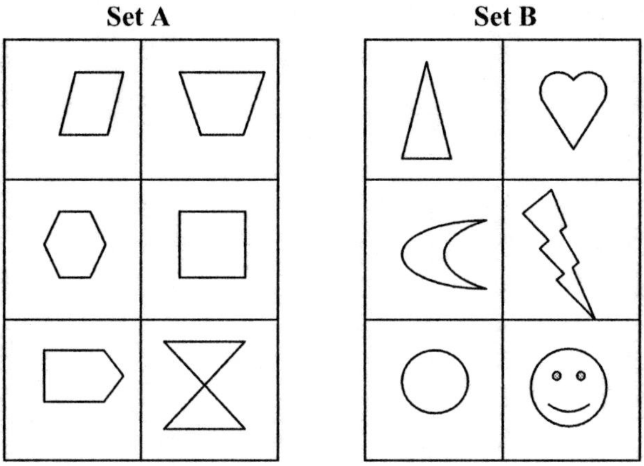

1. Which of the following belong to Set A?

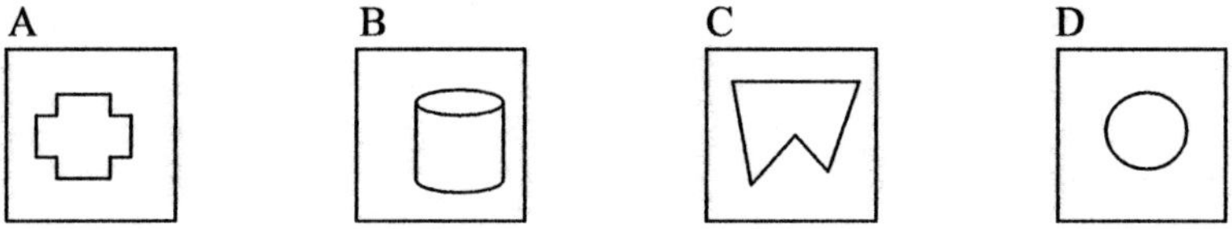

2. Which of the following belong to Set A?

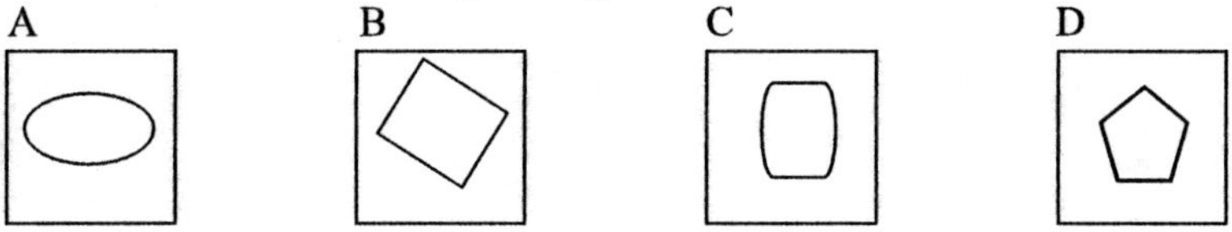

3. Which of the following belong to Set B?

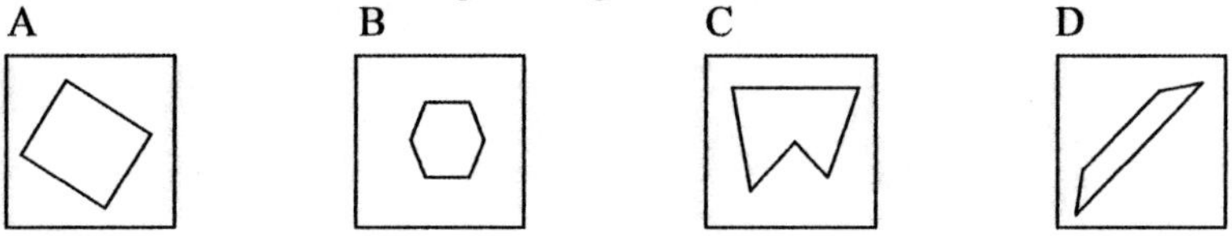

4. Which of the following belong to Set B?

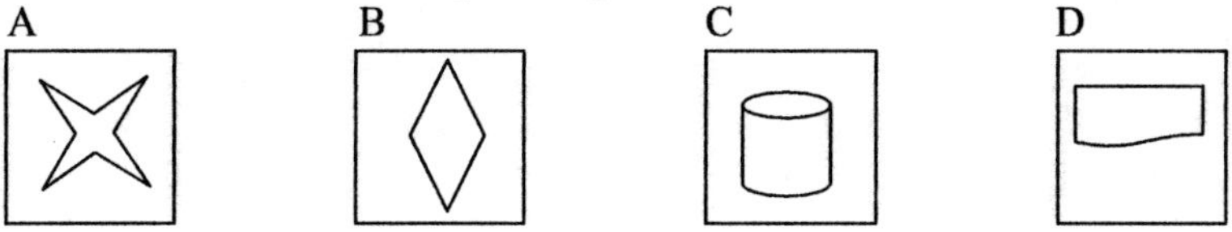

5. Which of the following belong to Set B?

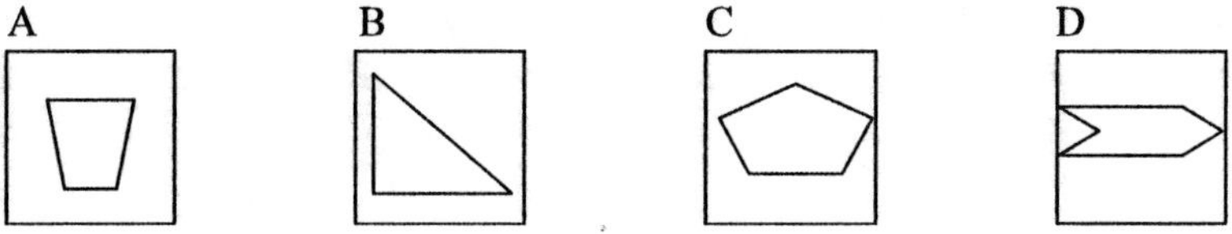

Question 6

Set A

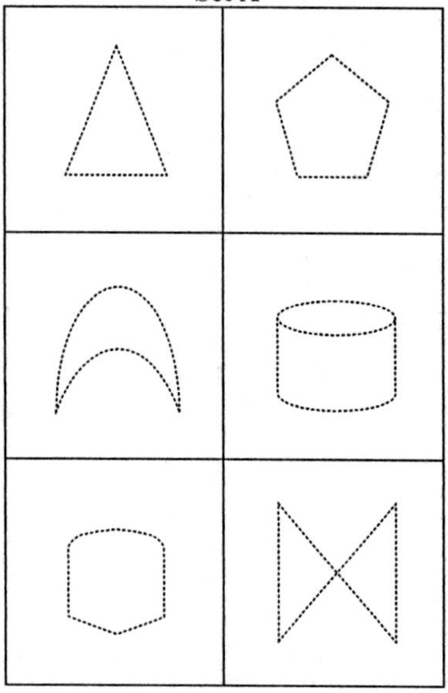

Set B

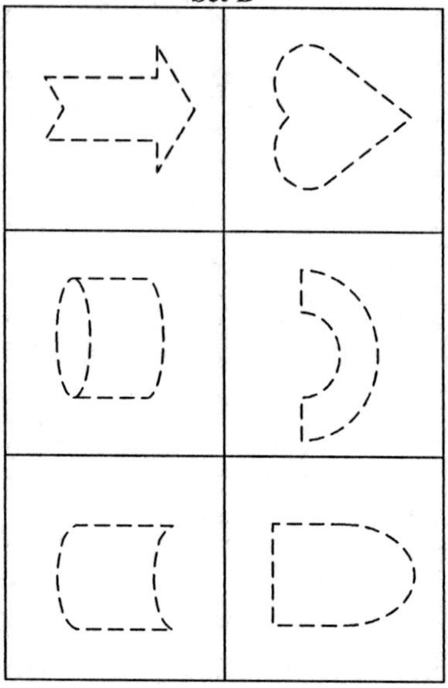

Test Shape 1

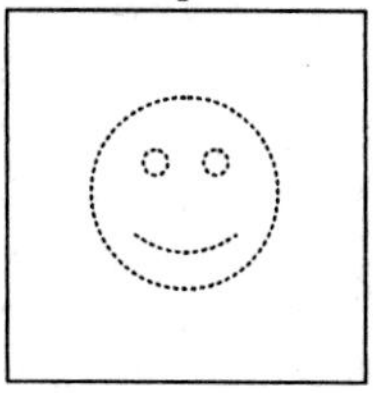

Set A

Set B

Neither

Test Shape 2

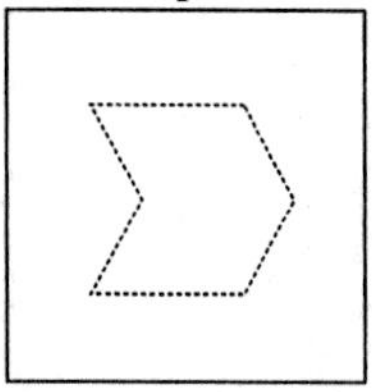

Set A

Set B

Neither

Test Shape 3

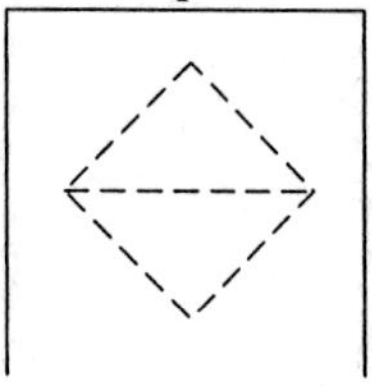

Set A

Set B

Neither

Test Shape 4

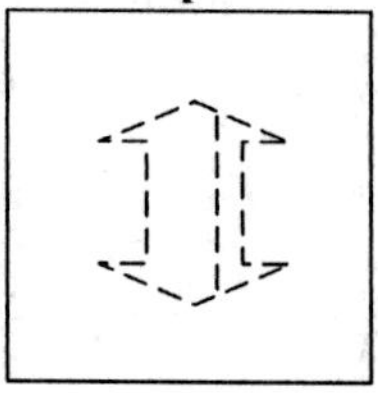

Set A

Set B

Neither

Test Shape 5

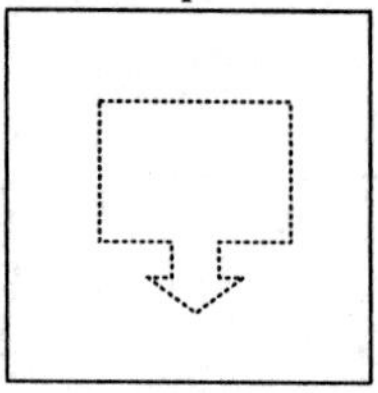

Set A

Set B

Neither

Question 7

Set A **Set B**

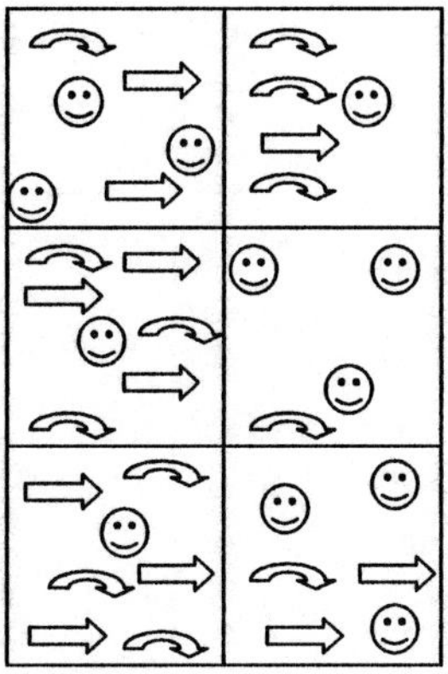

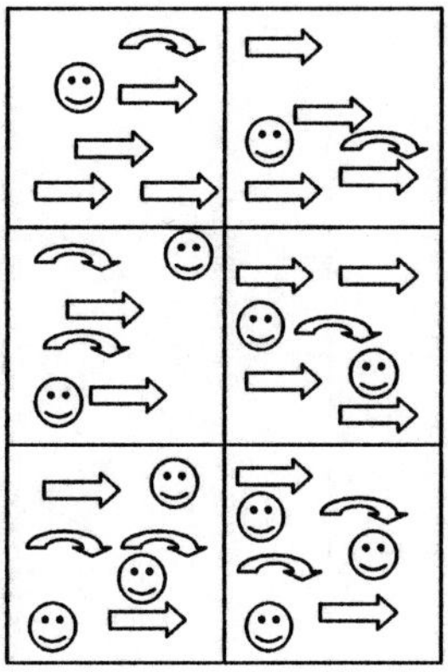

1. Which of the following belong to Set A?

A B C D

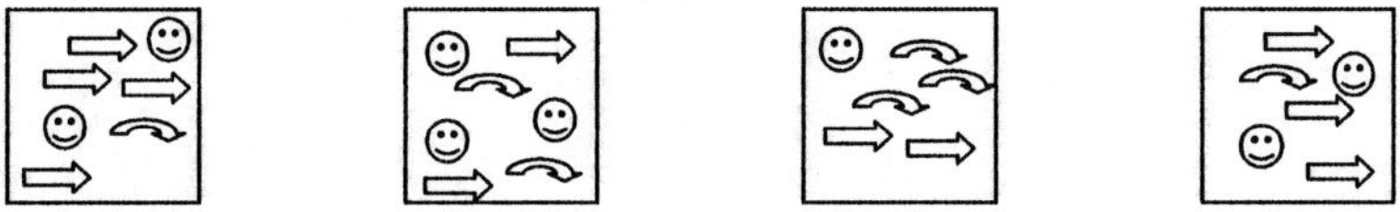

2. Which of the following belong to Set A?

A B C D

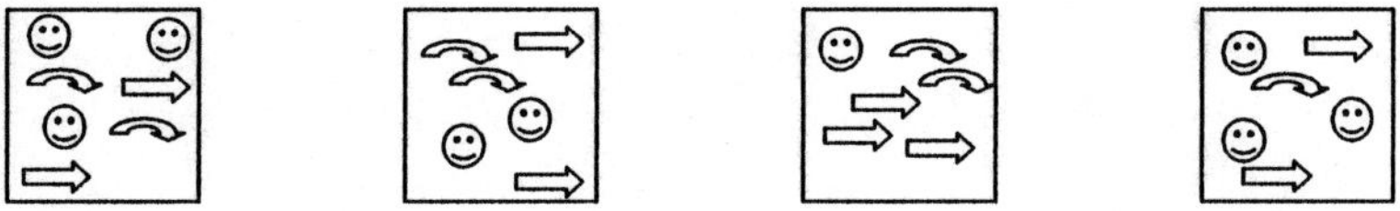

3. Which of the following belong to Set A?

A B C D

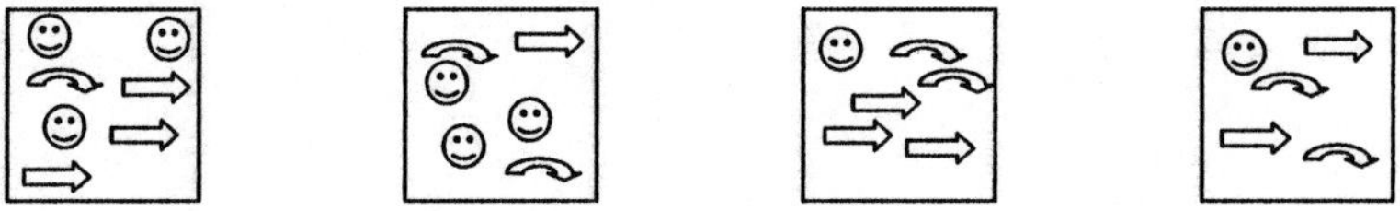

4. Which of the following belong to Set A?

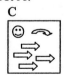

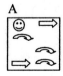

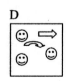

A B C D

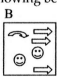

5. Which of the following belong to Set A?

A B C D

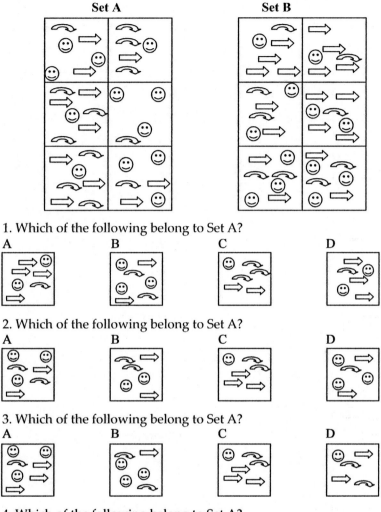

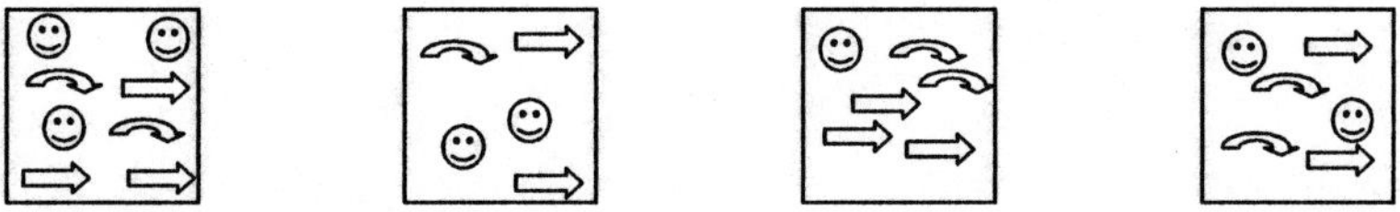

YOU ARE NOW OVER THE HALFWAY STAGE OF THIS SECTION. IDEALLY YOU SHOULD HAVE APPROXIMATELY 7 MINUTES LEFT. (Please note this prompt will not be given in your actual test.)

Question 8

Set A

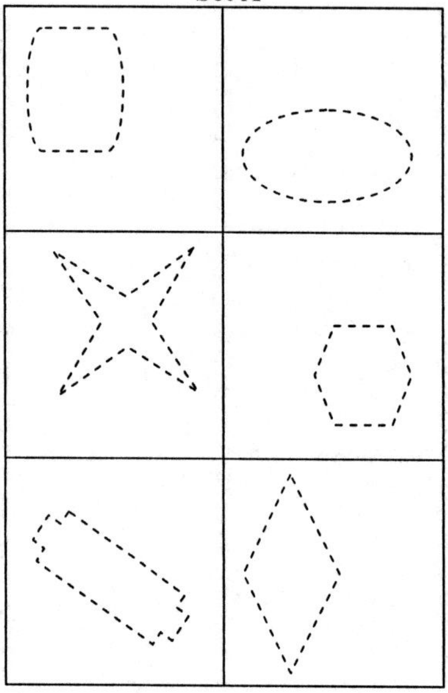

Set B

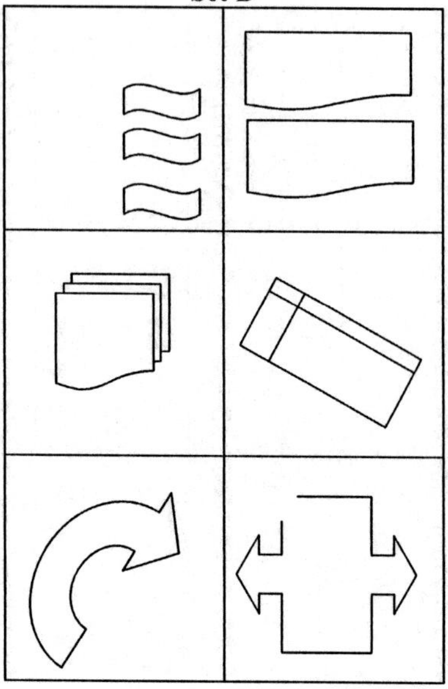

Test Shape 1

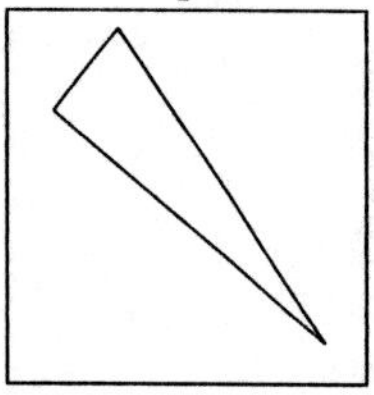

Set A

Set B

Neither

Test Shape 2

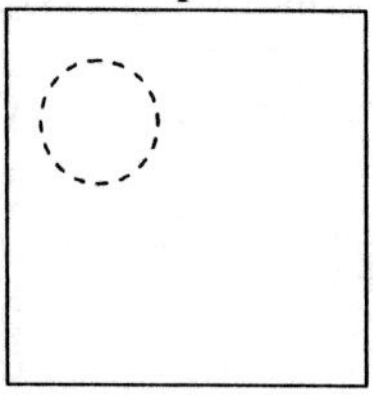

Set A

Set B

Neither

Test Shape 3

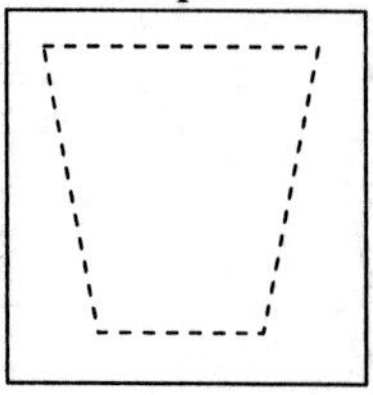

Set A

Set B

Neither

Test Shape 4

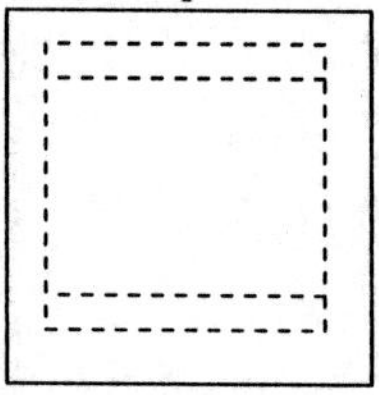

Set A

Set B

Neither

Test Shape 5

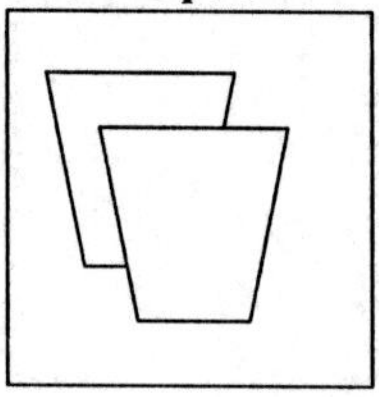

Set A

Set B

Neither

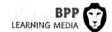

Question 9

Set A **Set B**

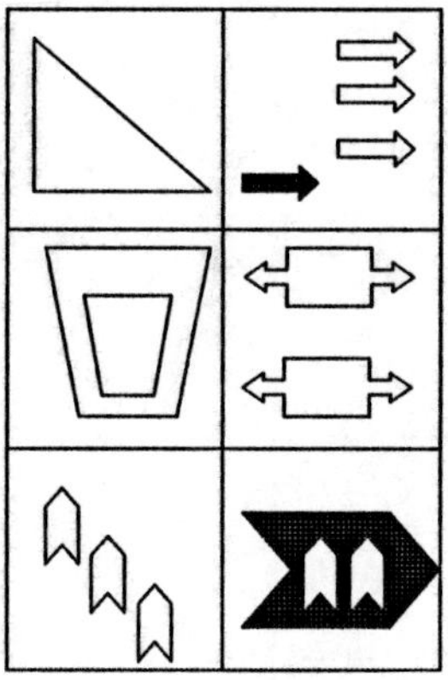

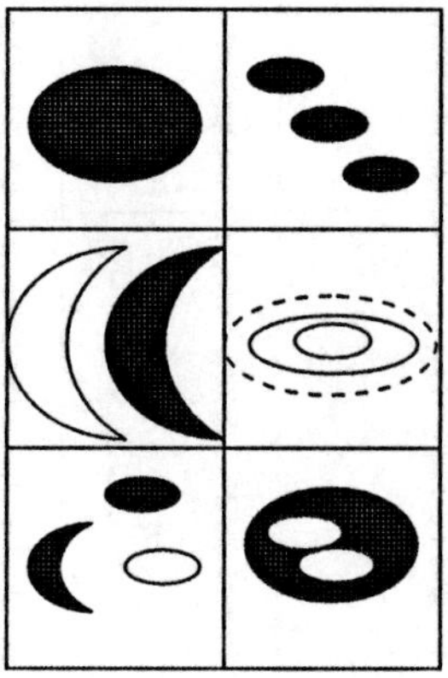

1. Which of the following belong to Set A?

A B C D

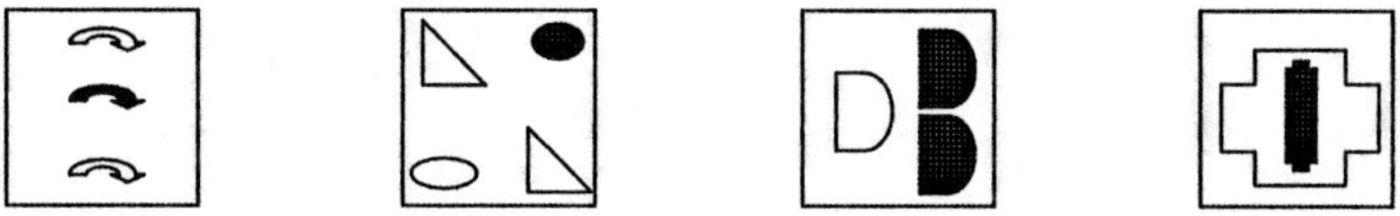

2. Which of the following belong to Set A?

A B C D

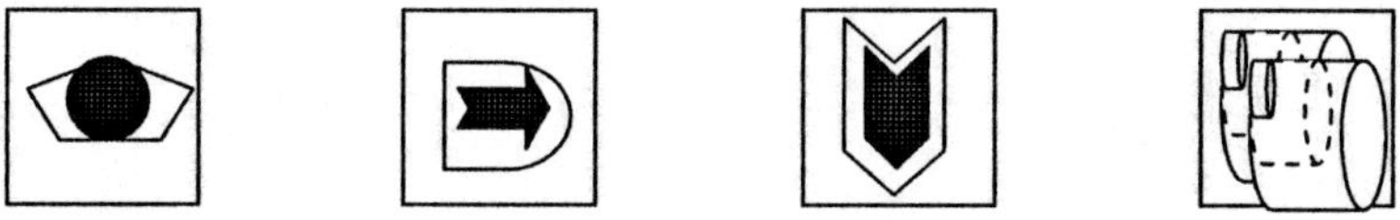

3. Which of the following belong to Set B?

A B C D

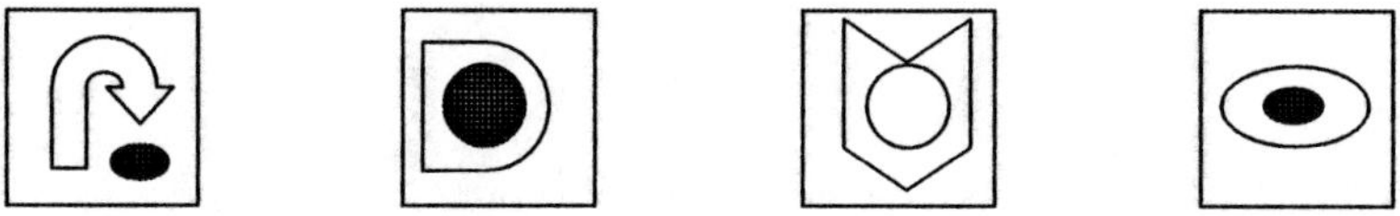

4. Which of the following belong to Set B?

A B C D

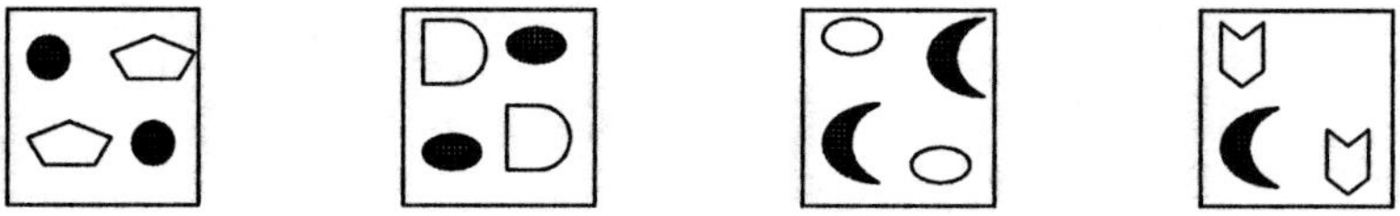

5. Which of the following belong to Set B?

A B C D

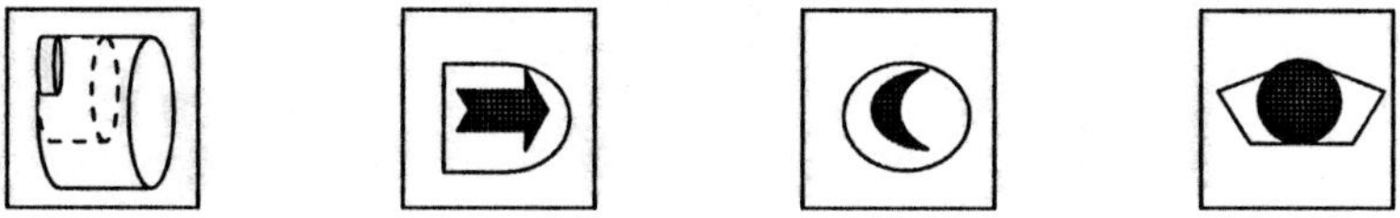

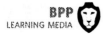

Question 10

Set A

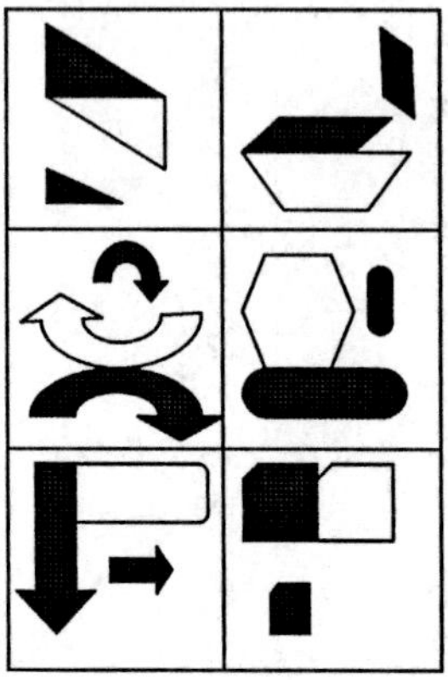

Set B

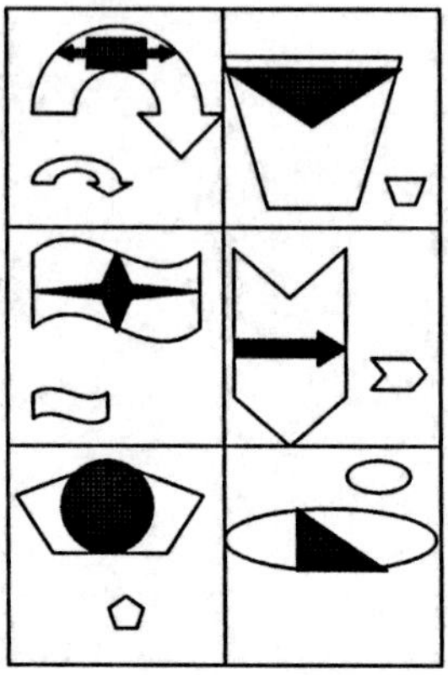

1. Which of the following belong to Set A?

A
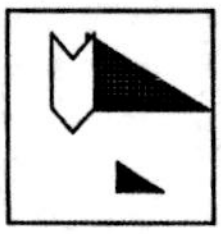

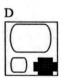

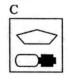

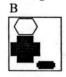

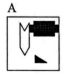

B
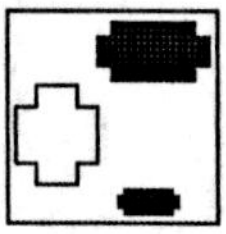

C

D
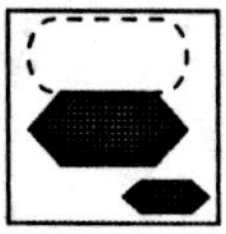

2. Which of the following belong to Set A?

A
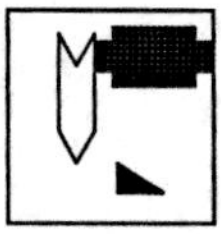

B

C
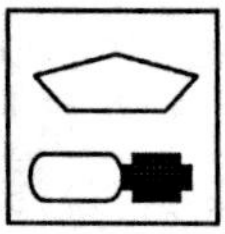

D
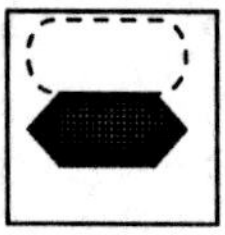

3. Which of the following belong to Set B?

A
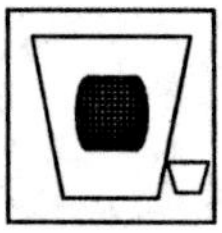

B
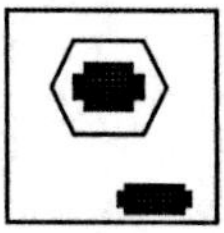

C
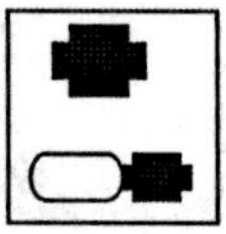

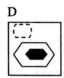

D

4. Which of the following belong to Set B?

A

B
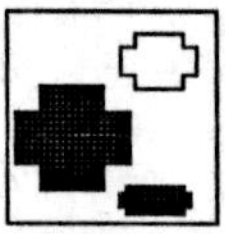

C
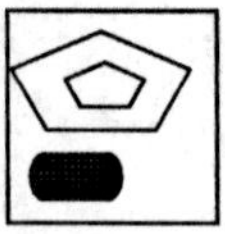

D
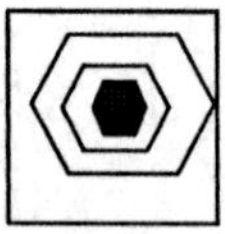

5. Which of the following belong to Set B?

A

B
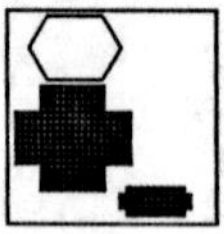

C

D

Question 11

Set A

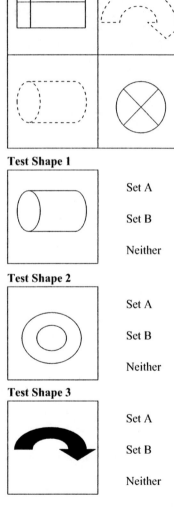

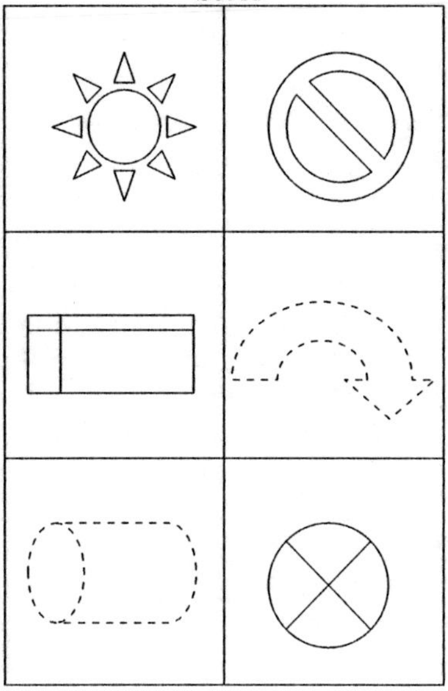

Set B

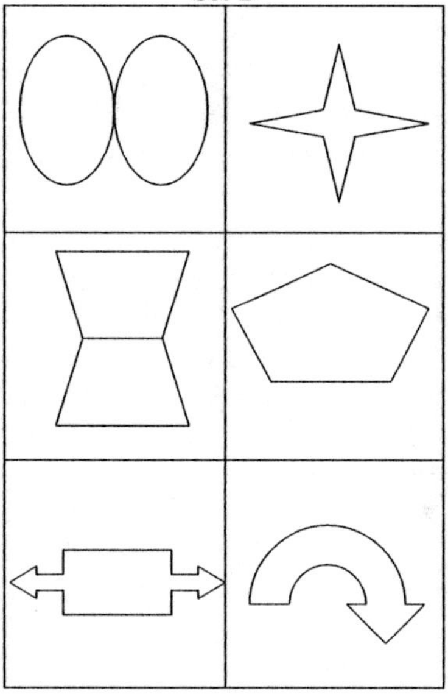

Test Shape 1

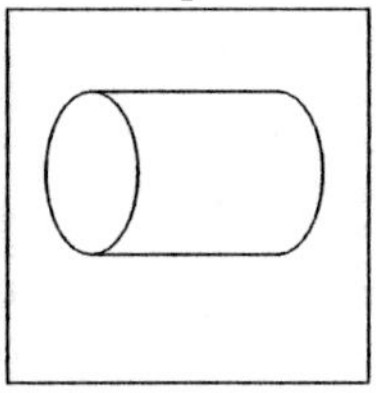

Set A

Set B

Neither

Test Shape 2

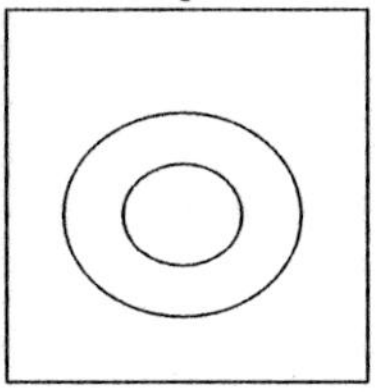

Set A

Set B

Neither

Test Shape 3

Set A

Set B

Neither

Test Shape 4

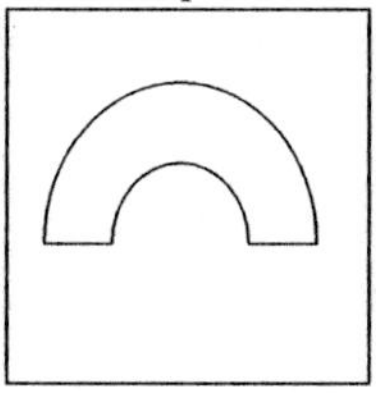

Set A

Set B

Neither

Test Shape 5

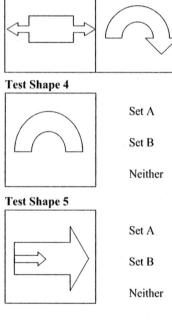

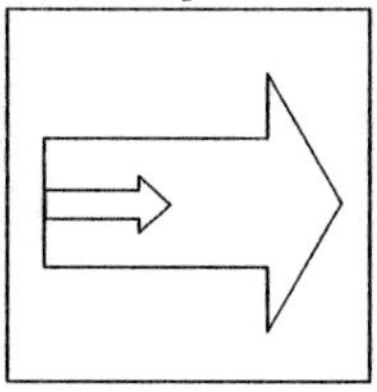

Set A

Set B

Neither

Decision Analysis – 32 minutes

Scenario

A group of linguists have developed a new language based upon a finite number of coded words, some of which are shown below. Your task is to examine particular codes or sentences and then choose the best interpretation of the code from one of five possible choices.

You will find that, at times, the information you have is either incomplete or does not make sense. You will then need to make your best judgement based on the codes rather than what you expect to see or what you think is reasonable. There will always be a best answer which makes the most sense based on all the information presented. It is important that you understand that this test is based on judgements rather than simply applying rules and logic.

Operating codes	Basic codes
1 = antonym	A = ocean
2 = decrease	B = intelligent
3 = closed	C = wind
4 = singular	D = sky
5 = negative	E = planet
6 = future	F = star
7 = drive	G = today
8 = present	H = tomorrow
9 = ascend	I = people
10 = walk	J = men
11 = conditional	K = adventure
12 = attribute	L = build
13 = plural	M = defeat
	N = sword
	O = building
	P = land
	Q = plant
	R = danger
	S = animals
	T = warm

Question 1

Examine the following coded message: **12(O, I), 3, H**

Now examine the following sentences and try to determine the most likely interpretation of the code.

A Tomorrow the office will be closed.
B The building will be closed to people tomorrow.
C The shops will be closed tomorrow.
D The school will be closed today.
E The office was closed.

Question 2

Examine the following coded message: **S, 10, P, (T, D), 8**

Now examine the following sentences and try to determine the most likely interpretation of the code.

A The hot animals were walking over great distances.
B The sun was too hot and the animals had to rest.
C The sun bathed the animals as they walked.
D The sun had been too hot for the animals to move.
E The camels are walking through the desert under the sun.

Question 3

Examine the following coded message: **G, (J, 4), 12(10), E, K**

Now examine the following sentences and try to determine the most likely interpretation of the code.

A Today the men set off on a great adventure.
B The man had set off on his planetary voyage.
C The spaceman had landed on a new planet.
D Man has discovered the planet over many adventures.
E Today he sets off on a world adventure.

Question 4

Examine the following coded message: **F(1, 4), 9, D, (1, G)**

Now examine the following sentences and try to determine the most likely interpretation of the code.

A There were many stars in the sky today.
B There are many stars in the sky tonight.
C The stars are high in the sky tonight.
D The North Star is high in the sky tonight.
E There is just one star in the sky tonight.

Question 5

Examine the following coded message: **I, 7, 12(O, S), 11, H, T**

Now examine the following sentences and try to determine the most likely interpretation of the code.

A The children will be driven to the zoo tomorrow providing the weather is warm.
B The animal sanctuary was only reachable by car, which was difficult in warm weather.
C The people had driven to the animal sanctuary but it was closed due to warm weather.
D The animals come out of their cages only if the weather is warm.
E The animal safari was planned for tomorrow providing the weather was warm.

Question 6

Examine the following coded message: **13(D, O), L, 9(1, 2), 6**

Now examine the following sentences and try to determine the most likely interpretation of the code.

A The soon to be built skyscraper will be much taller than any other.
B The skyscrapers of today are much taller than their predecessors.
C The skyscrapers will be built to accommodate more workers.
D The skyscrapers of the future will be built much taller.
E The skyscrapers were built to accommodate a larger future population.

Question 7

Examine the following coded message: **L(13, O), 12(B, I, 13), 6**

Now examine the following sentences and try to determine the most likely interpretation of the code.

A New universities will be built for the many students.
B The engineers were planning an exciting new city project.
C The new laboratory would be equipped with all the latest technology.
D Homes, offices and shops will be built in the new city.
E The academics of yesterday would attend university.

Question 8

Examine the following coded message: **(12, K), J, 12(N), (R, S), (1, 6)**

Now examine the following sentences and try to determine the most likely interpretation of the code.

A The expedition saw the men fight lions, tigers and bears.
B The adventure was fraught with dangerous battles.
C The challenge will see the adventurers battle difficult terrain and dangerous animals.
D The men had set off on their voyage only to be killed by dangerous seas.
E The discovery of skeletons suggested a large battle had occurred here.

Question 9

Examine the following coded message: **I, 9 (12, P), 11, (C, T), F, H**

Now examine the following sentences and try to determine the most likely interpretation of the code.

A The people are walking up the mountain in the beautiful weather.
B If the party could climb the mountain tomorrow they would witness the shooting stars.
C The group would arrive at the mountain summit tomorrow but only if the rain improved.
D The mountain ascent had been made easier by the calm winds and bright weather.
E Tomorrow the group will climb the mountain, providing the weather is calm and sunny.

Question 10

Examine the following coded message: **(13, Q), (1, R), (12, O), C(1, T), 6**

Now examine the following sentences and try to determine the most likely interpretation of the code.

A The plants will grow better this winter, as they will be placed indoors for shelter.
B The plants had been destroyed by cold winds this winter.
C Plants grow better indoors as they are protected from cold winds and bad weather.
D The greenhouse will protect the plants from the cold wind this winter.
E Next winter will destroy the plants as the perishing winds are too destructive.

Question 11

Examine the following coded message: **I, (1, G), (R, S), 5, 10, (1, 3), 8**
Now examine the following sentences and try to determine the most likely interpretation of the code.

A The tribe do not walk in the open at night for fear of predators.
B Today the tourists will not see the tigers because the zoo is closed.
C Only on the night safari can the tourists see the tigers and lions.
D Snakes are nocturnal creatures that slither along the open desert.
E The natives had hunted only at night because it was too dangerous to do so in the daylight.

Question 12

Examine the following coded message: **12(C, A), R, I, 12(13, O), (1, 6)**

Now examine the following sentences and try to determine the most likely interpretation of the code.

A The weather forecast predicts dangerous waves, and surfers should stay in their homes today.
B The ocean breeze was cooling and people did not stay indoors last weekend.
C The strong ocean currents were very dangerous and bathing had been forbidden.
D The ocean waves were very dangerous and people stayed within their homes.
E The beach was very windy but the sea was surprisingly calm.

Question 13

Examine the following coded message: **8, J, (1, J), 7, 12(O, 13), 10(1, 6)**

Now examine the following sentences and try to determine the **two most likely** interpretations of the code.

A These days men teach their sons to drive.
B Nowadays men and women drive to work whereas in the past they walked.
C In the past people tended to walk, however, today they drive.
D Men and women drive to the cities but walk in the countryside.
E Men and women have long driven to work but the congestion is forcing people to walk.

Scenario

The group of linguists have discovered another set of 'specialist' codes.

Operating codes	Basic codes	Specialist codes
1 = antonym	A = ocean	☹ = possess
2 = decrease	B = intelligent	✋ = unwell
3 = closed	C = wind	♌ = dream
4 = singular	D = sky	💣 = young
5 = negative	E = planet	✂ = anxious
6 = future	F = star	✈ = conquer
7 = drive	G = today	✡ = brave
8 = present	H = tomorrow	⌛ = test
9 = ascend	I = people	
10 = walk	J = men	
11 = conditional	K = adventure	
12 = attribute	L = build	
13 = plural	M = defeat	
	N = sword	
	O = building	
	P = land	
	Q = plant	
	R = danger	
	S = animals	
	T = warm	

Question 14

Examine the following coded message: **(💣, I, 4), ✂, (10, ⌛), 8**

Now examine the following sentences and try to determine the most likely interpretation of the code.

A The children are nervous about their exam.
B Yesterday's exam had left the young boy anxious.
C The teenager was scared about tomorrow's walking challenge.
D The toddler is nervous about attempting his first steps.
E The boy is whistling nervously.

YOU ARE NOW AT THE HALFWAY STAGE OF THIS SECTION. IDEALLY YOU SHOULD HAVE AROUND 14.5 MINUTES LEFT. (Please note that this prompt will not be given in your actual test.)

Question 15

Examine the following coded message: **💣(I, 4), ♌, K(E, F), 8**

Now examine the following sentences and try to determine the most likely interpretation of the code.

A The child is dreaming of adventures in fairytale lands.
B The girl is dreaming of being an astronaut.
C As a child you dream.
D Space adventure is every man's dream.
E The boy had once dreamed of growing up to be a space explorer.

Question 16

Examine the following coded message: **J, ☹, A, (T, G), ✋, (1, 6)**

Now examine the following sentences and try to determine the most likely interpretation of the code.

A They are drinking in the ocean as the weather is warm.
B The man had not meant to drink seawater and is feeling unwell.
C The weather was stifling yesterday and had given the men sunstroke.
D The ocean water is not for drinking as it can make you ill.
E The warm weather had made them drink seawater, which had made them ill.

Question 17

Examine the following coded message: **(I, 4), ✂, 7, ⌛, 5(C), H**

Now examine the following sentences and try to determine the most likely interpretation of the code.

A She was worried bad weather would make the journey difficult tomorrow.
B His driving test was cancelled because of bad weather.
C The lack of wind made flying his kite difficult.
D The side winds made him nervous about driving.
E Tomorrow's strong wind would make driving difficult and they were very nervous.

Question 18

Examine the following coded message: **(✡, J), ✈, (O, 13), P, ☹, (1, 8)**

Now examine the following sentences and try to determine the **two most likely** interpretations of the code.

A The soldiers were captured and their city destroyed.
B The army had been beaten in a huge battle.
C The city stronghold had been taken and its people killed.
D The warriors had conquered the city and ruled its land.
E The army are leaving their city to conquer new lands.

Question 19

Examine the following coded message: **💣(4, J), (1, ✡), (1, ✈), (1, 6)**

Now examine the following sentences and try to determine the most likely interpretation of the code.

A The cowardly warriors were easily defeated.
B The brave gladiator has never been defeated.
C The man has been both a coward and a loser.
D The young man was not strong enough to win this battle.
E The cowardly young man was captured.

Question 20

Examine the following coded message: **11, H, T(1, 2), (💣, I), A, (1, ✂)**

Now examine the following sentences and try to determine the most likely interpretation of the code.

A The youngsters are anxious that if it is not warmer tomorrow, they will not visit the ocean.
B Tomorrow's warm weather means the beach will be busy with children.
C If tomorrow is warmer, the relaxed teenagers will go to the seaside.
D The children would visit the ocean only if the weather improved.
E If the weather is warmer tomorrow, the children will go surfing in the ocean.

Question 21

Examine the following sentence: **'The land of the rising sun'**.

Now examine the following codes and try to determine the most likely interpretation of the sentence.

A (9, F), P
B (9, F), D, P
C 9, P
D 9, F, P, T
E (9, F)

Question 22

Examine the following sentence: **'The shops were closed due to bad weather'**.

Now examine the following codes and try to determine the most likely interpretation of the sentence.

A 3, (12, C), I(13, O), 6
B 13, O, I, 3, C, 1, 6
C I(13, O), 3, (1, 6), (12, C), ✡
D 3, 12, C, (1, 6), I(13, O)
E I(13, O), 3, (12, C), (1, 6)

Question 23

Examine the following sentence: **'The children are playing with the animals in the garden'**.

Now examine the following codes and try to determine the most likely interpretation of the sentence.

A 12(💣, I), 12(Q, P), S
B 12(💣, I), S, K, 12(Q, P), 8
C 12(💣, I), 12(Q, P), 8
D 12(💣, I), S, 12(Q, P), 8
E 12, 💣, I, S, 12, Q, P, 8

Question 24

Examine the following sentence: **'The old man is dreaming of an old adventure'**.

Now examine the following codes and try to determine the most likely interpretation of the sentence.

A (1, 💣), (J, 4), ♌, (K, 13), (1, 8), 8
B (1, 💣), (J, 4), ♌, K(1, 💣), 8
C ♌, K(1, 8), 8, (J, 4)
D (1, 💣), (J, 4), ♌, K(1, 8), 6
E 💣, (J, 4), (1,♌), K(1, 8), 8

Question 25

Examine the following sentence: **'The architects are constructing a new hospital'**.

Now examine the following codes and try to determine the most likely interpretation of the sentence.

A (B, J), O, (I, ✋, O), 8
B (✋, J), O, 6(I, ✋, O)
C (B, J), O, P, 6(I, ✋, O), 8
D (O, B, J), O, 6(I, ✋, O), 8
E (B, J), O, 6, I, ✋, O, 8

Question 26

Examine the following sentence: **'The hurricane had destroyed the city and countryside'.**

Now examine the following codes and try to determine the most likely interpretation of the sentence.

A (A, C, E), (1, L), (O, 13), 8
B (A, C, E), (1, L), (O, 13), (O, 13), P, (1, 8)
C (A, C, E), (O, 13), (1, ✈), P, (1, 8)
D (1, L), A, C, E, (O, 13), P, (1, 8)
E (A, C, E), (1, L), (O, 13), P, (1, 8)

Question 27

Examine the following coded message: Y B (4,I) Q H E

Now examine the following sentences and try to determine the most likely interpretations of the code.

A Victory for the brave man will happen later today
B The battle will be won tomorrow to conquer the planet
C The future of the town rests on the shoulders of a brave man
D An intelligent and brave individual will conquer the planet in the future
E A brave and smart person will conquer the village today

Question 28

Examine the following coded message: A, I, 2, E, R, Q

Now examine the following sentences and try to determine the most likely interpretations of the code.

A Rainfall has caused disease in the ocean but it is increasing in size
B Rainforests are decreasing due to illness in the water
C The ocean is increasing due to the growth of the plants across the earth
D The land mass is reducing due to illness in the plantlife across the globe
E The sea is decreasing due to illness and placing plantlife in danger across the globe

Situational Judgement Test – 27 Minutes

Scenario 1

A dental student called Alliaya is leading a fellow group of students on a research project into how modern lifestyles impact on public health, especially with regards to dentistry. Whilst working on the project it becomes apparent that another member of the group is falsifying data in relation to interviewing members of the public.

How **appropriate** is each of the following responses by **Alliaya** in this situation:

1. **Challenge the member of the group stating that it is unethical to falsify research data.**
   A. A very appropriate thing to do
   B. Appropriate but not ideal
   C. Inappropriate but not awful
   D. A very inappropriate thing to do

2. **Canvas the opinion of the other members of the group as to what should be done.**
   A. A very appropriate thing to do
   B. Appropriate but not ideal
   C. Inappropriate but not awful
   D. A very inappropriate thing to do

3. **Immediately post a message on the individual's Facebook page challenging them as to why they are falsifying data.**
   A. A very appropriate thing to do
   B. Appropriate but not ideal
   C. Inappropriate but not awful
   D. A very inappropriate thing to do

4. **Omit the falsified data and say nothing.**
   A. A very appropriate thing to do
   B. Appropriate but not ideal
   C. Inappropriate but not awful
   D. A very inappropriate thing to do

Scenario 2

A medical student, Alfred, is half way through his placement on a geriatric ward and feels that one of his fellow medical students is not really pulling their weight which is impacting on Alfred's performance and effecting the standard of care being provided.

How **appropriate** is each of the following responses by **Alfred** in this situation:

1. **Do nothing as there is only a week to go before the placement finishes.**
   A. A very appropriate thing to do
   B. Appropriate but not ideal
   C. Inappropriate but not awful
   D. A very inappropriate thing to do

2. **Ring the Human Resources department and ask to discuss the medical student's performance with someone.**
   A. A very appropriate thing to do
   B. Appropriate but not ideal
   C. Inappropriate but not awful
   D. A very inappropriate thing to do

3. **Confront the medical student in an angry manner and ask to speak to them in private to tell them how cross they are regarding their performance.**
   A. A very appropriate thing to do
   B. Appropriate but not ideal
   C. Inappropriate but not awful
   D. A very inappropriate thing to do

4. **Speak to the medical student in private in an empathetic manner regarding their performance and advise them that they think it wise that they discuss the problems they are having with the supervising Registrar.**
   A. A very appropriate thing to do
   B. Appropriate but not ideal
   C. Inappropriate but not awful
   D. A very inappropriate thing to do

5. **Confide in the supervising Registrar at the earliest opportunity.**
   A. A very appropriate thing to do
   B. Appropriate but not ideal
   C. Inappropriate but not awful
   D. A very inappropriate thing to do

Scenario 3

Zebedee, a second year dental student, is at a party attended by a large number of students from his class. Whilst at the party he sees another of his fellow students appearing to prepare a cannabis cigarette and proceed to smoke it.

How **appropriate** is each of the following responses by **Zebedee** in this situation:

1. **To leave the party.**
   A. A very appropriate thing to do
   B. Appropriate but not ideal
   C. Inappropriate but not awful
   D. A very inappropriate thing to do

2. **To seek guidance from his tutor on what to.**
   A. A very appropriate thing to do
   B. Appropriate but not ideal
   C. Inappropriate but not awful
   D. A very inappropriate thing to do

3. **To start complaining openly at the party to anyone who will listen that drug taking is disgraceful.**
   A. A very appropriate thing to do
   B. Appropriate but not ideal
   C. Inappropriate but not awful
   D. A very inappropriate thing to do

4. **To ask to speak to the student outside and air their concerns that what they are doing is wrong.**
   A. A very appropriate thing to do
   B. Appropriate but not ideal
   C. Inappropriate but not awful
   D. A very inappropriate thing to do

Scenario 4

James is a junior doctor currently working on his final rotation before applying for his specialty training. He is currently preparing his application form for this and has come across a number of model answers on the internet that if he included in his application form would strengthen his application.

How **appropriate** is each of the following responses by **James** in this situation:

1. **To copy and paste the model answers into his application.**
   A. A very appropriate thing to do
   B. Appropriate but not ideal
   C. Inappropriate but not awful
   D. A very inappropriate thing to do

2. **To use the model answers for guidance purposes.**
   A. A very appropriate thing to do
   B. Appropriate but not ideal
   C. Inappropriate but not awful
   D. A very inappropriate thing to do

3. **To arrange an appointment with his supervisor to ask for guidance with the application form.**
   A. A very appropriate thing to do
   B. Appropriate but not ideal
   C. Inappropriate but not awful
   D. A very inappropriate thing to do

4. **Accept an offer from a friend to write his application for him.**
   A. A very appropriate thing to do
   B. Appropriate but not ideal
   C. Inappropriate but not awful
   D. A very inappropriate thing to do

5. **Ask a friend to proof read his application for spelling, grammar and formatting.**
   A. A very appropriate thing to do
   B. Appropriate but not ideal
   C. Inappropriate but not awful
   D. A very inappropriate thing to do

Scenario 5

A junior doctor is on a geriatric rotation when a patient approaches them to administer their daily medication injection as the nurse is off sick. The junior doctor has never given this particular type of injection before but has given other types of injections on numerous occasions.

How **appropriate** is each of the following responses by the **junior doctor** in this situation:

1. **Tell the patient that they will have to wait until tomorrow when the nurse is back at work to receive their injection.**
   A. A very appropriate thing to do
   B. Appropriate but not ideal
   C. Inappropriate but not awful
   D. A very inappropriate thing to do

2. **Apologise to the patient that they are unable to administer the injection and reassure them that they will seek assistance promptly from someone who can.**
   A. A very appropriate thing to do
   B. Appropriate but not ideal
   C. Inappropriate but not awful
   D. A very inappropriate thing to do

3. **Ask the patient to return to their bed.**
   A. A very appropriate thing to do
   B. Appropriate but not ideal
   C. Inappropriate but not awful
   D. A very inappropriate thing to do

4. **Attempt to administer the injection himself.**
   A. A very appropriate thing to do
   B. Appropriate but not ideal
   C. Inappropriate but not awful
   D. A very inappropriate thing to do

5. **Ignore the patient because they are too busy but ask one of the other nurses to attend the patient.**
   A. A very appropriate thing to do
   B. Appropriate but not ideal
   C. Inappropriate but not awful
   D. A very inappropriate thing to do

Scenario 6

A GP working in general practice sees a 26-year old businessman for his routine blood results. Although his cholesterol is entirely normal and he has no risk factors for heart disease he is demanding quite insistently that he is prescribed medication to treat high cholesterol to lower his risk despite there being no evidence that it will do so.

How **appropriate** is each of the following responses by the <u>**GP**</u> in this situation:

1. **Explore his reasons behind why he feels he needs to be prescribed medication and try to address his health beliefs, explain that there is no evidence that taking the medication will reduce the risk of cholesterol and that on this basis it is therefore not appropriate to prescribe the medication.**
   A. A very appropriate thing to do
   B. Appropriate but not ideal
   C. Inappropriate but not awful
   D. A very inappropriate thing to do

2. **Prescribe the patient 4-weeks' worth of medication and arrange to see him in a month's time.**
   A. A very appropriate thing to do
   B. Appropriate but not ideal
   C. Inappropriate but not awful
   D. A very inappropriate thing to do

3. **Offer the patient a consultation with another GP to discuss the matter.**
   A. A very appropriate thing to do
   B. Appropriate but not ideal
   C. Inappropriate but not awful
   D. A very inappropriate thing to do

4. **Simply tell the patient that he does not need a statin and refuse to prescribe it.**
   A. A very appropriate thing to do
   B. Appropriate but not ideal
   C. Inappropriate but not awful
   D. A very inappropriate thing to do

Scenario 7

A dentist working in a busy partnership received a box of chocolates from an elderly patient for putting her at ease during a long procedure three months ago. The dentist graciously accepted the gift. Since then during her last two visits the elderly patient has given the dentist chocolates both times. The patient now attends for her routine appointment again with chocolates to give to the dentist.

How **appropriate** is each of the following responses by **Dentist** in this situation:

1. **Accept the chocolates thanking the elderly patient.**
   A. A very appropriate thing to do
   B. Appropriate but not ideal
   C. Inappropriate but not awful
   D. A very inappropriate thing to do

2. **Explain to the patient that they do not need to keep providing gifts and graciously refuse the gift.**
   A. A very appropriate thing to do
   B. Appropriate but not ideal
   C. Inappropriate but not awful
   D. A very inappropriate thing to do

3. **To suggest that if the patient feels it vital that they express their gratitude then a donation to the practice's designated charity would be more appropriate.**
   A. A very appropriate thing to do
   B. Appropriate but not ideal
   C. Inappropriate but not awful
   D. A very inappropriate thing to do

Scenario 8

An on-call doctor is on duty to cover all the wards in the hospital after 5pm. They have to look after patients that may not necessarily be theirs. A nurse bleeps to ask them to speak to a patient's relatives who are very angry that the patient has not been transferred to the local residential home. This is due to there being no room and the patient is still on the busy ward despite being told they would be transferred a week ago. The on-call doctor has never seen this patient before and has no clue about any details pertaining to them since their admission.

How **appropriate** is each of the following responses by the **on-call doctor** in this situation:

1. **Apologise and state that they will arrange for the patient to be transferred immediately.**
   A. A very appropriate thing to do
   B. Appropriate but not ideal
   C. Inappropriate but not awful
   D. A very inappropriate thing to do

2. **Ring the Consultant on call and ask their advice.**
   A. A very appropriate thing to do
   B. Appropriate but not ideal
   C. Inappropriate but not awful
   D. A very inappropriate thing to do

3. **Escort the relatives to a quiet room, listen to their concerns and then assure them they will look into this matter as soon as possible.**
   A. A very appropriate thing to do
   B. Appropriate but not ideal
   C. Inappropriate but not awful
   D. A very inappropriate thing to do

Scenario 9

A routine chest X-ray a Consultant has requested for a well 54-year-old female patient with a cough comes back showing a 'shadow' on the lung. The radiologist comments that he cannot ascertain the nature of the shadow so suggests a referral to the chest clinic. The patient asks the Consultant 'Is it cancer doctor'?

How **appropriate** is each of the following responses by the Consultant in this situation:

1. **Explain to the patient that although the shadowing could represent cancer it could also represent other possibilities, for example old scarring or infection and that is the reason additional tests are required.**
   A. A very appropriate thing to do
   B. Appropriate but not ideal
   C. Inappropriate but not awful
   D. A very inappropriate thing to do

2. **Explain sensitively that the shadowing could represent cancer but that they are referring her for more tests to find out for certain.**
   A. A very appropriate thing to do
   B. Appropriate but not ideal
   C. Inappropriate but not awful
   D. A very inappropriate thing to do

3. **Tell her that it is likely to be cancer so she can be prepared.**
   A. A very appropriate thing to do
   B. Appropriate but not ideal
   C. Inappropriate but not awful
   D. A very inappropriate thing to do

Scenario 10

During a nightshift a junior doctor is called to see an elderly dehydrated patient whose blood pressure has dropped. They prescribe IV fluids and tell the nurse looking after the patient that they should be started immediately. However, when the junior doctor returns to review the patient 30 minutes later the IV fluids have still not been started and the patient's blood pressure is even lower.

How appropriate is each of the following responses by junior doctor in this situation:

1. **Call the nurse to one side on the ward whilst no one is around and express their dissatisfaction with the situation.**
   A. A very appropriate thing to do
   B. Appropriate but not ideal
   C. Inappropriate but not awful
   D. A very inappropriate thing to do

2. **Contact their supervising Registrar and ask for advice.**
   A. A very appropriate thing to do
   B. Appropriate but not ideal
   C. Inappropriate but not awful
   D. A very inappropriate thing to do

Scenario 11

A student is mountain biking at the weekend when they fall off and seriously injure their arm. It becomes immediately clear that the injury is going to impede their upcoming clinical placement. If the student misses this placement it is going to result in having to defer their studies by six months.

How **important** to take into account are the following factors for the student when considering how to respond to the situation?

1. **The injury will impede their ability to perform in a clinical placement.**
   A. Very important
   B. Important
   C. Of minor importance
   D. Not important at all

2. **No one witnessed the accident.**
   A. Very important
   B. Important
   C. Of minor importance
   D. Not important at all

3. **As a result of the accident the student will not be able to work part time to fund their studies.**
   A. Very important
   B. Important
   C. Of minor importance
   D. Not important at all

Scenario 12

A junior doctor is nearing the end of a very tedious shift when they realise that the medication they administered to their last patient was incorrect, resulting in a mild overdose.

How **important** to take into account are the following factors for the junior doctor when considering how to respond to the situation?

1. **That the shift is about to end and they have a social engagement they need to attend.**
   A. Very important
   B. Important
   C. Of minor importance
   D. Not important at all

2. **A mild overdose of the medication in question is likely to have no effect on the patient.**
   A. Very important
   B. Important
   C. Of minor importance
   D. Not important at all

3. **That it is hospital policy that all errors of this kind are recorded in an incident book.**
   A. Very important
   B. Important
   C. Of minor importance
   D. Not important at all

4. **The junior doctor feels that the ward is understaffed and that this is what contributed to the error.**
   A. Very important
   B. Important
   C. Of minor importance
   D. Not important at all

Scenario 13

A newly qualified dentist has been ask to take some notes about a recent patient to one of the partners to discuss possible treatment option. As the dentist walks into the partner's office they see them putting a bottle of whisky into their office drawer. It is obvious from the smell that the partner has been drinking the whisky.

How **important** to take into account are the following factors for the **newly qualified dentist** when considering how to respond to the situation?

1. **That they are due to go on holiday tomorrow for a week.**
   A. Very important
   B. Important
   C. Of minor importance
   D. Not important at all

2. **The partner has always been incredibly kind and supportive to the newly qualified dentist.**
   A. Very important
   B. Important
   C. Of minor importance
   D. Not important at all

3. **The partner is due to begin their afternoon clinic in 30 minutes.**
   A. Very important
   B. Important
   C. Of minor importance
   D. Not important at all

4. **The practice manager is off that day.**
   A. Very important
   B. Important
   C. Of minor importance
   D. Not important at all

Scenario 14

Carly is a senior doctor working on a hospital ward when a senior nurse comes to her and asks her to speak to one of the junior doctors about her dress code. The nurse has noted that the junior doctor is wearing a short skirt that she feels is inappropriate and asks Carly to discuss this matter with her.

How **important** to take into account are the following factors for **Carly** when considering how to respond to the situation?

1. **A number of patients on the ward have complained about the short skirt.**
   A. Very important
   B. Important
   C. Of minor importance
   D. Not important at all

2. **That the senior nurse in question does not get on with the colleague wearing the short skirt.**
   A. Very important
   B. Important
   C. Of minor importance
   D. Not important at all

3. **That in the past the colleague wearing the short skirt responds very badly to criticism.**
   A. Very important
   B. Important
   C. Of minor importance
   D. Not important at all

4. **That Carly has not observed for herself what the colleague is wearing.**
   A. Very important
   B. Important
   C. Of minor importance
   D. Not important at all

Scenario 15

Amelia has been asked to conduct an audit for her department regarding reviewing waiting times in the main clinic. She is required to show the raw data to her supervisor tomorrow afternoon. She still has to look through ten more patient notes in order to complete the data but it is 3am and she is exhausted and falling asleep. The notes are quite large and it will take her at least an hour to look through the remaining notes properly. She also has to be at work later that morning for her shift which starts at 9am.

How **important** to take into account are the following factors for <u>Amelia</u> when considering how to respond to the situation?

1. **The impact having little sleep will have on her ability to practice as a doctor.**
   A. Very important
   B. Important
   C. Of minor importance
   D. Not important at all

2. **That her supervisor will be cross if she does not have the audit ready for her meeting.**
   A. Very important
   B. Important
   C. Of minor importance
   D. Not important at all

3. **Successful completion of the audit will help to improve the quality of care provided to patients in the clinic.**
   A. Very important
   B. Important
   C. Of minor importance
   D. Not important at all

Scenario 16

Jessica is approaching the end of her second year at university and her educational supervisor has requested a meeting with her to discuss her persistently submitting coursework late together with her not attending seminars on time.

How **important** to take into account are the following factors for **Jessica** when considering how to respond to the situation?

1. That she is feeling very anxious about failing her studies.
   A. Very important
   B. Important
   C. Of minor importance
   D. Not important at all

2. **That she knows of other students who are far worse than she is.**
   A. Very important
   B. Important
   C. Of minor importance
   D. Not important at all

3. **That whatever the outcome she must heed the advice of the tutor.**
   A. Very important
   B. Important
   C. Of minor importance
   D. Not important at all

Scenario 17

Eleanor is a junior doctor working on a paediatric ward. A young couple who are of Mexican descent are staying with their 2-year old son who has been admitted with a severe infection and is very poorly. Eleanor is preparing to do the ward round when she overhears one of the nurses complaining to another nurse about how rude the couple have been and that foreigners are a nuisance and should not be allowed to use the hospital.

How **important** to take into account are the following factors for Eleanor when considering how to respond to the situation?

1. **That the nurse was not overheard by the young couple.**
   A. Very important
   B. Important
   C. Of minor importance
   D. Not important at all

2. **That the nurse in question is one of the best nurses on the ward.**
   A. Very important
   B. Important
   C. Of minor importance
   D. Not important at all

3. **The nurse in question has been known to not respond to criticism well in the past.**
   A. Very important
   B. Important
   C. Of minor importance
   D. Not important at all

Scenario 18

Nicola is a third year dentist currently on placement. Today she is observing a root canal and the patient is noticeably nervous prior to the dentist commencing the procedure. However the surgery is running behind and currently the delay is 40 minutes.

How **important** to take into account are the following factors for Nicola when considering how to respond to the situation?

1. **The patient appears noticeably nervous.**
   A. Very important
   B. Important
   C. Of minor importance
   D. Not important at all

2. **The dental assistant appears to have a significant cough.**
   A. Very important
   B. Important
   C. Of minor importance
   D. Not important at all

3. **The dentist is not making any time to discuss any concerns the patient may have together with allaying any fears.**
   A. Very important
   B. Important
   C. Of minor importance
   D. Not important at all

4. **The surgery is running late.**
   A. Very important
   B. Important
   C. Of minor importance
   D. Not important at all

Scenario 19

Janice is a junior doctor working on a night shift. She is reviewing the patient notes of an elderly gentleman when she realises that according to the notes recorded consent has not been obtained by the Consultant for the scan the patient will be receiving tomorrow.

How **important** to take into account are the following factors for **Jack** when considering how to respond to the situation?

1. **The Consultant is now on holiday for a week.**
   A. Very important
   B. Important
   C. Of minor importance
   D. Not important at all

2. **That it is almost the end of his shift.**
   A. Very important
   B. Important
   C. Of minor importance
   D. Not important at all

Chapter 9

Entire mock UKCAT exam 1 answers

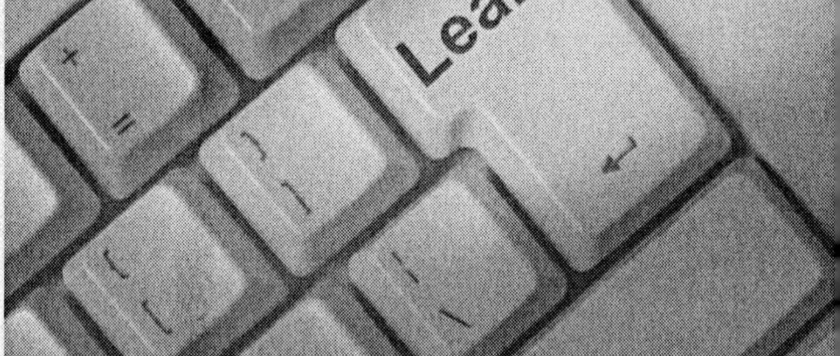

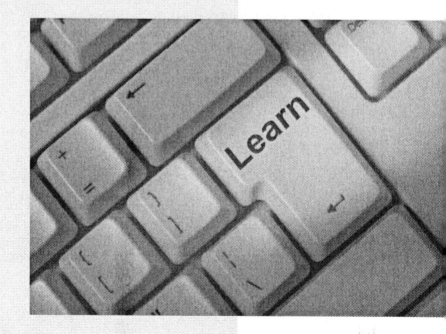

Entire mock UKCAT exam 1 answers

Verbal Reasoning answers and justifications

Question 1

1. **True.** This statement is confirmed by the following in the passage: *'However, if the criminal issue compromises patient safety or if it involves the work ethic of a colleague, it is necessary to involve someone more senior and escalate the matter to a higher level. This is the case in a scenario where a colleague is stealing prescription drugs or viewing child pornography, as obviously patients may be at risk in these cases'.*
2. **False.** This statement is contradicted by the following in the passage: *'Although there may be a criminal issue at hand and the police may need to be involved at some point, you are only a foundation doctor, and thus it may be sensible to go to your Registrar or Consultant first before contacting the police yourself'.*
3. **True.** This is confirmed by the following in the passage: *'You must also be able to use your common sense to assess the severity of the crime and use your judgement in when to involve more senior authorities. For example, although all theft is illegal it may not be necessary to involve the police for a minor theft, and thus you must show that you are able to apply common sense to individual situations'.*
4. **Can't tell.** Though the passage states that it preferred to deal with matters involving colleagues locally first, the passage neither confirms nor denies that the views of the colleague should be requested in writing: *'As previously stated, it is common courtesy when dealing with conduct issues in colleagues to deal with the matter locally first'.*

Question 2

1. **The correct answer is A.** 'Arimaa is a two-player board game', 'but about 900 games are played on-line every week'.
2. **The correct answer is C.** It can also be played on-line at the arimaa. com gameroom.
3. **The correct answer is C.** In 2002 Syed published the rules to Arimaa and announced a $10,000 prize, available through 2020, for the first computer program to win matches against top-ranked human players. David Wu's bot Sharp accomplished this in 2015.
4. **The correct answer is B.** Syed has released an experimental license called 'The Arimaa Public License', with the declared intent to 'make Arimaa as much of a public domain game as possible while still protecting its commercial usage'.

Question 3

1. **Can't tell.** It is not possible from the passage to confirm or deny whether this was true and therefore it is not possible to confirm whether this statement is true or false.
2. **False.** The statement is contradicted by the fact that the passage states they are similar but not the same: *'However, what you should not delegate is accountability for the task. Accountability is a similar term to responsibility, so how may accountability be accurately defined?'*
3. **True.** This statement is confirmed by the following in the passage; *'You must also be prepared to deal with the consequences of problems which may arise'.*
4. **False.** This is false. The passage states that instilling confidence is key to delegation; *'Confidence is key to all performance issues and once you have instilled it in your colleagues you will be able to delegate to them on a regular basis'.*

Question 4

1. **The correct answer is C.** It is believed Polynesian settlers used subtropical weather systems to find their way from their native islands, in Polynesia to New Zealand. As the settlers colonised the country, they developed their distinctive Maori culture
2. **The correct answer is A.** According to Maori, the first Polynesian explorer to reach New Zealand was Kupe, who travelled across the Pacific in a Polynesian-style voyaging canoe.
3. **The correct answer is B.** The current understanding is that they migrated from East Polynesia, the Southern Cook and Society islands region. They migrated deliberately, at different times, in different canoes, first arriving in New Zealand in the late 13th Century.
4. **The correct answer is C.** The passage states that the Polynesians first started to arrive in the 13th Century (which began in 1201) 13th Century – to the present day is greater than 800 years.

Question 5

1. **Can't tell.** Although in theory this statement would not save an individual any more time, the passage does not make any reference to this and therefore it is not possible to confirm or deny the statement.
2. **False.** This statement is incorrect based on following in the statement: *'When long discussions ensue it can be difficult for someone to judge accurately. As Chair, you should decide which points are pertinent to capture. This will include all actions'.*

3. **Can't tell.** Although reference is made to following the agenda, the passage makes no reference to points being discussed as part of an Any Other Business section in the meeting and therefore the passage neither confirms or contradicts the statement.
4. **True.** This statement is confirmed by the following in the passage: *'Could you obtain all the information you need from reading a copy of the minutes? If the answer is yes then consider removing the meeting from your diary'.*

Question 6

1. **The correct answer is B.** Innovation and invention in 19th century America has been said to be attributed to the development of the patent system.
2. **The correct answer is B.** Everyone has the right to the protection of the moral and material interests resulting from any scientific, literary or artistic production of which he is the author.
3. **The correct answer is A.** Natural Rights/Justice Argument: this argument is based on Locke's idea that a person has a natural right over the labour and/or products which is produced by his/her body. Appropriating these products is viewed as unjust.
4. **The correct answer is D.** Natural Rights/Justice Argument, Utilitarian-Pragmatic Argument, Personality Argument.

Question 7

1. **True.** The passage says that it is possible to apply with a science or a non-science degree: *'Both science and non-science graduates may be accepted, but this varies according to the institution'.*
2. **Can't tell.** Although the passage refers to the entire GAMSAT taking five hours to complete the passage does not confirm the timings of each section therefore it is not possible to confirm or deny this statement: *'It comprises an arduous set of three exams over five hours'.*
3. **Can't tell.** It is not possible to tell from the passage what exact score is required in the GAMSAT: *'Some GEPs specify A level requirements too, but the main factor that determines whether or not you get an interview is your score on the GAMSAT or other entrance exam'.*
4. **True.** This statement is confirmed by the following: *'Most of these dedicated courses are accelerated and take four years in total. Typically, the pre-clinical part of the course is separate from that of the undergraduate course of five years. For the clinical years, graduate entry courses and undergraduate courses are often the same'.*

Question 8

1. **True.** This statement is confirmed by the following in the passage: *'If there are gaps in your CV after your previous positions, then take steps to remedy this as quickly as possible. These steps can be relatively easy (eg expand outside interests, book on to relevant courses, involve yourself in an audit) or may require more commitment (volunteer to teach anatomy / physiology at the university, book a college exam and start revising, register for a distance learning qualification)'.*
2. **True.** This statement is confirmed by the following in the passage: *'Compare yourself with your peers and their achievements, as unfortunately these are the people you are competing with. If there are large gaps in your CV, think practically with the resources you have and the time left that you have to prepare'.*
3. **False.** This statement is contradicted by the following in the passage: *'If there are gaps in your CV after your previous positions, then take steps to remedy this as quickly as possible. These steps can be relatively easy (eg expand outside interests, book on to relevant courses, involve yourself in an audit) or may require more commitment (volunteer to teach anatomy / physiology at the university, book a college exam and start revising, register for a distance learning qualification). Some of these steps take more time than others to complete, and it depends on how committed you are to following that specialty, and how much time you have before the application deadline, as to what you can achieve'.*
4. **Can't tell.** Although a sensible statement it is not possible to confirm from the passage whether this statement is true or false: *'Early planning of how to improve and develop your CV for a given post is well advised and a friendly Consultant is invaluable in this quest. Approach your Consultant, particularly your educational supervisor, with a copy of your CV and ask if they will go through it with you to see where there are areas you could improve'.*

Question 9

1. **The correct answer is D.** These connections should have led to a political career for Plato but at some stage for reasons unknown he made a decision not to enter political life.
2. **The correct answer is C.** Perictione's cousin Critias and her brother Charmides are known to have been friends with Socrates and they themselves were part of the oligarchic leadership of 404 BC.
3. **The correct answer is A.** Plato is regarded by many to be one of the West's greatest ancient philosophers. The student of Socrates and teacher of Aristotle, he wrote many books in his life time.
4. **The correct answer is C.** Perictione's cousin Critias and her brother Charmides are known to have been friends with Socrates.

Question 10

1. **True.** This statement is confirmed by the following in the passage: *'The more senior you become the more you will be expected to manage a team of people, directing their actions in the most productive way for your service. You will be actively involved in the mentoring of junior staff'.*
2. **True.** This statement is confirmed by the following in the passage: *'You will often find yourself in situations that require you to negotiate with others to achieve your outcomes. You may need to persuade and convince other people that your plan is the best one'.*
3. **Can't tell.** Although this would be a reasonable task to expect as part of a mentoring role the passage neither confirms nor contradicts this statement. Though it confirms, *'You will be actively involved in the mentoring of junior staff'*, it does not say whether this means appraising them.
4. **True.** This statement is confirmed by the following in the passage; *'As you can see, the more senior you become, the more you are drawn away from clinical responsibilities'.*

Question 11

1. **False.** This statement is false based on the following in the passage: *'Specialist nurses are highly trained in a single field, eg cardiac, endoscopy, diabetes, cancer (MacMillan nurses)'.*
2. **False.** This statement is false based on the following in the passage: *'You must get nurses to complete your Mini-Peer Assessment Tool (Mini-PAT), and they can also observe you completing DOPS assessments'.*
3. **Can't tell.** Although the passage outlines some of the ways pharmacists can assist doctors it neither confirms nor contradicts that they are involved with budgeting. The relevant section is: *'The ward pharmacist knows the dosages and indications for drugs, and they can also tell you if a drug you want to prescribe is in the hospital formulary. Ask them if you are unsure. Pharmacists can also work directly with the hospital pharmacy, to get medications for your patients quickly, especially in emergency situations and prior to discharges'.*
4. **False.** Green ink is used by pharmacists, not physiotherapists: *'Pharmacists can also work directly with the hospital pharmacy, to get medications for your patients quickly, especially in emergency situations and prior to discharges. Look out for their green ink on your drug charts'.*

Quantitative Reasoning answers and justifications

1. The correct answer is C.

The mean is worked out by adding the prices of all the items together and dividing by the number of items:

(3.20 + 1.20 + 1.00 + 2.00 +1.00 + 2.39) ÷ 6 = **£1.80** (to the nearest penny)

2. The correct answer is C.

The median is a value which divides a sample of numbers into two equal parts.

In order to find out the median of the price list, we need to arrange all of the prices in ascending order and then find the middle value or pair. If there is a pair of values, we add the two values together and divide by two.

3.20, 2.39, **2.00, 1.20,** 1.00, 1.00.

(£2.00 + £1.20) ÷ 2 = **£1.60**

3. The correct answer is C.

The range is found by subtracting the lowest priced item on the list from the highest priced item in the list:

£3.20 – £1.00 = **£2.20**

4. The correct answer is D.

Add the totals of the range, the median and the mean, which have all been worked out in the previous questions within this section:

1.80 + 1.60 + 2.20 = **£5.60**

5. **The correct answer is D.**

Look under the heading which provides information regarding % breakdown of adults in 1998.

13% of females and 10% of males read **'Alive in the Past'**. Therefore this book was read by a higher percentage of females than males in 1998.

6. **The correct answer is B.**

Add up the total readership of the following books in 1981:

(Alive in the Past) 6.9 + (A Warm Day) 2.2 + (My Best Friend) 2.9 = **12 million readers.**

7. **The correct answer is A.**

Find the difference between the two readership figures:

6.9 million (1981) – 4.8 million (1998) = 2.1 million

Find the percentage decrease, which is calculated by dividing the difference by the original number of readers (ie 6.9 million):

2.1 ÷ 6.9 × 100 = **30.43%**

8. **The correct answer is B.**

In 1998 the table indicates that there were 8.9 million readers, and a total of 22% of the readership were male adults and read the book in that year.

Calculate how many adult males read the book as follows:

8,900,000 × 0.22 = **1,958,000 male readers**

9. **The correct answer is E.**

(54 × 44) + 77 = **2,453**

10. **The correct answer is D.**

(312 × 22)/(28 + 27) = 124.8 or **125** (to 3 significant figures)

11. The correct answer is E.

432 ÷ 62 = 6.9677419

Therefore 432:62 = **7:1** to the nearest whole number.

12. The correct answer is D.

23 + 34 + 21 + 23 + 56 + 54 + 45 + 126 = 382 ÷ 8 = 47.75 or **47.8** to one decimal place.

13. The correct answer is C.

4,356/(935 + 4,356 + 2,345 + 94) × 100 = **56.35%**

14. The correct answer is C.

Total number of votes in Nottingham East:
6,345 + 2,432 + 890 + 125 = 9,792

This number represents 37% of the total population, therefore to obtain the total population figure:

(9,792 ÷ 37) × 100 = 26,465

Total number of votes in Nottingham South:

8,733 + 7,822 + 1,352 + 61 = 17,968

This number represents 37% of the total population, therefore to obtain the total population figure:

(17,968 ÷ 37) × 100 = 56,150

To obtain the total population for both regions:

26,465 + 56,150 = **82,615**

15. The correct answer is B.

Conservative: 8,546 + 6,345 + 935 + 3,627 + 8,733 = 28,186

Labour: 3,672 + 2,432 + 4,356 + 3,328 + 7,822 = 21,610

28,186 + 21,610 = **49,796**

16. The correct answer is B.

Labour won the vote with 4,356 votes.

17. The correct answer is E.

The question asks how many garage doors are ≤ than 6.9 metres. The ≤ symbol means 'equal to or less than'.

There are 4 doors which are 5–5.9 metres and 12 doors which are 6–6.9 metres, giving a total of **16 doors** which are less than or equal to 6.9 metres.

18. The correct answer is D.

There are a total of 92 doors in the table. Of these, 32 have a height of less than or equal to 7.9 metres.
As a fraction this can be written as 32/92.

However, we can still reduce this fraction to its simplest form by dividing it by 4:

$32 \div 4 = 8$

$92 \div 4 = 23$

The fraction can therefore be written as **8/23**.

19. The correct answer is C.

There are 12 doors in the range of 6–6.9 metres and 24 in the range 8–8.9 metres. Hence the ratio is 12:24.

However, as ratios are customarily written in their simplest form, each number can be divided by 12 to show a ratio of **1:2**.

20. The correct answer is C.

In 1 metre there are 100 cm. Therefore in 12.9 metres there are 1,290 cm (12.9 × 100).

The question states that there are 5 garage doors, therefore we need to multiply the above total by 5:

1,290 × 5 = **6,450 cm**

21. The correct answer is E.

Rifle F is 1.5 cm calibre. Rifle B is 0.45 cm calibre.

1.5 cm – 0.45 cm = **1.05 cm**

22. The correct answer is A.

To calculate the Effectiveness Quotient of Rifle B:

0.45 × 435 × 150 × 4 = 117,450
To calculate the Effectiveness Quotient of Rifle F:

1.5 × 567 × 600 × 2 = 1,020,600

To calculate the difference:

1,020,600 – 117,450 = 903,150 or **903,200** (to 4 significant figures).

23. The correct answer is A.

500 + 435 + 650 + 900 + 760 + 567 = 3,812 ÷ 6 = **635 m/s** (to the nearest whole number).

24. The correct answer is E.

Rifle F has the lowest value of 2 and therefore the highest accuracy.

25. The correct answer is B.

Make **C** the subject of both equations 1 and 2 and equate. Then solve to find A with respect to D:

C = 4B + 2D (equation 1, where C is already the subject)

C = A + 4B (equation 2 with C as the subject)

A + 4B = 4B + 2D (equating the two equations)

A = **2D** (taking away 4B from both sides gives the required answer).

26. The correct answer is C.

Rearrange the equation to make B the subject:

4B + 2D = C (minus 2D from both sides)

4B = C – 2D (then divide both sides by 4)

B = (C – 2D)/4 (leaving you with the final answer).

27. The correct answer is E.

Substitute the given values for B and D into equation 1 and calculate.
C = 4B + 2D (put in the values for B and D)

C = 4(1.25) + 2(3) (calculate)

C = 11

28. The correct answer is C.

Rearrange equation 1 to make **B** the subject then substitute the given values for **C** and **D**.

4B + 2D (rearrange to make B the subject)

B = (C – 2D)/4 (substitute the values for C and D)

B = (8 – 2(2))/4 (calculate)

B = 1

29. The correct answer is D.

The percentage of Business A is split evenly between Businesses D and C. So add half of the percentage held by Business A onto Business D.

38% ÷ 2 = 19%

20% + 19% = **39%**

30. The correct answer is D.

With Business B gone, the remaining 68% becomes the new 100% so the other percentages must be adapted. Do this by dividing the original percentage by 0.68.

Eg For Business A:

38% ÷ 0.68 = **55.88%**

31. The correct answer is D.

Find the value of Business C in 2010 and 1990. Then take the value in 1990 away from the value in 2010.

Value in 1990 = £15bn × 0.1 = £1.5bn
Value in 2010 = £23bn × 0.1 = £2.3bn

Difference = £2.3bn – £1.5bn = **£0.8bn**

32. The correct answer is D.

Find the value of 1% in 1990 and then in 2010. Then take the value in 1990 away from the value in 2010.

1990: £15bn × 0.01 = £0.15bn

2010: £23bn × 0.01 = £0.23bn

Difference = £0.23bn – £0.15bn = **£0.08bn**

33. The correct answer is E.

Find the total income of Bubble inc. Then divide Electronics income by the total income and multiply by 100 to convert into a percentage.
Total income: (80 + 60 + 30 + 20 +15) = 205

80 ÷ 205 = 0.39 × 100 = **39%**

34. The correct answer is A.

Calculate the increase in income/year:

20% of 60 million = (60 ÷ 100) × 20 = 12 million/year

An investment of 600 million would take 600 ÷ 12 = **25 years to recoup**

35. The correct answer is D.

Take away the yearly expenses from the yearly income to find the yearly profits.

£205 million – £100 million = **£105 million**

36. The correct answer is B.

Identify the loss that the Services sector is making by finding the difference between income and expenses. Then add this difference on to the original total profits of Bubble inc.
The cost of running the Services sector = £15 million × 1.25 = £18.75 million

The loss of running the Services sector = £18.75 million – £15 million = £3.75 million

Therefore the new profit = £105 million + £3.75 million = **£108.75 million**

Abstract Reasoning answers and justifications

Question 1

Set A

In this set there are always two shapes. One of the shapes is large and the other shape is small. The shapes are always positioned in opposing diagonal corners.

- The rule in this set is that if the large shape possesses a curved line, it is positioned in the top left hand corner and the smaller shape is positioned in the bottom right hand corner.
- However, if the large shape does not possess any curved lines, it is positioned in the bottom right hand corner and the small shape is positioned in the top left hand corner.

Set B

As above, in this set there are always two shapes. One of the shapes is large and the other shape is small. The shapes are always positioned in opposing diagonal corners.

- The rule in this set is that if the large shape possesses a curved line, it is positioned in the bottom right hand corner and the smaller shape is positioned in the top left hand corner.
- However, if the large shape does not possess any curved lines, it is positioned in the top left hand corner and the small shape is positioned in the bottom right hand corner.

Test Shape 1 Answer: Neither
Both Set A and Set B require the shapes to be diagonally aligned from top left to bottom right. However, this test shape does not have this alignment. Therefore, the test shape does not belong to either set.

Test Shape 2 Answer: Set B
The large heart is positioned in the bottom right hand corner and the arch is positioned in the top left hand corner. The heart contains two curves, therefore it is correctly positioned for the test shape to belong to Set B.

Test Shape 3 Answer: Set A
The triangle is positioned in the bottom right hand corner. The triangle does not contain any curved lines, therefore, it is correctly positioned for the test shape to belong to Set A.

Test Shape 4 Answer: Neither
Both Set A and Set B require the shapes to be diagonally aligned from top left to bottom right, however, this test shape has a vertical alignment. Therefore, the test shape does not belong to either set.

Test Shape 5 Answer: Set B
The arrow is positioned in the top left hand corner and the star is positioned in the bottom right hand corner. The arrow does not contain any curved lines, therefore it is correctly positioned for the test shape to belong to Set B.

Question 2

Set A

In this set there is a mix of arrows, chevrons and pentagons directed left and right.

- The rule in this set is that each box must contain five shapes.
- Also, within the five shapes there must be two arrows pointing right.

Set B

As with Set A, there is a mix of arrows, chevrons and pentagons directed left and right.

- The rule in this set is there must be five shapes.
- Also, within the five shapes there must be two chevrons pointing left.

1. **Correct answer A:** The box contains five shapes, with two arrows pointing right, therefore it belongs to set A.
2. **Correct answer D:** The box contains five shapes, with two arrows pointing right, therefore it belongs to set A.
3. **Correct answer C:** The box contains five shapes, with two arrows pointing right, therefore it belongs to set A.
4. **Correct answer D:** The box contains five shapes, with two chevrons pointing left therefore it belongs to set B.
5. **Correct answer B:** The box contains five shapes, with two chevrons pointing left therefore it belongs to set B.

Question 3

Set A

In this set there are two shapes with the same outline in each box. Some of the shapes are shaded and others are unshaded.

- The rule in this set is that the two shapes must have identical outlines.
- Also, the two shapes must touch at one apex, or face.

Set B

In this set there are two shapes with the same outline in each box. Some of the shapes are shaded and others are unshaded.

- The rule in this set is that the shapes must have identical outlines.
- Also, the two shapes must touch at either two apices, or two faces.
- Also, one shape must be shaded and one must be unshaded.

Test Shape 1 Answer: Neither
Although the shapes are touching at one apex, the shapes do not have identical outlines. Therefore, the test shape does not fit into either set.

Test Shape 2 Answer: Set A
The shapes touch at one point, therefore the test shape belongs to Set A.

Test Shape 3 Answer: Neither
The shapes are not touching, therefore, the test shape does not fit into either set.
Test Shape 4 Answer: Set B
The test shape contains two shapes with identical outlines, one of which is shaded. The shapes are touching at two points. Therefore the test shape belongs to Set B.

Test Shape 5 Answer: Set A
The shapes are touching at one point. Therefore the shape belongs to Set A.

Question 4

Set A

In this set there are always four shapes, comprising arches, doughnuts and stop sign shapes.

- The rule in this set is that there must always be an upright arch shape in the top left hand corner and a stop sign (with the line orientated downward and right) in the bottom right hand corner of the box, or vice versa.

Set B

In this set there are always four shapes, comprising arches, doughnuts and stop sign shapes.

- The rule in this set is that there must always be an inverted arch shape in the top right hand corner and a stop sign (with the line orientated downward and left) in the bottom left hand corner of the box, or vice versa.

Test Shape 1 Answer: Neither
The test shape contains a correctly orientated stop sign in the top left hand corner to belong to Set A. However, the arch shape is inverted. The test shape also contains a correctly orientated stop sign in the bottom left hand corner to belong to Set B. However, there is no inverted arch shape in the top right hand corner. Therefore, the test shape does not fit into either set.

Test Shape 2 Answer: Set A
The test shape contains a correctly orientated stop sign in the top left hand corner to belong to Set A. In addition, there is a correctly positioned arch shape. Therefore the shape belongs to Set A.

Test Shape 3 Answer: Neither
The test shape contains a correctly orientated stop sign in the top right hand corner to belong to Set B. However, the arch shape is not inverted which is a requirement to belonging to Set B. The test shape does not have any of the defining characteristics to belong to Set A.

Test Shape 4 Answer: Set B
The test shape contains a correctly orientated stop sign in the bottom left hand corner to belong to Set B. The arch shape is also correctly positioned and orientated to belong to Set B.

Test Shape 5 Answer: Set A
The test shape contains a correctly orientated stop sign in the bottom right hand corner to belong to Set A. The arch shape is also correctly positioned and orientated to belong to Set A.

Question 5

Set A

In this set there is one shape per box.

- The rule in this set is that the shape must be made of straight lines.
- Also, there must be at least one set of parallel lines.

Set B

In this set there is one shape per box.

- The rule in this set is that there cannot be any parallel lines.
- Also, there cannot be any right angles.

1. **Correct answer A:** The shapes all contain straight sides and at least one contains parallel sides, therefore it belongs to set A.
2. **Correct answer B:** The shapes all contain straight sides and at least one contains parallel sides, therefore it belongs to set A.
3. **Correct answer C:** No sides of the shape are parallel and it does not contain any right angles, therefore it belongs to set B.
4. **Correct answer A:** No sides of the shape are parallel and it does not contain any right angles, therefore it belongs to set B.
5. **Correct answer C:** No sides of the shape are parallel and it does not contain any right angles, therefore it belongs to set B.

Question 6

Set A

In this set there is one shape per box.

- The rule in this set is that the shape must be composed of dots
- Also, each shape must have a vertical line of symmetry and no others.

Set B

In this set there is also one shape per box.

- The rule in this set is that the shape must be composed of long dashes.
- Also, the shape must have a horizontal line of symmetry and no others.

Test Shape 1 Answer: Set A
The shape has a vertical line of symmetry and is also composed of dots, the shape therefore belongs to Set A.

Test Shape 2 Answer: Neither
The shape has a horizontal line of symmetry, which is a prerequisite to belong to Set B. However, it is composed of dots, rather than long dashes. Therefore the shape belongs to neither set.

Test Shape 3 Answer: Neither
At first glance the shape appears to belong to Set B as it is composed of long dashed lines and has a horizontal line of symmetry. However, on closer inspection we can see the shape also has a vertical line of symmetry. Therefore it does not fit into either set.

Test Shape 4 Answer: Set B
The shape has a horizontal line of symmetry but no vertical line of symmetry. Also the shape consists of long dashes. Therefore it belongs to Set B.

Test Shape 5 Answer: Set A
The shape consists of dots and there is a vertical line of symmetry. Therefore, the shape belongs to Set A.

Question 7

Set A

In this set there are three shapes: faces, curved arrows and straight arrows with the following rules:

- When there are three faces there must only be one curved arrow
- When there is only one face there must only be three curved arrows.
- The straight arrows are distracters.

Set B

Again, this set contains the same three shapes: faces, curved arrows and straight arrows. However, the rules differ as follows:

- When there are four straight arrows there must be only one curved arrow.
- When there are two straight arrows there must be only two curved arrows.
- The faces are used as distracters.

1. **Correct answer C:** There is one face and three curved arrows present, therefore it belongs to set A.
2. **Correct answer D:** There are three faces and one curved arrow present, therefore it belongs to set A.
3. **Correct answer A:** There are three faces and one curved arrow present, therefore it belongs to set A.
4. **Correct answer C:** There are four straight arrows and one curved arrow, therefore it belongs to set B.
5. **Correct answer D:** There are tow straight arrows and two curved arrows, therefore it belongs to set B.

Question 8

Set A

This set contains a single shape with dashed lines. Each shape may have curved or straight lines, or a combination of both. The orientation, position and size of the shapes follow no pattern.

- The rule in this set is that each shape must have two or more lines of symmetry.

Set B

This set contains shapes with solid lines only. There may be one or more shapes in each box with either straight or curved lines. All of the shapes are large but their positioning is random.

- The rule is that the shapes must contain no lines of symmetry.

Test Shape 1 Answer: Set B
This test shape is large and has no lines of symmetry.

Test Shape 2 Answer: Set A
This test shape has dashed lines with infinite lines of symmetry.

Test Shape 3 Answer: Neither
While this test shape has dashed lines it has only one line of symmetry and does not satisfy the rules of Set A.

Test Shape 4 Answer: Set A
This test shape has dashed lines with two lines of symmetry.

Test Shape 5 Answer: Set B
This test shape is large with no lines of symmetry.

Question 9

Set A

The shapes in Set A include circles, arrows and trapezoids that may be shaded or unshaded. The size, placement and number of each shape may vary.

- The rule in this set is that all the shapes must have straight edges.

Set B

Set B includes ovals and ellipses, which may be shaded or unshaded. Again, the size, placement and number of each shape may vary.

- The rule in this set is that all the shapes must contain curved lines only.

1. **Correct answer D:** All the shapes have straight sides, therefore it belongs to set A.
2. **Correct answer C:** All the shapes have straight sides, therefore it belongs to set A.

3. **Correct answer D:** All the shapes have curved sides, therefore it belongs to set B.
4. **Correct answer C:** All the shapes have curved sides, therefore it belongs to set B.
5. **Correct answer C:** All the shapes have curved sides, therefore it belongs to set B.

Question 10

Set A

This set contains three shapes: two large and one small. The two large shapes are touching; one is shaded while the other is unshaded.

- The rule in this set is that the third shape, which is smaller, is a smaller version of the larger shaded shape.
- Also, all shapes consist of solid lines.

Set B

This set also contains three shapes: a large, medium and small. The large shape is unshaded and contains the medium size shape.

- The rule in this set is that the small shape is unshaded and corresponds to the large shape.
- Also, all shapes consist of solid lines.

1. **Correct answer A:** All shapes consist of solid sides, the smallest shape is a copy of the largest shape, therefore it belongs to set A.
2. **Correct answer B:** All shapes consist of solid sides, the smallest shape is a copy of the largest shape, therefore it belongs to set A.
3. **Correct answer A:** All shapes consist of solid lines, the smallest shape is unshaded and is the same as the largest shape, therefore it belongs to set B.
4. **Correct answer C:** All shapes consist of solid sides, the smallest shape is a copy of the largest shape, therefore it belongs to set A.
5. **Correct answer D:** All shapes consist of solid sides, the smallest shape is a copy of the largest shape, therefore it belongs to set A.

Question 11

Set A

The set contains triangles, circles, squares and rectangles with straight or curved lines. Shapes possess either solid or dashed lines and are unshaded.

- The rule in this set is that each shape must be composed of two or more individual lines that cannot be drawn without lifting the pen off the page, or drawing over the same line twice.

Set B

Set B contains circles, stars, arrows, hexagons and adjacent quadrilateral shapes with straight or curved edges.

- The rule in this set is that each shape must possess only solid lines and be unshaded.
- Also, all the shapes must be able to be drawn without lifting the pen off the page.

Test Shape 1 Answer: Set B
This test shape contains an unshaded cylinder with solid lines, features of both Set A and B. The shape can be drawn without lifting the pen and therefore belongs to Set B.

Test Shape 2 Answer: Set A
This test shape contains two circles, the smaller of which lies within the larger one. Both are unshaded and do not touch. It is not possible to draw them both without lifting the pen off the page, a feature of Set A.

Test Shape 3 Answer: Neither
The shaded arrow is similar to that of Set B, however, it is shaded which is a feature of neither set.

Test Shape 4 Answer: Set B
This test shape contains a single solid line that can be drawn without lifting the pen off the page. Therefore the test shape belongs to Set B.

Test Shape 5 Answer: Set B
This test shape contains two straight, unshaded arrows with solid lines, features of Set B. At close inspection we can see that the arrows can be drawn from a single line without lifting the pen off the page. Therefore, the test shape belongs to Set B.

Decision Analysis answers and justifications

Question 1

Answer: A

12(O, I), 3, H

The code combines the words: attribute (building, people), closed, tomorrow.

A **Is the correct answer as it uses all the codes and the rules within the brackets. 'Attribute (building, people)' is taken to mean 'office'.**
B Incorrect as it ignores the code 'attribute (building, people)' and instead uses the words directly.
C Incorrect as the word 'shops' implies more than one shop, while the code – 'attribute (building, people)' – implies only one.
D Incorrect as it ignores the word 'tomorrow' and instead introduces 'today'.
E Incorrect as it ignores the word 'tomorrow'.

Question 2

Answer: E

S, 10, P, (T, D), 8

The code combines the words: animals, walk, land, (warm, sky), present.

A Incorrect as it introduces the words 'great distances' and ignores '(warm, sky)'.
B Incorrect as it ignores the coded words 'walk' and 'land' and introduces the word 'rest'. The statement is also set in the past.
C Incorrect as it ignores the word 'land' and sets the statement in the past.
D Incorrect as it is set in the past tense and ignores the word 'present'.
E **Is the correct answer as it uses all the codes and the rules within the brackets. 'Camels' is substituted for 'animals', while 'desert' is substituted for 'land'. '(Warm, sky)' is combined to give 'sun'. The sentence is set in the present tense.**

Question 3

Answer: E

G, (J, 4), 12(10), E, K

The code combines the words: today, (men, singular), attribute (walk), planet, adventure.

A Incorrect as it ignores the combined code '(men, singular') and code word for 'planet'.
B Incorrect as it ignores the code word for 'today' and is set in the past tense.
C Incorrect as introduces the word 'spaceman' and ignores the code 'attribute (walk)'.
D Incorrect as it introduces the word 'many' when only one adventure is described by the code.
E **Is the correct answer as it uses all the codes and the rules within the brackets. (Men, singular) are combined to give 'he'. 'Attribute (walk)' is combined to give 'sets off' while 'world' is substituted for 'planet'. The sentence is correctly phrased in the present tense.**

Question 4

Answer: C

F(1, 4), 9, D, (1, G)

The code combines the words: star (antonym, singular), ascend, sky, (antonym, today).

A Incorrect as it does not combine '(antonym, today)' and ignores the word 'ascend'.
B Incorrect as it ignores the word 'ascend'.
C **Is the correct answer as it uses all the codes and the rules within the brackets. Combines 'star (antonym, singular)' as 'the stars'. 'High' is substituted for 'ascend', while '(antonym, today)' is combined to give 'tonight'.**
D Incorrect as it introduces the word 'North'.
E Incorrect as it ignores the code '(antonym, singular)', which implies more than one star.

Question 5

Answer: A

I, 7, 12(O, S), 11, H, T

The code combines the words: people, drive, attribute (building, animals), conditional, tomorrow, warm.

A **Is the correct answer as it uses all the coded words and combines 'attribute (building, animals)' as 'zoo'. The code for 'people' is substituted for 'children', and the sentence is correctly phrased in the future tense, which is implied from the code 'tomorrow'. The statement also correctly uses the conditional code as 'provided', and 'drive' and 'warm'.**

B Incorrect as it introduces the word 'difficult'.

C Incorrect as it is set in the past tense and introduces the word 'closed'.

D Incorrect as it ignores the words 'people, drive and tomorrow' and introduces 'cages'.

E Incorrect, as although it introduces 'animal safari', the sentence ignores the code for 'attribute (building, animals)'. Therefore it is not the best fit.

Question 6

Answer: D

13(D, O), L, 9(1, 2), 6

The code combines the words: plural (sky, building), build, ascend (antonym, decrease), future.

A Incorrect as it ignores the word plural as it describes only one 'skyscraper'.

B Incorrect as it ignores the word 'future'. It also ignores the word 'build'.

C Incorrect as it introduces the word 'workers' and ignores combining 'ascend (antonym, decrease)'.

D **Is the correct answer as it uses all the codes and the rules within the brackets. 'Plural' and '(sky, building)' are combined to imply 'the skyscrapers'. 'Ascend (antonym, decrease)' is combined to imply 'much taller'. The sentence is set in the future tense.**

E Incorrect as it introduces the word 'population' and does not combine 'ascend (antonym, decrease)'.

Question 7

Answer: A

L(13, O), 12(B, I, 13), 6

The code combines the words: build (plural, building), attribute (intelligent, people, plural), future.

A **Is the correct answer as it uses all the codes and the rules within the brackets. It is set in the future tense and combines 'attribute (intelligent, people, plural)' as 'many students'. In this context, 'build (plural, building)' is combined to mean 'new universities'.**

B Incorrect as it ignores the word 'future'. It also introduces the word 'exciting'.

C Incorrect as it ignores the code 'attribute (intelligent, people, plural)' and 'build (plural building)'. Also it introduces 'laboratory' and 'latest technology'.

D Incorrect as it ignores the code 'attribute (intelligent, people, plural)'.

E Incorrect as it ignores the word 'future' and introduces 'yesterday'.

Question 8

Answer: A

(12, K), J, 12(N), (R, S), (1, 6)

The code combines the words: (attribute, adventure), men, attribute (sword), (danger, animals), (antonym, future).

A **Is the correct answer as it uses all the codes and the rules within the brackets. It combines '(attribute, adventure)' as 'expedition'. 'Attribute (sword)' is combined to imply 'fight'. Although not explicitly mentioned in the code, 'lions, tigers and bears' is substituted for the code '(danger, animals)' and is the best fit. '(Antonym, future)' implies the past tense.**

B Incorrect as it ignores the codes for '(danger, animals)' and 'men'.

C Incorrect as it is set in the future tense and introduces the word 'terrain' and ignores 'men'.

D Incorrect as it ignores the code for '(danger, animals)' and introduces the word 'seas'.

E Incorrect as it ignores the code for '(danger, animals)'.

Question 9

Answer: E

I, 9 (12, P), 11, (C, T), F, H

The code combines the words: people, ascend (attribute, land), conditional, (wind, warm), star, tomorrow.

A Incorrect as it is set in the present tense and ignores the codes for 'tomorrow' and 'star'.

B Incorrect as it ignores the code '(wind, warm)'.

C Incorrect as it ignores combining 'wind' and 'warm'. It also ignores 'star' and introduces the words 'rain' and 'improve' which cannot be implied in any of the code.

D Incorrect as it is set in the past tense and ignores the codes for 'people' and 'conditional'.

E **Is the correct answer as it uses all the codes and the rules within the brackets. It is set in the future tense 'tomorrow' and substitutes 'people' for 'group' and combines 'ascend (attribute, land)' as 'climb the mountain'. The code for 'conditional' is implied in 'providing', while '(wind, warm)' are combined to form 'calm', and 'star' is replaced with 'sunny'.**

Question 10

Answer: D

(13, Q), (1, R), (12, O), C(1, T), 6

The code combines the words: (plural, plant), (antonym, danger), (attribute, building), wind (antonym, warm), future.

A Incorrect as it ignores the code 'wind (antonym, warm)'.

B Incorrect as it ignores the word 'future' and is set in the past tense. It also ignores the code '(attribute, building)' and '(antonym, danger)'.

C Incorrect as it is set in the present and introduces the words 'bad weather'.

D **Is the best answer as it uses all the codes and the rules within the brackets. It combines '(plural, plant)' as 'the plants' with '(attribute, building)' which implies 'the greenhouse'. 'Protect' is substituted for '(antonym, danger)' whilst 'wind' is combined with '(antonym, warm)' to mean 'cold wind'. The sentence introduces 'this winter' which, though not specifically mentioned in the code, is implied by the word 'future'.**

E Incorrect as it ignores the codes '(attribute, building)' and '(antonym, danger)'. Also, the statement introduces the word 'destructive'.

Question 11

Answer: A

I, (1, G), (R, S), 5, 10, (1, 3), 8

The code combines the words: people, (antonym, today), (danger, animals), negative, walk, (antonym, closed), present.

- A **Is the correct answer as it uses all the codes and the rules within the brackets. 'People' is substituted for 'tribe'. 'Open' is implied from the combined code '(antonym, closed)'. 'Night' is implied from '(antonym, today)' and '(danger, animals)' is combined to give 'predators'. The sentence is correctly set in the present tense.**
- B Incorrect as it introduces the word 'zoo' and ignores the codes '(antonym, today)', 'negative', 'walk', '(antonym, closed)'.
- C Incorrect as it ignores the codes 'negative', '(antonym, closed)' and 'walk'.
- D Incorrect as it ignores the words 'people', 'negative' and 'walk'.
- E Incorrect as it is set in the past tense and ignores several elements of the code.

Question 12

Answer: D

12(C, A), R, I, 12(13, O), (1, 6)

The code combines the words: attribute (wind, ocean), danger, people, attribute (plural, building), (antonym, future).

- A Incorrect as it introduces the words 'weather forecast predicts' and is set in the present tense.
- B Incorrect as it ignores the word 'danger'.
- C Incorrect as it does not combine 'plural' and 'building'. Also, 'people' has been ignored.
- D **Is the correct answer as it uses all of the words in the code. It correctly combines '(antonym, future)' to be set in the past tense. An attribute of 'wind' and 'ocean' is 'waves', while an attribute of '(plural, buildings)' is taken to imply 'homes'. 'Dangerous' is used in the correct tense and 'people' is correctly used.**
- E Incorrect as it ignores most of the code and combined words.

Question 13

Answers: B & C

8, J, (1, J), 7, 12(O, 13), 10(1, 6)

The code combines the words: present, men, (antonym, men), drive, attribute (building, plural), walk (antonym, future).

A Incorrect as it ignores the code '(antonym, men)' as well as 'attribute (building, plural)' and 'walk (antonym, future)'.

B Is a correct answer as it uses all the codes and the rules within the brackets. It uses 'nowadays' to suggest the present tense and combines '(antonym, men)' as 'women'. An attribute of '(building, plural)' in this context implies 'work'. 'Walk' is combined with 'antonym' and 'future' to imply 'in the past they walked'. 'Drive' is also used in the statement.

C Is also a correct answer. Although this sentence does not expressly state 'men and women', it instead uses the combined noun 'people'. In all other respects the rules in sentence B apply.

D Incorrect as it ignores the code '(antonym, future)', which should be combined with 'walk'. The statement also ignores combining 'attribute' with 'building' and 'plural'. It also introduces the word 'countryside'.

E Incorrect as it introduces the word 'congestion' and ignores the code '(antonym, future)'.

Question 14

Answer: D

(💣, I, 4), ✂, (10, ⌛), 8

The code combines the words: (young, people, singular), anxious, (walk, test), present.

A Is incorrect as it refers to plural children.

B Is incorrect as it is set in the past tense and ignores the combination of '(walk, test)'.

C Is incorrect as it is set in the past tense.

D Is the correct answer as it uses all the codes and the rules within the brackets. The statement combines '(young, people, singular)' as 'the toddler', 'anxious' is substituted for 'nervous' while '(walk, test)' implies 'attempting his first steps'. The sentence is correctly set in the present tense.

E Is incorrect as it ignores the words '(walk, test)'.

Question 15

Answer: B

💣(I, 4), ♌, K(E, F), 8

The code combines the words: young (people, singular), dream, adventure (planet, star), present.

A Is incorrect as it introduces the word 'fairytale' and ignores combining adventure '(planet, star)'.

B Is the correct answer as it uses all the codes and the rules within the brackets. 'The girl' is implied by combining 'young (people, singular)'; 'dreaming' replaces 'dream', while 'adventure (planet, star)' is substituted for 'astronaut' in this context. The statement is also set in the present tense.

C Is incorrect as it ignores 'adventure (planet, star)'.

D Is incorrect as it ignores the word 'young'.

E Is incorrect as it ignores the word 'present' and is set in the past tense.

Question 16

Answer: E

J, ☹, A, (T, G), ✋, (1, 6)

The code combines the words: men, possess, ocean, (warm, today), unwell, (antonym, future).

A Is incorrect as it is set in the present tense and ignores the code '(antonym, future)'.

B Incorrect as it ignores the code '(warm, today)' and also describes only one 'man'.

C Is incorrect as it ignores the word 'ocean'.

D Is incorrect as it ignores the words 'men', '(warm, today)' and is set in the present.

E Is the best answer as it uses all the codes and the rules within the brackets. '(Warm, today)' is combined to give 'warm weather'. 'Men' is substituted with 'them', 'seawater' is substituted for 'ocean' and 'unwell' is substituted for 'ill'. '(Antonym, future)' implies the past, which is the correct tense of the sentence. The code for 'possess' is understood as 'drink' in this context.

Question 17

Answer: A

(I, 4), ✂, 7, ⌛, 5(C), H

The code combines the words: (people, singular), anxious, drive, test, negative (wind), tomorrow.

A **Is the correct answer as it uses all the codes and the rules within the brackets. '(People, singular)' is taken to mean 'she', while 'anxious' is substituted for 'worried'. 'Negative (wind)' implies 'bad weather' while 'drive' is substituted for 'journey' and 'difficult' is another word for test.**
B Is incorrect as it introduces the word 'cancelled' and ignores the words 'anxious' and 'tomorrow'.
C Is incorrect as it introduces the word 'kite' and ignores the words 'anxious', 'drive', and 'tomorrow'. Also, the statement ignores combining '(people, singular)'.
D Is incorrect as it ignores the words 'tomorrow' and 'test'.
E Is incorrect as it ignores '(people, singular)' and uses 'they'.

Question 18

Answers: A & D

(✡, J), ✈, (O, 13), P, ☹, (1, 8)

The code combines the words: (brave, men), conquer, (building, plural), land, possess, (antonym, present).

A **Is the correct answer. It makes use of '(brave, men)' in 'the soldiers'. 'Possess' is substituted for 'captured' while '(building, plural)' is combined to give 'city'. 'Conquer' is similar to 'destroyed' and the sentence is set in the past tense: '(antonym, present)'. Although the sentence ignores the word 'land' it is the second best match.**
B Is incorrect as it does not mention buildings.
C Is incorrect as it ignores combining '(brave, men)', 'land' and 'possess'. Also, the statement introduces the word 'killed'.
D **Is also the correct answer as it is set in the past tense, which is implied by '(antonym, present)'. 'Warriors' derives from '(brave, men)' while '(building, plural)' is combined to give 'city'. 'Possess' is substituted for 'ruled'.**
E Is incorrect as it is set in the present tense and introduces 'leaving'.

Question 19

Answer: E

💣(4, J), (1, ✡), (1, ✈), (1, 6)

The code combines the words: young (singular, men), (antonym, brave), (antonym, conquer), (antonym, future).

A Is incorrect as it introduces the word 'warriors' and ignores combining 'young (singular, men)'.

B Is incorrect as it ignores combining 'young (singular, men)' and '(antonym, brave)'. Also, it is set in the present and not the past tense.

C Is incorrect as it ignores the word 'young'.

D Is incorrect as it introduces the words 'battle' and 'strong' and ignores combining '(antonym, brave)' and '(antonym, conquer)'.

E **Is the correct answer as it uses all the codes and the rules within the brackets. It correctly combines 'young, (singular, men)' to give 'the young man'. The antonym of 'conquer' is 'defeat', or in this context, 'captured'. 'Antonym (brave)' is combined to give 'cowardly'. The sentence is set in the past tense, as implied by '(antonym, future)'.**

Question 20

Answer: C

11, H, T(1, 2), (💣, I), A, (1, ✂)

The code combines the words: conditional, tomorrow, warm (antonym, decrease), (young, people), ocean, (antonym, anxious).

A Is incorrect as it ignores combining '(antonym, anxious)'.

B Is incorrect as it ignores the words 'conditional' and 'ocean'. Also the statement ignores combining 'warm (antonym, decrease)' and '(antonym, anxious)'. It also introduces the word 'busy'.

C **Is the correct answer as it uses all the codes and the rules within the brackets. The sentence is based on a condition, 'if'. 'Warmer' is implied from 'warm (antonym, decrease)', while '(antonym, anxious)' means 'relaxed'; '(young, people)' is combined to give 'teenagers'. The word 'ocean' is substituted for 'seaside'. 'Tomorrow' is also used.**

D Is incorrect as it ignores 'tomorrow' and ignores combining 'warm (antonym, decrease)' and '(antonym, anxious)'.

E Is incorrect as it introduces the word 'surfing' and ignores '(antonym, anxious)'.

Question 21

Answer: A

(9, F), P

The code combines the words: (ascend, star), land.

A **Is the best interpretation as it conveys the sentence in its simplest form. '(Ascend, star)' gives 'rising sun'.**
B Is incorrect as it introduces the word 'sky' unnecessarily.
C Is incorrect as it does not use the code to describe a star.
D Is incorrect as it introduces the code word for 'warm'.
E Is incorrect as it does not use the code word for 'land'.

Question 22

Answer: E

I(13, O), 3, (12, C), (1, 6)

The code combines the words: people (plural, building), closed, (attribute, wind), (antonym, future).
A Is incorrect as it introduces a code for 'future'.
B Is incorrect as it does not use brackets to give specific meaning to pairs of codes.
C Is incorrect as it introduces a code for the word 'brave'.
D Is incorrect as it does not use brackets to give specific meaning to the code 'attribute, wind'.
E **Is the correct answer. 'The shops' is implied by the code 'people (plural, building)'. 'Were closed' is in the past tense, which is implied by the code '(antonym, future)', while 'due to bad weather' is implied by the code '(attribute, wind)'.**

Question 23

Answer: D

12(💣, I), S, 12(Q, P), 8

The code combines the words: attribute (young, people), animals, attribute (plant, land), present.

A Is incorrect as it does not include a code to set it in the present tense.
B Is incorrect as it introduces a code for the word 'adventure'.
C Is incorrect as it does not include a code for the word 'animals'.

D **Is the correct answer: '(young, people)' suggests 'children' while combining this with the code for 'attribute' gives 'are playing'. 'Animals' is used directly, while 'in the garden' is implied from 'attribute (plant, land)'. The sentence is set in the present tense.**

E Is incorrect as it does not include appropriate use of brackets.

Question 24

Answer: B

(1, 💣), (J, 4), ♌, K(1, 💣), 8

The code combines the words: (antonym, young), (men, singular), dream, adventure (antonym, present), present.

A Is incorrect as it introduces the code for 'plural' with 'adventure' to imply more than one adventure.

B **Provides the best interpretation of the sentence. 'The old man' is implied by '(antonym, young)' and '(men, singular)'; '(antonym, young)' implies 'old' and is combined with 'adventure'. The sentence is set in the present tense.**

C Is incorrect as it does not include a code to describe the word 'old'.

D Is incorrect as it does not include a code to suggest the sentence is set in the present tense. Instead, the code for 'future' is used.

E Is incorrect as it does not include a code for 'old', '(antonym, young)'. It also combines 'antonym' and 'dream', which incorrectly implies a nightmare.

Question 25

Answer: D

(O, B, J), O, 6(I, ✋, O), 8

The code combines the words: (building, intelligent, men), building, future (people, unwell, building), present.

A Is incorrect as it does not include a code to describe the word 'new'.

B Is incorrect as it does not include a code for 'intelligent' and instead combines 'unwell' with 'men'.

C Is incorrect as it unnecessarily includes an extra code for the word 'land'.

D **Is the best interpretation as it combines '(building, intelligent, men)' to give 'the architects', the word 'building' is replaced with 'constructing', and 'future (people, unwell, building)' is combined to give 'a new hospital'. The sentence is correctly set in the present tense.**

E Is incorrect as although this code uses the same symbols as that of D, it does not use brackets to combine 'future (people, unwell, building)'. Without the use of brackets, 'new hospital' cannot be implied.

Question 26

Answer: E

(A, C, E), (1, L), (O, 13), P, (1, 8)

The code combines the words: (ocean, wind, planet), (antonym, build), (building, plural), land, (antonym, present).

A Is incorrect as it does not include a code to describe the word 'countryside' and is also set in the present tense.
B Is incorrect as it unnecessarily repeats the following code.
C Is incorrect as it does not use a code to describe the word 'destroyed' and instead introduces the code for 'conquer'.
D Is incorrect as it does not include brackets to give specific meanings for 'hurricane'.
E **Is the correct answer. 'The hurricane' is inferred from '(ocean, wind, planet)' while '(antonym, build)' implies 'destroyed'. 'City' is implied by combining '(building, plural)' and 'countryside' is used instead of the word 'land'. The sentence is also based in the past tense '(antonym, present)'.**

Question 27

Answer D

Y B (4,I) Q H E

The code combines the words: Brave, intelligent, (singular, people), conquer, planet, tomorrow,

A Incorrect as it ignores the words tomorrow and intelligent.
B Incorrect as it ignores the words person, brave and intelligent.
C Incorrect as it ignores the words planet, tomorrow and intelligent and introduces the word town and shoulders.
D **Is the correct answer as it uses all the codes and the rules within the brackets.**
E Incorrect as it ignores the word planet and tomorrow and introduces the word village.

Question 28

Answer E

A, I, 2, E, R, Q

The code combines the words Ocean, unwell, decreasing, planet, danger, plants

A This is incorrect as it does not use all of the words in the code and introduces rainfall.
B This is incorrect as it does not use all of the words in the code and introduces reference to rainforests.
C This is incorrect as it does not use all of the words in the code and introduces growth.
D This is incorrect as it does not use all of the words in the code and references landmass as decreasing.
E **This is the correct answer as it uses all of the words, or iterations of them, in the code.**

Situational Judgement answers and justifications

Scenario 1

1. **A very appropriate thing to do** – as the group leader this would be a very appropriate thing to do. Falsifying research data in any way is very unethical and a serious fitness to practice concern.
2. **Appropriate but not ideal** – it would not be inappropriate to seek the opinion of the other members of the group and would demonstrate good team working and communication skills. However as the leader of the group the most appropriate action is to address the matter directly with the individual falsifying the data.
3. **A very inappropriate thing to do** – clear communication in healthcare is key and posting a message on a person's social media page would not be conducive to remedying the situation in any way.
4. **A very inappropriate thing to do** – this is not addressing the situation in any way. As the team leader Alliaya needs to be assertive and address the situation so that the group member is made aware that this is not acceptable.

Scenario 2

1. **A very inappropriate thing to do** – the fact that the behaviour is impacting on the standard of care and therefore effecting patients means that taking no action would be a very inappropriate thing to do. The care of patients and anything impacting upon it must always be of primary concern to a healthcare professional.
2. **Appropriate but not ideal** – although this would not be inappropriate it would be more appropriate to speak to someone directly involved in the supervision of the medical student to air their concerns first to enable the issue to be resolved locally.
3. **A very inappropriate thing to do** – confronting the medical student in an aggressive manner would be a very inappropriate thing to do. Treating colleagues with dignity and respect is just as important as doing the same with patients.
4. **Appropriate but not ideal** – this would be appropriate to do however the ideal response would be to raise the matter with a senior.
5. **A very appropriate thing to do** – this would be an ideal response so that the situation is dealt with at a local level as soon as possible and no patients are put at risk.

Scenario 3

1. **Appropriate but not ideal** – leaving the party so as not to be associated with any drug taking would be an appropriate thing to do however it does not address the fact that a fellow student is taking illegal drugs which is a serious fitness to practice matter.
2. **A very appropriate thing to do** – seeking advice from his tutor would be a very appropriate thing to do as illegal drug use is a serious fitness to practice issue.
3. **Inappropriate but not awful** – although not completely inappropriate addressing the situation in this way is not a constructive approach to dealing with the situation.
4. **Appropriate but not ideal** – asking to speak to the fellow student to air concerns would be appropriate and certainly more appropriate that challenging them openly in front of other people.

Scenario 4

1. **A very inappropriate thing to do** – submitting an application containing model answers would be very inappropriate. This course of action would be dishonest and fraudulent and in direct odds with fitness to practice guidelines.
2. **Appropriate but not ideal** – although this would be an appropriate thing to do sources on the internet cannot always be trusted and there are far better ways to seek guidance and advice on preparing application forms such as from his supervisor.
3. **A very appropriate thing to do** – seeking guidance and advice from James supervisor would be very constructive in helping to compose his application form.
4. **A very inappropriate thing to do** – an application should always be completed by the individual applying and submitting an application that is not would be very unethical
5. **A very appropriate thing to do** – this would be a very appropriate thing to do to ensure there are no simple mistakes contained in the application form.

Scenario 5

1. **A very inappropriate thing to do** – the needs of a patient must always come first. The patient has made it clear that it is a daily injection and waiting until tomorrow to receive the injection could put the patient at serious risk.
2. **A very appropriate thing to do** – realising that the junior doctor would be acting outside of their competency and seeking assistance from someone who can give the injection would be a very appropriate course of action to take.
3. **Inappropriate but not awful** – simply instructing the patient to return to their bed with no offers of assurance that they will resolve the matter does not demonstrate good empathy and communication skills but would not result in serious harm to the patient if the matter is addressed subsequently.
4. **A very inappropriate thing to do** – acting outside of his competency is very dangerous and can put the welfare and safety of the patient at risk. This would be a very inappropriate course of action.
5. **Inappropriate but not awful** – ignoring the patient does not demonstrate good communication skills and empathy and is therefore inappropriate. However by ensuring another nurse attends to the patient will mean that the injection is administered.

Scenario 6

1. **A very appropriate thing to do** – seeking to understand the concerns of the patient and explaining to the patient that there is no evidence that taking medication reduces risk and refusing to prescribe would be a very appropriate course of action.
2. **A very inappropriate thing to do** – prescribing the medication for no medical need and against the evidence base would be a very inappropriate thing to do and could put the health of the patient at risk.
3. **Inappropriate but not awful** – although patients have the right to seek a second opinion in this case there is no basis that could change the outcome by seeing another GP based on the facts and could mislead the expectations of the patient.
4. **Appropriate but not ideal** – although this approach is direct it is appropriate but it would be better to seek to understand the patient's motivation for wanting the medication and allay any concerns he may have.

Scenario 7

1. **A very inappropriate thing to do** – creating the perception that patients must constantly provide gifts to healthcare professionals is unethical and not in the spirit of providing an unbiased standard of care to all.
2. **A very appropriate thing to do** – making it clear that the patient should not keep providing gifts would be a very appropriate course of action to take here.
3. **Appropriate but not ideal** – A donation to the practice's designated charity would be more appropriate. However it is important to remember that some elderly patients can be lonely and vulnerable. It is important to not make the patient feel as if she is expected to do this every time she attends the practice.

Scenario 8

1. **A very appropriate thing to do** – it is clear that there is no room at the residential for the patient to be transferred so it would be inappropriate to provide false hope that the patient will be transferred immediately.
2. **Inappropriate but not awful** – it would be better to take steps to establish the facts before troubling the on-call Consultant for a matter that is not life threatening.

3. **A very appropriate thing to do** – showing compassion to relatives and understanding their concerns is a key skill and providing a private room to do so away from the busy ward would be a very appropriate thing to do.

Scenario 9

1. **A very appropriate thing to do** – this course of action presents the facts that it may or may not be cancer and that further tests are require to ascertain.
2. **Appropriate but not ideal** – although showing compassion by being sensitive is important it is important not to draw premature conclusions without all of the facts and it is uncertain at this stage as to what the shadowing could be.
3. **A very inappropriate thing to do** – there is no basis to draw the conclusion that it is cancer at this stage and by taking this course of action it will create a great deal of unnecessary distress to the patient.

Scenario 10

1. **Appropriate but not ideal** – challenging the nurse as to why the fluids have not been started is appropriate however it would have better to have done this away from the ward and more importantly remedied the situation immediately.
2. **Appropriate but not ideal** – this would be an appropriate course of action although the ideal action would be to request the nurse begins the IV fluids immediately.

Scenario 11

1. **Very important** – accepting that a certain condition or situation will impact on an individual's ability to perform clinically is a very important factor to consider so as to not put patients at risk.
2. **Not important at all** – the fact that no one witnessed the accident has little bearing in how to address this situation.
3. **Important** – the effect of not being able to work to fund their studies is a longer term factor that must considered in order to ensure the wellbeing of the student.

Scenario 12

1. **Not important at all** – the fact that the junior doctor has a social engagement that they may be late for is of no significance in relation to remedying the situation.
2. **Of minor importance** – although this is of some consolation, regardless of what potential side effects it may have should not influence the immediate response to the situation and to ensure that the doctor learns from the experience to reduce the risk of it occurring again.
3. **Very important** – following hospital protocols and guidelines is very important and in this case recording medication errors helps to inform others to avoid similar errors occurring in the future.
4. **Important** –although not immediately related to remedying the current situation this is an important factor and should be raised with the junior doctor's supervisor.

Scenario 13

1. **Of minor importance** – the fact that the newly qualified dentist is going on holiday tomorrow is of minor importance as although this would not delay the need to report this matter immediately it may have some impact on availability for participating in the subsequent investigation into the matter.
2. **Not important at all** – the working relationship between the newly qualified dentist and the partner is of no importance at all in terms of the fact that observing the partner consuming alcohol in the workplace should be reported immediately.
3. **Very important** – performing clinically whist under the influence of alcohol is a serious fitness to practice issue and the partner must be prevented from potentially harming patients.
4. **Important** – although this is an important factor to consider in how best to report this matter there are other more senior individuals within the practice such as another partner that the incident can be reported to.

Scenario 14

1. **Very important** – the views of patients and how the behaviour and conduct of colleagues impacts on them is a very important factor to consider.
2. **Of minor importance** – although not of major importance this may have a bearing on the situation in terms of the facts not being truly represented.
3. **Important** – addressing this situation will require tact and empathy. Ensuring that a conversation around the dress of the fellow colleague is

conducted in a private manner away from the ward and constructively will ensure a positive outcome.

4. **Very important** – in any situation it is always important to establish the facts as the senior nurse's perception may differ to that of Carly's.

Scenario 15

1. **Very important** – ensuring that she is fit to practice and able to perform safely is very important and this should be her primary concern rather than completing the audit.
2. **Of minor importance** – although completing the audit is important putting her ability to practice safely is much more important.
3. **Important** – it is important to consider longer term that the audit will have a positive impact on the clinic but this must not be at the detriment of her ability to practice safely.

Scenario 16

1. **Very important** – being open and honest about what may be contributing to her failing to meet deadlines and be on time will empower her tutor to support her.
2. **Not important at all** – in this case whether or not other students are behaving the same way is irrelevant and she should focus on how she is going to address her own shortfalls.
3. **Very important**- accepting and following educational advice as part of a student's studies is vital to progressing successfully and failure to do so can lead to ejection from the course.

Scenario 17

1. **Of minor importance** – it is some consolation that the comments were not directed at the couple in question but this does not excuse the comments.
2. **Of minor importance** – discriminatory behaviour of any kind is unacceptable and although the nurse is one of the best on the ward and could be looked to as a role model for others, it does not excuse the comments.
3. **Important** – this is important to consider in how best to approach addressing the situation using good communication skills and avoiding a confrontation on the ward by conducting any discussion regarding the matter away from the ward.

Scenario 18

1. **Very important** – if a patient appears nervous then clear communication skills must be used to allay any fears the patient may have to put them at ease.
2. **Important** – although not directly related to the immediate problem of the very nervous patient the issue of the dental nurse not being fit for work and potentially passing on an illness to patients is of important consideration.
3. **Very important** – addressing the concerns of the patient and putting them at ease should be a priority in this case and the fact that the dentist does not appear to be doing so is an important factor to consider.
4. **Of minor importance** – although the impact of the surgery running late on other patients should be considered the most important factor in this situation is addressing the concerns and fears of the patient.

Scenario 19

1. **Of minor importance** – although this matter will need to be raised with the Consultant on his return it does not influence the immediate need to obtain the patient's consent for the scan.
2. **Of minor importance** – gaining consent is a critical in delivering high quality care. Ensuring that the matter is dealt with and corrected is the primary concern here.

Chapter 10

Entire mock UKCAT exam 2 questions

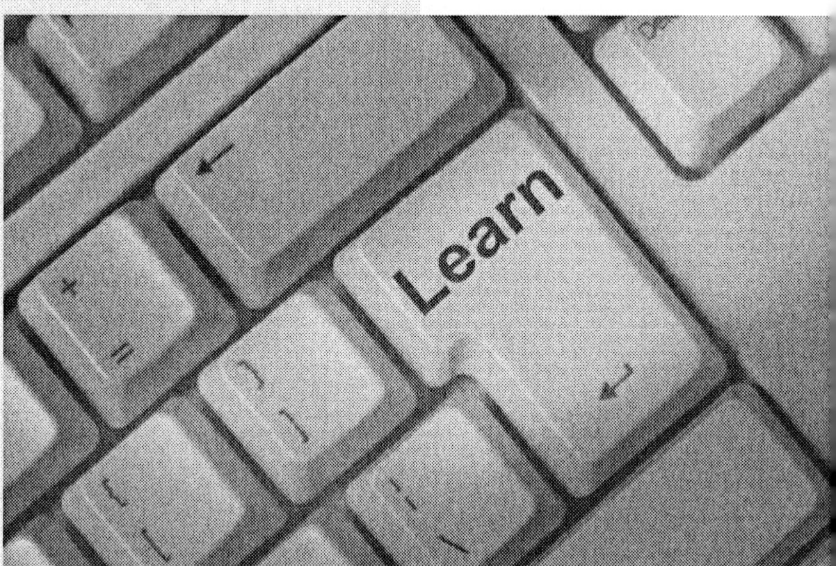

Entire mock UKCAT exam 2 questions

Verbal Reasoning – 22 minutes

Question 1

In December 1997, the idea for a commission for health improvement (CHI) was mooted in New Labour's first health policy white paper, *The New NHS*. It proposed an arm's length statutory body to 'monitor, assure and improve' clinical systems in NHS providers, with powers to intervene in failing trusts. In June 1998, yet another white paper, *A First Class Service – Quality in the NHS*, was published outlining further details of how CHI would work, including its role as a 'trouble-shooter'. By June 1999, the Health Act 1999 received Royal assent and CHI was created. Operations began in April 2000, and publications of the first routine clinical governance reviews were completed in December 2000.

Another landmark was August 2001, when Epsom and St Helier hospital's NHS trust was the subject of CHI's critical routine inspection report. It uncovered high death rates, 20-hour trolley waits, filthy toilets and patient complaints that took too long to resolve. The Trust Chief Executive became the first manager to resign directly as a result of a CHI report. In November 2001 the NHS reform bill was published.

This followed the recommendations of the July 2001 public inquiry into children's heart surgery at Bristol Royal Infirmary. The bill proposed new powers for an NHS inspectorate, including the ability to suspend services at failing trusts, to inspect private health facilities where NHS work was carried out and to publish an annual state-of-the-NHS report. In response to this the then chancellor, Gordon Brown, made a budget speech in April 2002, outlining a five-year 43% increase in NHS funding. He unveiled plans for a new super-inspectorate to keep track of NHS performance.

Subsequently the NHS Reform Act 2002 expanded the powers of CHI to include performance assessment of the NHS. This indicated that CHI would publish NHS star ratings in future. The performance ratings published by CHI in July 2003 (relating to 2002–3) covered all acute, specialist, ambulance and mental health Trusts – and all Primary Care Trusts (PCTs).

From *Succeeding in your Consultant Interview.*

1. **The NHS Reform Bill was published after the events that unfolded at the Royal Infirmary in Bristol.**
   A. True
   B. False
   C. Can't Tell

2. **The NHS Reform Act enabled the CHI to assess the performance of NHS organisations against five key criteria.**
   A. True
   B. False
   C. Can't Tell

3. **The passage indicates that the roles of the CHI include publishing a bi-annual performance report of the NHS and inspecting private healthcare providers.**
   A. True
   B. False
   C. Can't Tell

4. **The passage indicates that three key white papers influenced the set-up and future roles of the CHI.**
   A. True
   B. False
   C. Can't Tell

Question 2

Macroeconomics

Broadly, the objective of macroeconomic policies is to maximise the level of national income, providing economic growth to raise the utility and standard of living of participants in the economy. There are also a number of secondary objectives which are held to lead to the maximisation of income over the long run. While there are variations between the objectives of different national and international entities, most follow the ones detailed below:

1. **Sustainability** – a rate of growth which allows an increase in living standards without undue structural and environmental difficulties.
2. **Full employment** – where those who are able and willing to have a job can get one, given that there will be a certain amount of frictional, seasonal and structural unemployment (referred to as the natural rate of unemployment).
3. **Price stability** – when prices remain largely stable, and there is not rapid inflation or deflation. Price stability is not necessarily the

same as zero inflation, but instead steady levels of low-moderate inflation is often regarded as ideal. It is worth noting that prices of some goods and services often fall as a result of productivity improvements during periods of inflation, as inflation is only a measure of general price levels. However, inflation is a good measure of 'price stability'. Zero inflation is often undesirable in an economy.

4. **External Balance** – equilibrium in the Balance of payments without the use of artificial constraints. That is, the value of exports being roughly equal to the value of imports over the long run.
5. **Equitable distribution of income and wealth** – a fair share of the national 'cake', more equitable than would be in the case of an entirely free market.

http://en.wikibooks.org/wiki/Macroeconomics/Macroeconomic_Objectives.

1. **According to the passage Macroeconmics can be defined as:**
   A. The trading of shares on the open market
   B. How a government can guarantee a good quality of like for all.
   C. The approach taken by individuals to earn more money
   D. The measures adopted by a nation to improve income levels which will in turn improve the quality of life of those within the economy

2. **Which of the following statements best describes Price Stability as outlined in the passage:**
   A. When the price of items do not fluctuate significantly
   B. When inflation reaches a level of zero
   C. When pricing is increasing rapidly
   D. It is undesirable in a stable economy

3. **Most nations following the 5 principles outlined in the passage will:**
   A. Take measures to support those who are able or willing to work
   B. Raise taxes to combat zero inflation
   C. Embrace fully free markets to spread wealth
   D. Utilise artificial constraints to limit imports and exports

4. **Which of the following statements is true based on the passage:**
   A. A recession arise when inflation increases above 5%
   B. External balance takes into account both exports and imports
   C. Achieving sustainability results in an environment that is unpleasant to live in
   D. Steady inflation in an economy is damaging to a nation's growth

Question 3

Where the target population is particularly large, a sample of this would need to be extracted and audited. If, for example, the aim is to audit the management of hypertension in a district general hospital (DGH), it is likely that this would be too large an undertaking in itself. However, it may be a more practical and feasible option to audit the management of hypertension in a specific ward over a three-month period. By taking an appropriate subset of the population, the expectation is that generalisation will be possible, and that the results would give a good indication for those expected of the whole population. As an alternative, by taking a random sample of patients, one could also hope to achieve a representative result. Such random sampling may be carried out with the help of most statistical textbooks and a random numbers table, or alternatively using mathematical computer software.

Where random sampling is not a viable option, systematic samples can be employed. This technique involves the selection of units from an ordered sampling frame. For example if bookshop owners wanted to observe the buying habits of their customers, by using systematic sampling, they could choose every fifth or tenth customer entering the shop and conduct the study on this sample. However, if the audit is associated with a smaller population size, eg patients with pancreatic malignancy on the general surgical wards, it may well be possible to collect the relevant data from the complete population and, in so doing, provide an insight into a truer performance. A common example of sampling in use is at the time of an election. Here opinion polls are commonly constructed in an effort to select samples that are indicative of the population as a whole. The timing of sampling is critical. If a defined time period is not stated, there may be a huge discrepancy between the numbers and characteristics of patients involved during one set defined period compared with what you may expect at a different time of year. For example, if the prospective audit were based on the management and treatment of patients in a hospital presenting with pneumonia, you may be more likely to achieve a higher population over the winter months compared with what one would expect over summer.

From *Clinical Audit for Doctors.*

1. **One approach to random sampling is through the use of IT.**
   A. True
   B. False
   C. Can't Tell

2. **One way to manage a large target population in an audit is to sample over a period.**
   A. True
   B. False
   C. Can't Tell

3. **An opinion poll can be used to determine the opinion of a particular community.**
   A. True
   B. False
   C. Can't Tell

4. **Any statistical textbook will be able to assist an individual in random sampling.**
   A. True
   B. False
   C. Can't Tell

Question 4

The neurology of stuttering

This abnormal right-hemisphere activity has produced a variety of speculative hypotheses from researchers. According to one hypothesis, something is wrong with stutterers' left-brain speech areas, and so right-brain areas which are not developed for speech take over. This seems unlikely, given that most stutterers are capable of normal, fluent speech in certain conditions. In contrast, neurogenic speech disorders (resulting from head injuries, strokes, etc.) result in disordered speech under all conditions. Because stutterers sometimes speak fluently and sometimes stutter, it seems unlikely that stutterers have something wrong with their left-hemisphere speech areas.

Another hypothesis says that the right-hemisphere activity is the fears and anxieties that stutterers experience, generated by the limbic and paralimbic structures. But brain scans haven't shown these areas to be abnormally active during stuttering.

A third hypothesis suggests that stutterers' auditory processing underactivity reduces the left-brain communication of sensory information processed in the rear brain to frontal speech and language areas. The abnormal right-brain activity may be an alternative pathway for rear-brain sensory information to travel to the front of the brain.

http://en.wikibooks.org/wiki/Speech-Language_Pathology/Stuttering/Neurology_of_Stuttering

1. **Based on the passage which of the following statement is true:**
   A. Head injuries that cause neurogenic speech disorders result in disordered speech only some of the time
   B. It is clear what causes stuttering
   C. Multiple hypotheses have been proposed to explain why stuttering occurs
   D. Disruption of the thyroid can cause stuttering

2. **According to the passage it is unlikely the hypothesis of the right brain areas not being developed for speech taking over when there are problems with a stutterers' left brain speech areas because:**
   A. Those experiencing a stroke experience stuttering occasionally
   B. Stutterers do not experience stutter episodes all of the time
   C. Limbic structures are not active
   D. Sensory information is processed in rear brain

3. **According to the passage auditory processing underactivity in stutterers:**
   A. Increases Limbic and Paralimbic activity
   B. Reduces left brain information communication of sensory information
   C. Reduces right brain activity
   D. Increases left brain activity

4. **Based on the passage stuttering is caused by:**
   A. Defects in the brain
   B. Head injuries
   C. Disordered speech
   D. Strokes

Question 5

After the NHS Plan, the SHO position was scrutinised by Sir Liam Donaldson, the Chief Medical Officer (the most senior advisor to the government on health). His report, *Unfinished Business*, published in September 2002, signalled the beginning of the end of the SHO grade. It criticised the stand alone nature of over half of the posts, which forced SHOs to apply for new jobs every six months. It highlighted the lack of career guidance and the wide range in the quality of SHOs. The need to pass tough exams before becoming an SpR was leading to many SHOs not progressing as quickly as they would like, making the grade feel more like a detention camp than a desert island.

Perhaps the most significant part of *Unfinished Business*, however, was its advice regarding the Consultant grade. It argued that by the time doctors reach the level of Consultant, most are more specialised than they need to be to provide the services that the NHS needs. A more focused and structured junior doctor training programme was required to 'produce fully trained specialists with . . . skills more closely attuned to the current needs of the NHS'.

And so, the following year, MMC was launched. The first stage of the new career path, the Foundation Programme, launched in 2005. The next stage, Specialty Training was implemented in 2007 with the infamous Medical Training Application System (MTAS). The first doctors to achieve the end point of their training, the Certificate of Completion of Training (CCT), will begin to come through in the next couple of years.

From *Becoming a Doctor*.

1. **The main focus of the report *Unfinished Business* related to time spent at medical school.**
   A. True
   B. False
   C. Can't Tell

2. **The Foundation Programme has been running for over six years now.**
   A. True
   B. False
   C. Can't Tell

3. **The position of Senior House Officer became obsolete in September 2003.**
   A. True
   B. False
   C. Can't Tell

4. **Liam Donaldson was knighted in 2006.**
   A. True
   B. False
   C. Can't Tell

Question 6

Learning theories

Typical adult learning theories encompass the basic concepts of behavioural change and experience. From there, complexities begin to diverge specific theories and concepts in an eclectic barrage of inferences. Up until the 1950s basic definitions of learning were built around the idea of change in behaviour (Merriam and Caffarella, 1999). After this point more complexities were introduced "such as whether one needs to perform in order for learning to have occurred or whether all human behaviour is learned " (Merriam and Caffarella, 1999, p. 249).

Jean Piaget states that there are "four invariant stages of cognitive development that are age related" (Merriam & Caffarella, 1999, p. 139). According to the authors, Piaget contends that normal children will reach the final stage of development, which is the stage of formal operations, between the age of twelve and fifteen. As cited by Merriam and Caffarella (1999), Arlin (1975, 1984), established from the work of Gruber (1973)on the development of creative thought in adults, has attempted to identify a fifth stage of development, in addition to Piaget's formal operations. "She [Arlin] contends that formal thought actually consists of two distinct stages, not one, as Piaget proposed" (p. 141). Arlin (1975) proposes that Piaget's fourth stage, formal operations, be renamed the problem-solving stage. According to Merriam and Caffarella (1999), Arlin's hypothesised fifth stage was the problem-finding stage. This stage focuses on problem discovery. Though Arlin's proposed fifth stage produced more questions than answers, it opens the door to understanding the learning needs of adults; to be approached as thinkers.

http://en.wikibooks.org/wiki/Learning_Theories/Adult_Learning_Theories

1. **What conclusion can be drawn from the passage?**
   A. The 4th stage of can also be referred to as the 'bench-marking stage'
   B. Formal thought comprises of three stages
   C. A healthy individual should be fully developed by their 18th Birthday
   D. There are six stages of development

2. **Which of the following statements can be inferred from the passage:**
   A. Gruber built on the work of Arlin to develop a fifth stage of development
   B. Piaget developed the four invariant stage theory in the late 1800's
   C. Arlin first proposed in 1985 that the 4th stage proposed by Paiget should be split into 2 stages
   D. There is still much work to be done to explore the 5th Stage

3. **From the passage Learning Theories attempt to:**
   A. Attribute why individuals interact in social situations in a particular way
   B. Explain why adults commit crime
   C. Explain how human's develop physiologically
   D. Break down the progress of learning into stages

4. **It can be deduced from the passage that one of the following statements is False:**
   A. Piaget's theory was age related
   B. Arlin has contributed to the field of learning theories
   C. The identification of problems is not relevant
   D. The second half of the 20th century saw learning theories become more complicated

YOU ARE NOW OVER THE HALFWAY STAGE OF THIS SECTION. IDEALLY YOU SHOULD HAVE APPROXIMATELY 10 MINUTES LEFT.
(Please note this prompt will not be given in your actual test.)

Question 7

Psychiatry is the medical specialty that often arouses most curiosity in prospective doctors. Its reputation, after all, is laden with cultural myths. With its long heritage of colourful characters such as Freud, and coverage in the media and other cultural domains, preconceptions can fuel attitudes to it as a potential career path. While such views are still evident in society as a whole, they also continue in mainstream medicine. This can skew what advice or perspective you gain of psychiatry during medical school. Limited experience of dealing with mental illness and psychological distress means that many doctors are not skilled in dealing with the nuances of mental health problems.

Psychiatry in its most literal form is the study of the mind. However, much of the work of general psychiatrists deals with the assessment, treatment and long term management of individuals with what are termed 'severe and enduring' mental illnesses such as schizophrenia and bipolar disorder (previously known as manic depression). In the UK, to become a psychiatrist you must have been to medical school and completed your foundation year training. After this period, you are in a position to choose a specialty. It can seem a long time to wait before embarking on a specialty that is fundamentally different from other medical specialties. Why, you might ask, do I not train as a psychologist if I want to learn about the mind and deal with patients with pysychological difficulties?

This is valid question that you should ponder before you consider applying to medical school. It took me seven years from the start of medical school to start my psychiatric training. Could that time not have been better spent? The answer to this is that you are in a unique position if you have medical training behind you. It is then possible to integrate an understanding of psychology, psychotherapy and some of the other intellectual disciplines of psychiatry into the framework you have established over the preceding years.

From *Becoming a Doctor*.

1. **A psychiatrist does not necessarily need to attend medical school to become qualified.**
   A. True
   B. False
   C. Can't Tell

2. **Freud is responsible for formulating the theory of the unconscious mind.**
   A. True
   B. False
   C. Can't Tell

3. **Prospective psychiatrists gaining advice from doctors may receive information that is not necessarily accurate.**
   A. True
   B. False
   C. Can't Tell

4. **A psychologist may practise psychotherapy in some cases.**
   A. True
   B. False
   C. Can't Tell

Question 8

Scintillation Materials

Thallium-activated sodium iodide, NaI(Tl), is a crystalline material which is widely used for the detection of gamma-rays in scintillation detectors. Another crystalline material sodium-activated caesium iodide, CsI(Na), is widely used for X-ray detection in devices such as the X-ray image intensifier. Another one called calcium tungstate, CaWO4, has been widely used in X-ray cassettes although this substance has been replaced by other scintillators such as lanthanum oxybromide in many modern cassettes.

Some scintillation materials are activated with certain elements. What this means is that the base material has a small amount of the activation element present. The term doped is sometimes used instead of activated. This activating element is used to influence the wavelength (colour) of the light produced by the scintillator.

Silver-activated zinc sulphide is a scintillator in powder form and p-terphenyl in toluene is a liquid scintillator. The advantage of such forms of scintillators is that the radioactive material can be placed in close contact with the scintillating material. For example if a radioactive sample happened to be in liquid form we could mix it with a liquid scintillator so as to optimise the chances of detection of the emitted radiation and hence have a very sensitive detector.

A final example is p-terphenyl in polystyrene which is a scintillator in the form of a plastic. This form can be easily made into different shapes like most plastics and is therefore useful when detectors of particular shapes are required.

http://en.wikibooks.org/wiki/ Basic_Physics_of_Nuclear_Medicine/Scintillation_Detectors

1. **It can be inferred from the passage that:**
   A. The field of scintillators has advanced over the years
   B. All scintillation materials are activated with elements
   C. The use of plastic scintillators does not provide much flexibility
   D. NaI(TI) is a carbon material

2. **From the following which statement is correct:**
   A. Lanthanum oxybromide was present in the earliest X-ray cassettes
   B. Liquid scintillators are less accurate than those that measure solid samples
   C. Liquid scintillators provide very sensitive readings
   D. Silver activated zinc sulphide is a liquid scintillator that provides incredibly accurate readings

3. **Which of the following statements are supported by the passage:**
   A. X-Ray cassettes are a recent addition to the field of scintillation
   B. The use of P-terphenyl in polystyrene has enabled detection devices to be tailored to a particular design
   C. Doping in sport originates from the study of scintillation
   D. NMR imaging builds on the field of scintillation technology

4. **According to the passage some scintillation devices work by:**
   A. Activation occurs which alters the wavelength and it is this that is measured by the device
   B. Using the principles of Quantum Thermodynamics
   C. Immuno technology
   D. Radiowaves

Question 9

From the late 1980s onwards, concerns about the performance of the Bristol Paediatric Cardiothoracic Unit were increasingly expressed in a variety of contexts. Some of these concerns were from healthcare professionals working in the Unit, while others were expressed by individuals in a variety of contexts outside the Unit. Rumours were common, and some appeared in the form of unattributed reports in the media. An operation performed on Joshua Loveday on 12 January 1995 proved to be the catalyst for further action. Joshua died on the operating table, and an external review was instituted. Complaints were subsequently made to the GMC concerning the conduct of two cardiac surgeons and of the Chief Executive of the Trust. They were charged and found guilty in 1998 of serious professional misconduct by the GMC. A group of parents of children who had undergone cardiac surgery at the BRI organised themselves to provide mutual support. In June 1996 the group first called for a Public Inquiry into the Paediatric Cardiothoracic services at the BRI.

The Kennedy report was published by the Bristol Royal Infirmary Inquiry in July 2001. The remit was:

- To inquire into the management of the care of children receiving complex cardiac surgical services at the Bristol Royal Infirmary between 1984 and 1995 and relevant related issues.
- To make findings as to the adequacy of the services provided.
- To establish what action was taken both within and outside the hospital to deal with concerns raised about the surgery.
- To identify any failure to take appropriate action promptly.
- To reach conclusions from these events.
- To make recommendations which could help to secure high quality care across the NHS.

From *Succeeding in your Consultant Interview.*

1. **The GMC has the power to charge doctors with professional misconduct.**
   A. True
   B. False
   C. Can't Tell

2. **The aims for the Kennedy report included helping to improve the NHS as a whole.**
   A. True
   B. False
   C. Can't Tell

3. **The public enquiry was initiated by a parental support group.**
   A. True
   B. False
   C. Can't Tell

4. **The report investigated services provided at the Bristol Royal Infirmary during two different decades.**
   A. True
   B. False
   C. Can't Tell

Question 10

The aim of the Foundation Programme is to form a stepping stone between medical school and specialty training – it's a big step up, so that can only be a good thing! It's much more structured than the old pre-registration house officer (PRHO) position. For instance, you must complete various assessments and you have a supervisor who sets objectives with you and monitors your progress.

During this time, various clinical and non-clinical skills (or 'competencies') are assessed. This is done using four types of assessment: DOPS, mini-CEX, CBDs and mini-ePATs. **DOPS** stands for Directly Observed Procedural Skills. Examples include taking blood or inserting a catheter. A senior doctor will watch you and score you against certain criteria. A **mini-CEX** is a mini-Clinical Evaluation Exercise. It assesses doctor-patient interactions. Examples include taking a history or giving some bad news to a patient. Again, this is done on the ward with one of your seniors. **CBDs**, or Case Based Discussions, involve presenting a case and answering questions about the diagnosis and management. A **mini-ePAT**, or 360 degree assessment, looks at how well those who work with you think you're doing. They rate your ability across a range of skills including communication, timekeeping and attitude.

Each foundation year (FY1 and FY2) is divided into three or four blocks, known as 'firms'. FY1 jobs range from general medicine or surgery to ENT or renal medicine. FY2 jobs can also include A&E and general practice. On a day-to-day level, the job of a foundation year trainee is very similar to that of the old PRHO or SHO. FY1 doctors do many of the basic tasks that keep the firm ticking over. Most days start with a ward round, usually with a Registrar or Consultant. Your job is to know where all the patients are, write in their notes, and make a list of all the things that need doing for each patient that day – and then do them.

From *Becoming a Doctor*.

1. **The Foundation Year involves undertaking various assessments which include a 360-degree assessment, a clinical evaluation exercise and presenting cases while answering questions relating to the diagnosis and management.**
   A. True
   B. False
   C. Can't Tell

2. **The old PRHO position used to run for a period of 12 months.**
   A. True
   B. False
   C. Can't Tell

3. **One way an individual can be assessed during the Foundation Programme is to evaluate the way in which they record a patient's history.**
   A. True
   B. False
   C. Can't Tell

4. **The Foundation Programme comprises two years where individuals complete at least three different jobs during each year.**
   A. True
   B. False
   C. Can't Tell

Question 11

The PCTs receive 75% of the NHS budget. (The remainder of the monies are distributed to bodies and institutions, including arm's length bodies). For services which cannot be provided directly by the PCT, 'service level agreements' (SLAs) are arranged with providers; these arrangements deal with quantity and quality of provision, and are legally binding. Historically, hospitals were paid according to 'block contracts' – a fixed sum of money for a broadly specified service – or 'cost and volume' contracts which attempted to specify in more detail the activity and payment. But there was no incentive for providers to increase throughput, since they received no additional funding.

Subsequently the government, through the NHS Plan, signalled its intention to link the allocation of funds to hospitals to the activity they undertook. It stated that in order to get the best from extra resources there would need to be some differentiation between incentives for routine surgery and those for emergency admissions. Hospitals would be paid for the elective activity they undertook. This in theory offered the right incentives to reward good performance, to support sustainable reductions in waiting times for patients and to make the best use of available capacity. The aim of Payment by Results (PbR) would be to provide a transparent, rules based system for paying trusts. It would reward efficiency, support patient choice and diversity and encourage activity for sustainable waiting time reductions. Payment would be linked to activity and adjusted for case mix.

Importantly, this system would ensure a fair and consistent basis for hospital funding rather than being reliant principally on historic budgets and the negotiating skills of individual managers. Competition between providers would also be encouraged by this system.

From *Succeeding in your Consultant Interview*.

1. **Block contracts ensure consistency and fairness in funding of SLAs.**
   A. True
   B. False
   C. Can't Tell

2. **PbR stemmed from the NHS Plan.**
   A. True
   B. False
   C. Can't Tell

3. **Of the 25% NHS budget that goes towards SLAs, 18% is now allocated on a PbR basis.**
   A. True
   B. False
   C. Can't Tell

4. **One of the aims of PbRs is to reducing waiting times of patients.**
   A. True
   B. False
   C. Can't Tell

Quantitative Reasoning – 25 minutes

Here is a recipe for making chocolate biscuits for four people:

Weight	Ingredient
689 grams	Self-raising flour
100 grams	Sugar
124 grams	Margarine
256 grams	Chocolate

1. **Bars of chocolate are sold in 200 g blocks. How many bars would you need to buy to make biscuits for 11 people?**
   A 2 bars
   B 3 bars
   C 4 bars
   D 5 bars
   E 6 bars

2. **If 1,705 grams of margarine are used in the recipe, how many servings is this recipe now based on?**
   A 12
   B 45
   C 66
   D 56
   E 55

3. **What is the percentage content of sugar in the recipe? (Give your answer to 2 decimal places.)**
   A 8.55%
   B 8.14%
   C 85.5%
   D 11.25%
   E 0.85%

4. **What is the ratio of margarine to chocolate?**
   A 62:128
   B 1:64
   C 64:31
   D 31:64
   E 32:64

Ian is trying to change his diet. The recommended daily calorie intake for a man is 2,000 kcal. He is starting a weights programme, so he needs more protein, but wants to keep down his fat intake. Below is a table of the nutritional content of a selection of meats.

Per 100g	Fat (g)	Protein (g)	Calories (kcal)	Cholesterol (mg)	Iron (mg)	Vitamin B-12(mcg)
Bison	2.42	28.44	143	82	3.42	2.86
Beef (choice)	18.54	27.21	283	87	2.72	2.50
Beef (select)	8.09	29.89	201	86	2.99	2.64
Pork	9.66	29.27	212	86	1.10	0.75
Chicken (skinless)	7.41	28.93	190	89	1.21	0.33
Sockeye salmon	10.97	27.31	216	87	0.55	5.80

5. **What is the approximate ratio of fat to protein in pork?**
   A 3:2
   B 1:2
   C 4:2
   D 1:3
   E Can't tell

6. **Which meat has the best protein-to-calorie ratio?**
   A Bison
   B Beef (choice)
   C Pork
   D Chicken (skinless)
   E Sockeye salmon

7. **It is said that 1/5th of your daily calorie intake should be from meat. How much chicken does Ian have to eat to do this?**
   A 105 g
   B 300 g
   C 211 g
   D 330 g
   E 250 g

8. **What meat contains the most iron?**
   A Bison
   B Beef (choice)
   C Pork
   D Chicken (skinless)
   E Sockeye salmon

Below is a pie chart showing the sales of product Y by region. There is also a product X, which is worth 75% more than Y.

Sales of product Y by Region

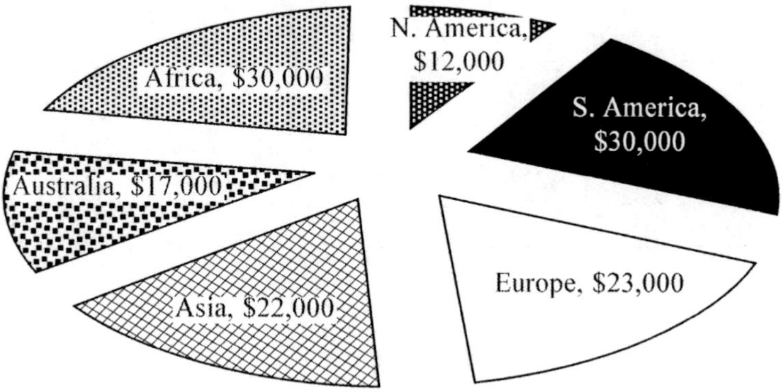

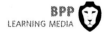

9. What fraction of the total sales are made in Asia and Australia?

A 2/7
B 3/8
C 4/11
D 1/2
E 1/4

10. What percentage of total sales are made in Asia and Australia?

A 41%
B 12%
C 35%
D 29%
E 24%

11. What is the average sales value for a region?

A $22,000
B $12,000
C $30,000
D $24,000
E $19,000

12. If product X sells as many units as Y in South America, what will be the value of the sales?

A $43,500
B $55,500
C $22,500
D $60,000
E $52,500

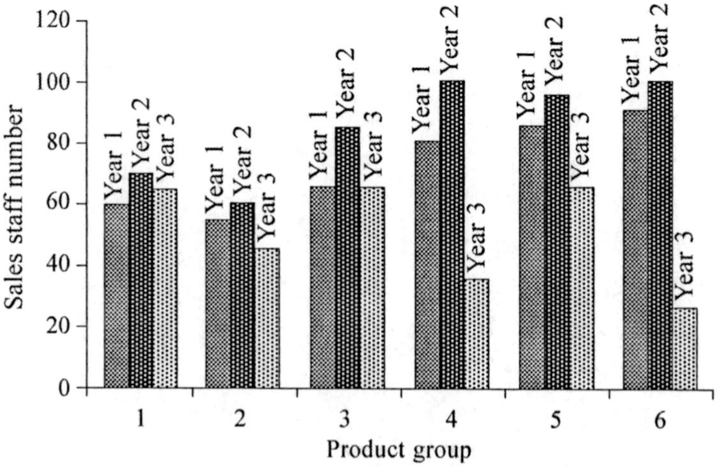

The graph above shows the number of sales staff in six different Product groups for years 1 – 3.

13. Which year had the greatest staff numbers?

A Year 3
B Year 2
C Year 1
D Can't tell
E Year 4

14. What was the total number of staff in Year 3?

A 200
B 300
C 350
D 240
E 500

15. What was the percentage decrease from Year 1 to Year 3, for the staff members in Product group 4?

A 33.7%
B 23.9%
C 39.13%
D 45.75%
E 56.25%

16. What is the mean for the total staff members in Year 1?

A 72.1
B 78.2
C 72.5
D 79.5
E 74.0

Washing machine brands	Wholesale price for a lot of 13 (£)	Recommended Retail Price (RRP) per unit (£)
A	6,789	732.13
B	7,685	699.29
C	8,786	875.85
D	8,790	723.12
E	9,009	932.45
F	5,789	678.92
G	9,843	923.40

17. A store buys 11 'Brand G' washing machines at the wholesale price and sells them all at the recommended retail price. How much profit did the store make?

A £1,838.29
B £1,828.90
C £1,768.90
D £1,828.75
E £1,829.60

18. A store sold 7 'Brand D' washing machines with 25% off the recommended retail price. What loss did the store make?

A £938.98
B £1,000.98
C £3,796.38
D £936.67
E £937.60

THIS IS THE HALFWAY STAGE OF THIS SECTION. IDEALLY YOU SHOULD HAVE APPROXIMATELY 11 MINUTES LEFT. (Please note this prompt will not be given in your actual test.)

19. By how much does the recommended retail price for 'Brand B' differ when compared to the wholesale price? Please give your answer as a percentage.

A 16%
B 18.3%
C 25.3%
D 15.3%
E 15.9%

20. If a 'Brand C' washing machine was sold at 5/8 of the recommended retail price, what is the price decrease expressed as a percentage?

A 30%
B 36%
C 47.5%
D 37%
E 37.5%

Here is a liquid measures equivalent table, and a recipe for a tomato cocktail. Lloyd wants to make the cocktail but needs some conversions done. Lloyd has 1 gallon of tomato juice to use.

American standard (cups & quarts)	American standard (ounces)	Metric (millilitres & litres)
2 tbsp	1 fl oz	30 ml
1/4 cup	2 fl oz	60 ml
1/2 cup	4 fl oz	125 ml
1 cup	8 fl oz	250 ml
1 1/2 cups	12 fl oz	375 ml
2 cups or 1 pint	16 fl oz	500 ml
4 cups or 1 quart	32 fl oz	1,000 ml or 1 litre
1 gallon	128 fl oz	4 litres

Tomato cocktail recipe

- 4 cups tomato juice
- 5 fluid ounces of lemon juice
- 60 ml Worchester sauce
- 2 tablespoons Tabasco

21. How many tablespoons of Worchester sauce are needed?

A 2
B 1/4
C 3
D 4
E 1

22. What is the ratio of Worchester sauce to Tabasco?

A 2:1
B 3:1
C 1:2
D 1:3
E 2:2

23. How many times could Lloyd perform this recipe with his 1 gallon of tomato juice?

A 1 time
B 2 times
C 3 times
D 4 times
E 5 times

24. How many cups is the complete recipe in total?

A 3
B 4
C 5
D 6
E 7

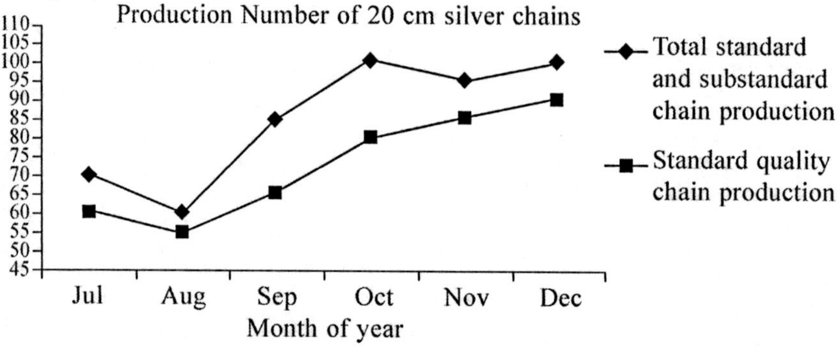

The graph shows the total number of silver chains and the proportion of silver chains that were of standard quality. Sales price for standard quality chains is £5.70 per 100. Sales price for substandard chains is £2.85 per 100.

25. What percentage of the total chain production was classed as substandard in September?

A 13.5%
B 16.5%
C 17.5%
D 22.0 %
E 23.5%

26. By how much did the total sales value of November's chain production vary from October?

A Decrease of £0.1425
B Decrease of £1,425.00
C Increase of £25.00
D No change
E Increase of £5.00

27. What is the ratio of substandard to standard chains in October (in its simplest form)?

A 80:20
B 20:80
C 2:8
D 8:2
E 1:4

28. What was the percentage of substandard chains produced in July?

A 15.28
B 14.39
C 14.19
D 12.89
E 14.29

Below is a straight line graph. The standard equation for a straight line graph is: y = mx + c, where m is the gradient and c is the y intercept.

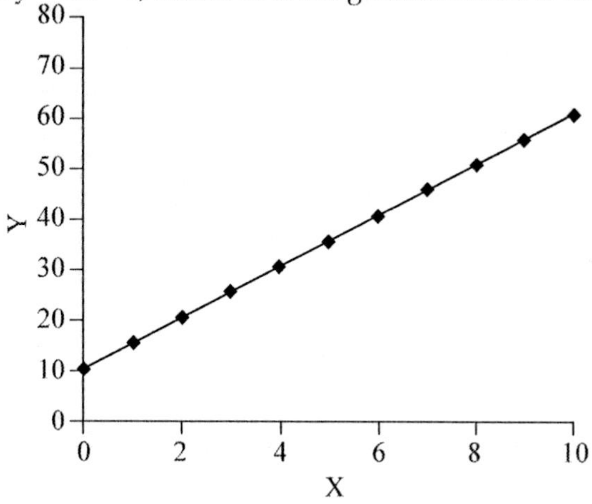

29. From the graph, what is the value of c?

A Can't tell
B 20
C 5
D 15
E 10

30. What is the gradient (m) of the graph?

A Can't tell
B 20
C 5
D 15
E 10

31. Using the formula: if y = 3, m = 2 and c = 0, what is the value of x?

A 0.5
B 1.5
C 2
D 3
E 1

32. Using the formula: if y = 9, x = 12 and c = 3, what is the value of m?

A 0.5
B 1.5
C 2
D 3
E 1

Country/currency	Rate of exchange
USA – US Dollar	1.29 USD = £1.00
Afghanistan – Afghani	2.98 AFA = £1.00
Cuban – Cuban Peso	213 CUP = £1.00
Bangladesh – Taka	2.4 BDT = £1.00
Bulgaria – Lev	21 BGL = £1.00

33. How many Bulgarian Levs are you able to exchange for £45.00?

A 678.00 Levs
B 945.00 Levs
C 4,521.00 Levs
D 1,000 Levs
E 950 Levs

34. How much is 677 Bangladeshi Takas worth in Pounds Sterling?

A £1,624.80
B £1,367.00
C £200.00
D £282.10
E £277.92

35. If the exchange rate for the Cuban Peso increases by 10%, how many Cuban Pesos (CUPs) would you need to make £45.00?

A 234 CUPs
B 456 CUPs
C 105.43 CUPs
D 1,054.3 CUPs
E 10,543.5 CUPs

36. A traveller exchanges 6,790.00 French Francs for £1,900.00. What is the exchange rate (to one decimal place)?

A 2.2
B 6.1
C 3.6
D 3.0
E 0.3

Abstract Reasoning – 14 minutes

Question 1

Set A

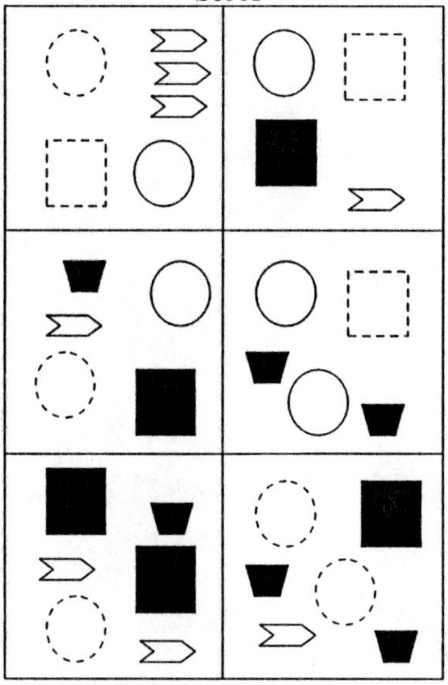

Set B

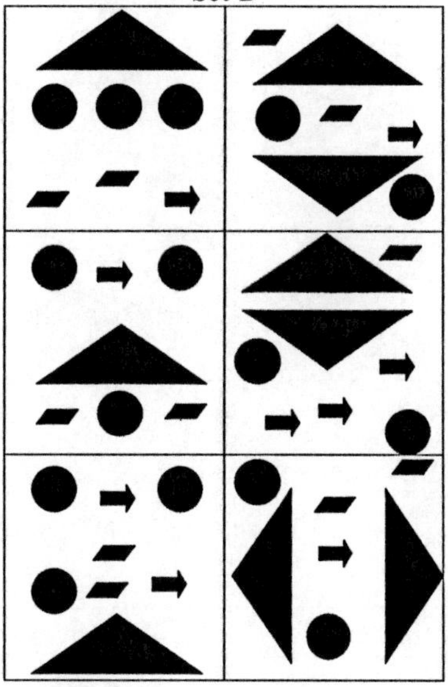

Test Shape 1

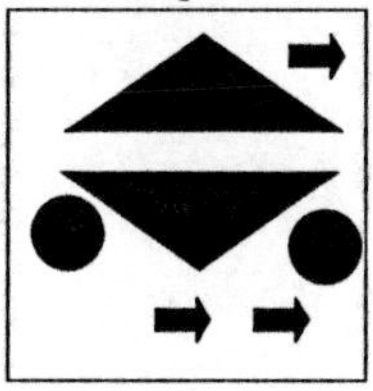

Set A

Set B

Neither

Test Shape 2

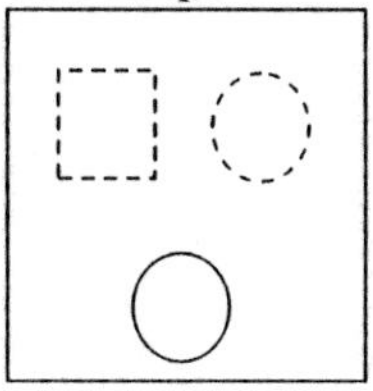

Set A

Set B

Neither

Test Shape 3

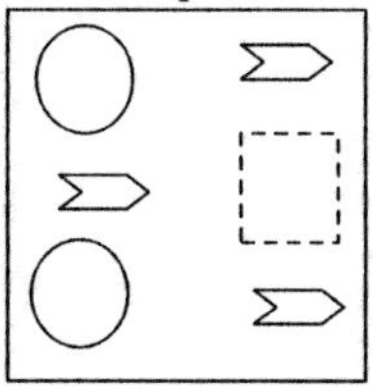

Set A

Set B

Neither

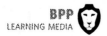

Test Shape 4

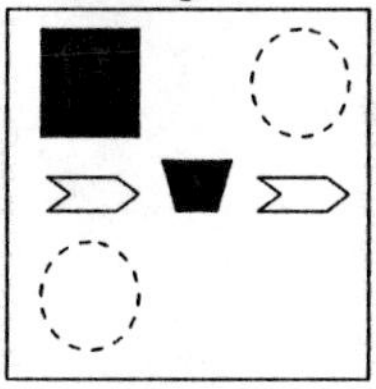

Set A

Set B

Neither

Test Shape 5

Set A

Set B

Neither

Question 2

Set A

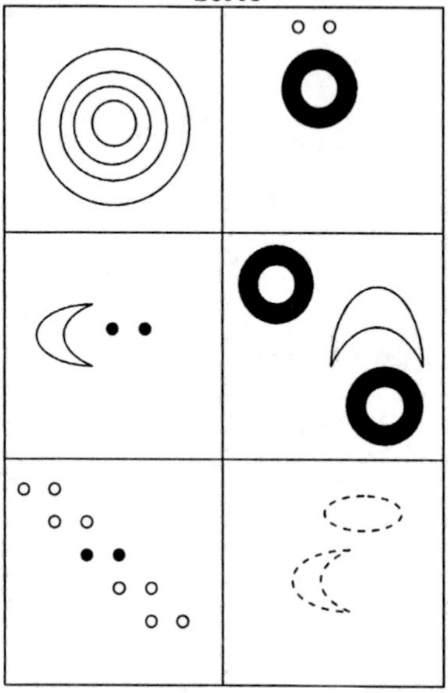

Set B

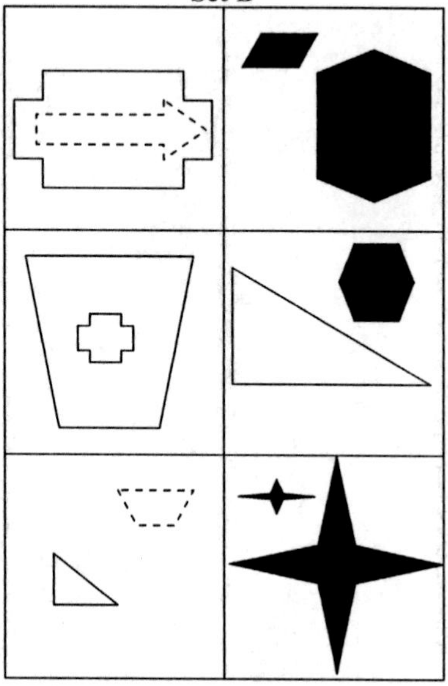

Test Shape 1

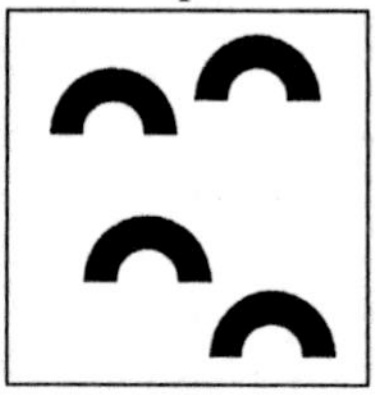

Set A

Set B

Neither

Test Shape 2

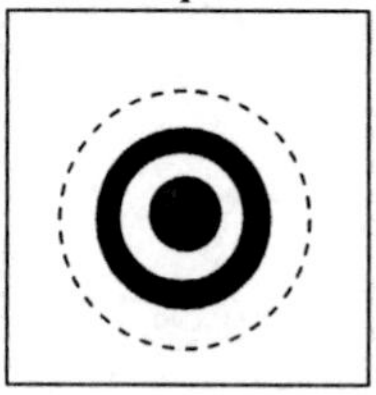

Set A

Set B

Neither

Test Shape 3

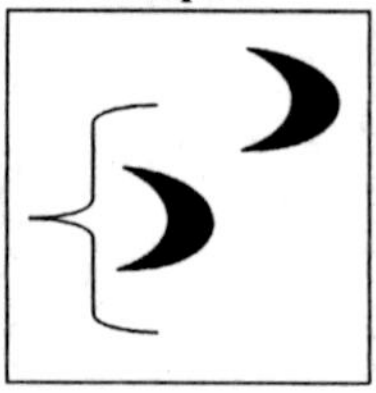

Set A

Set B

Neither

Test Shape 4

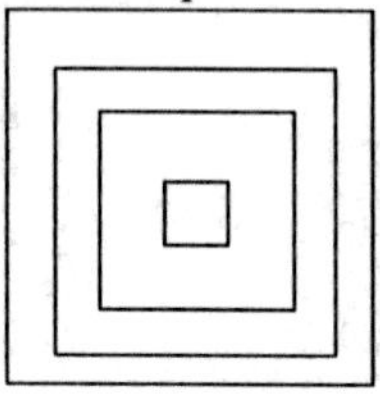

Set A

Set B

Neither

Test Shape 5

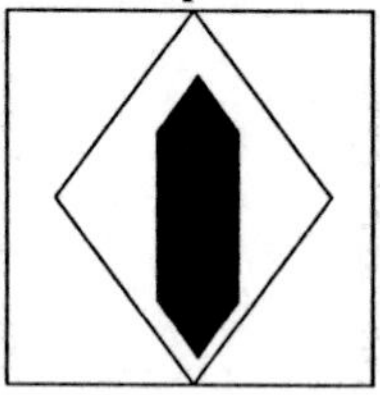

Set A

Set B

Neither

Question 3

Set A

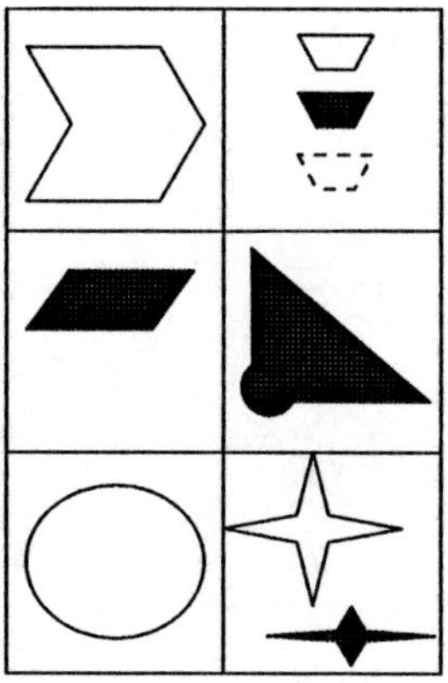

Set B

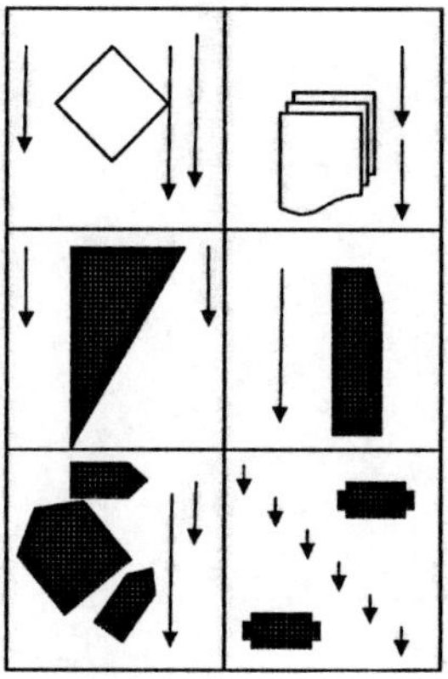

1. Which of the following belong to Set A?

A

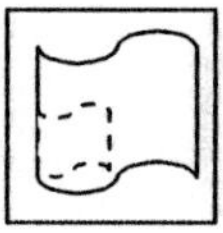

B

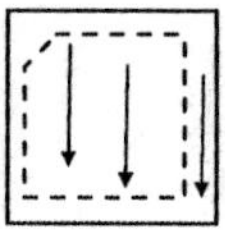

C

D

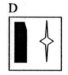

2. Which of the following belong to Set A?

A

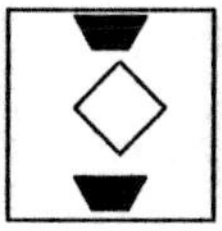

B

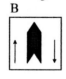

C

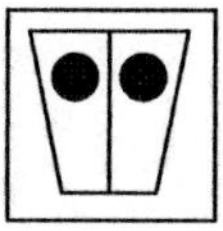

D

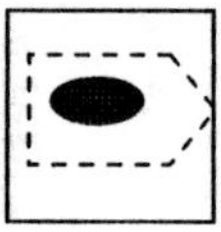

3. Which of the following belong to Set B?

A

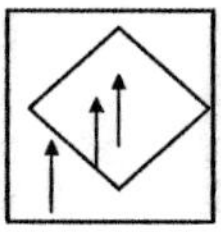

B

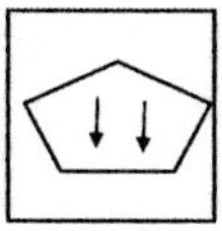

C

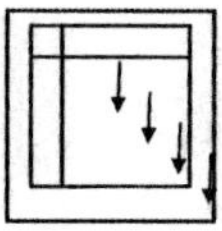

D

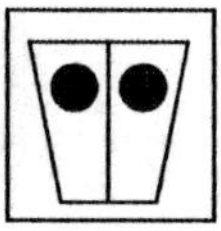

4. Which of the following belong to Set B?

A

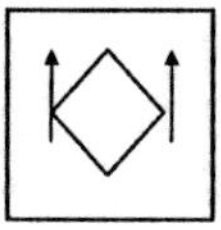

B

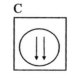

C

D

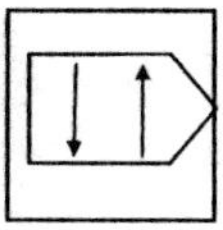

5. Which of the following belong to Set B?

A

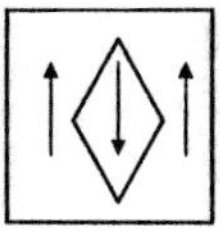

B

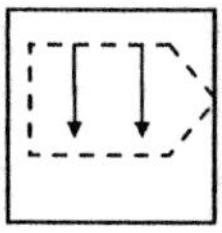

C

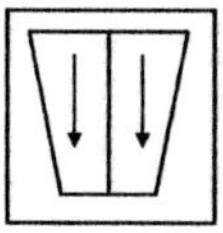

D

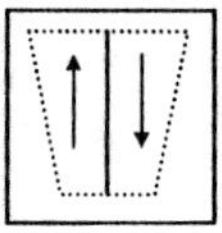

Question 4

Set A

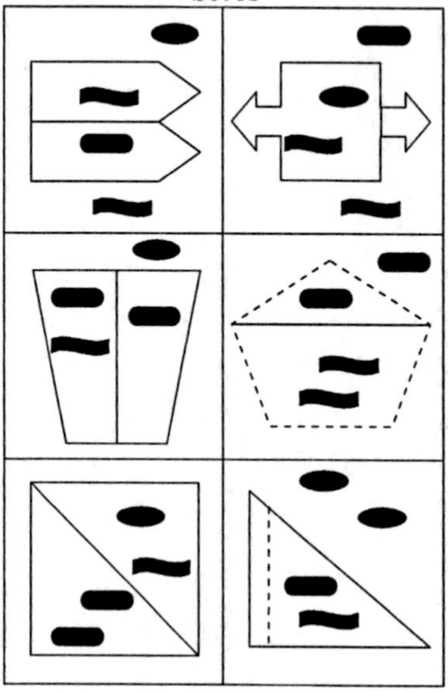

Set B

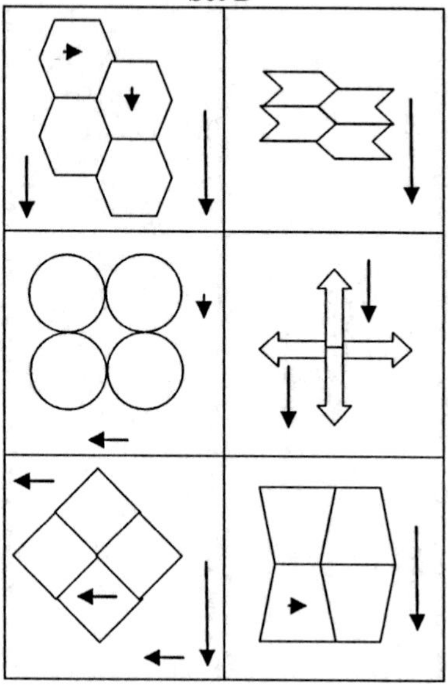

Test Shape 1

Set A

Set B

Neither

Test Shape 2

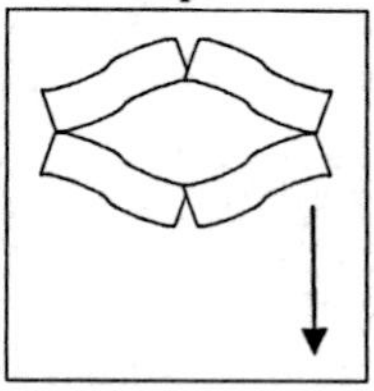

Set A

Set B

Neither

Test Shape 3

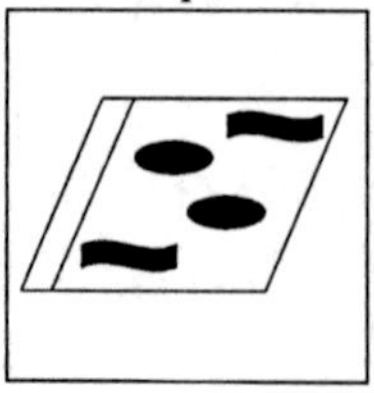

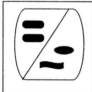

Set A

Set B

Neither

Test Shape 4

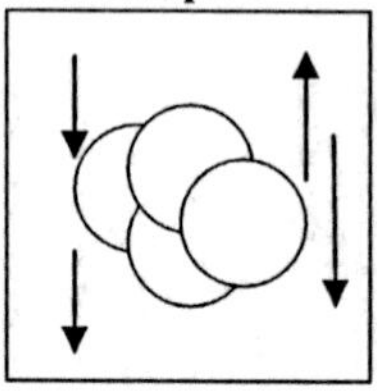

Set A

Set B

Neither

Test Shape 5

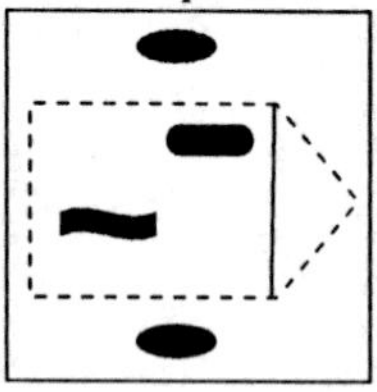

Set A

Set B

Neither

Question 5

Set A **Set B**

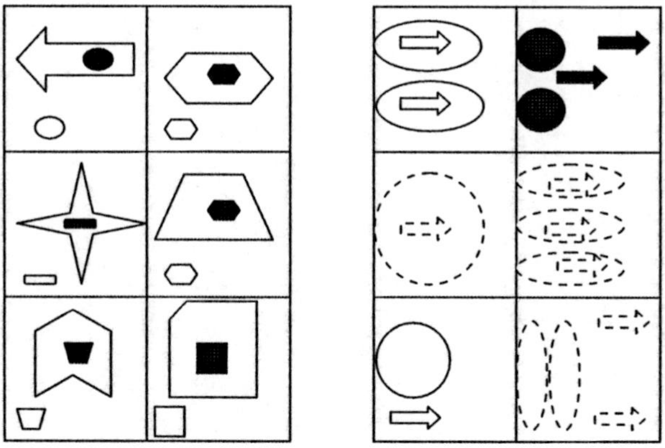

1. Which of the following belong to Set A?

A B C D

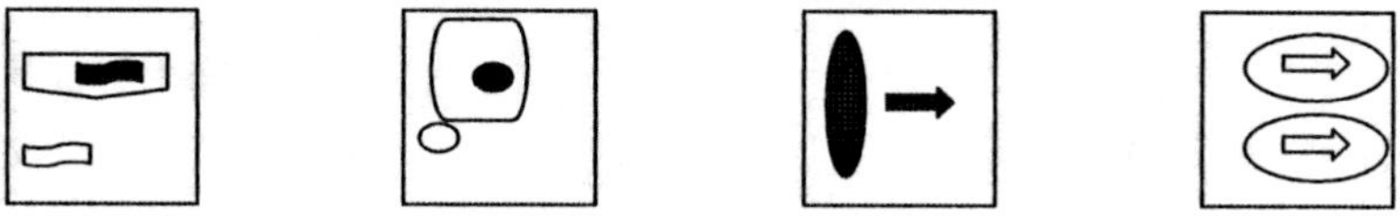

2. Which of the following belong to Set A?

A B C D

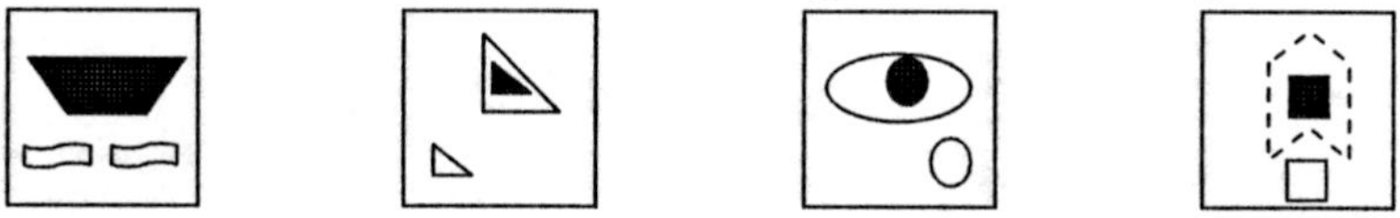

3. Which of the following belong to Set A?

A B C D

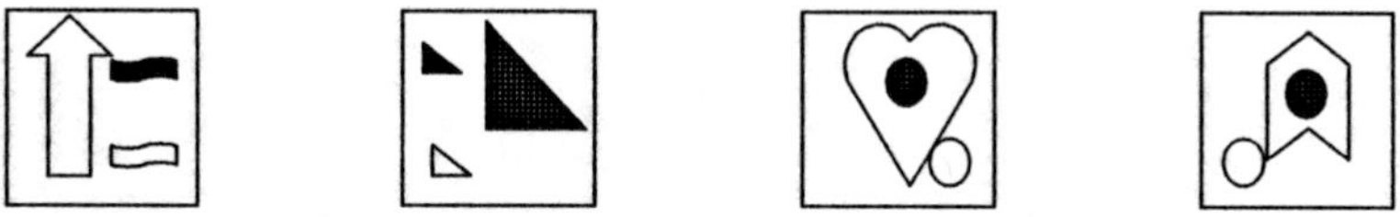

4. Which of the following belong to Set B?

A B C D

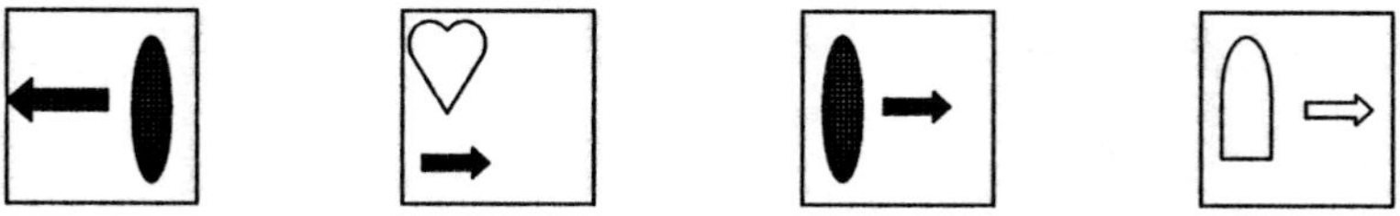

5. Which of the following belong to Set B?

A B C D

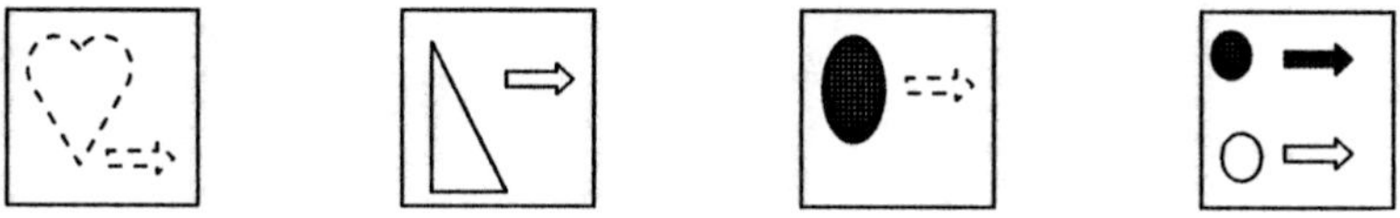

Question 6

Set A

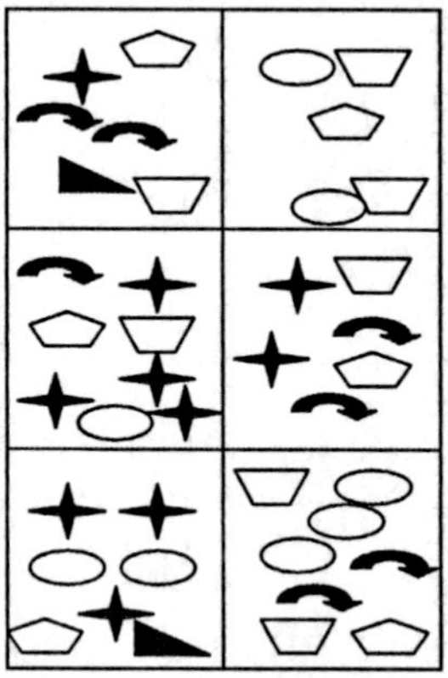

Set B

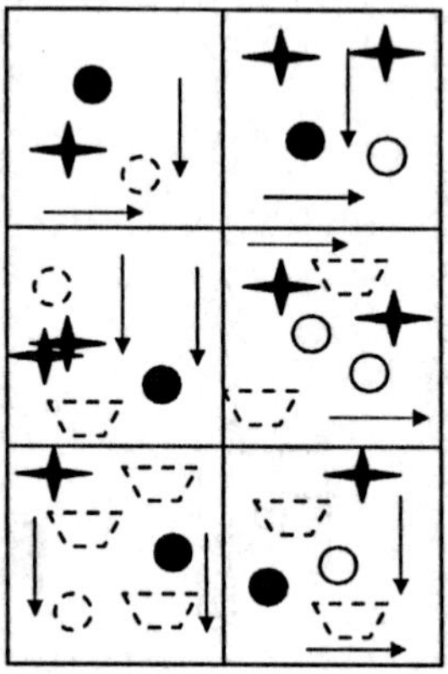

1. Which of the following belong to Set A?

A B C D

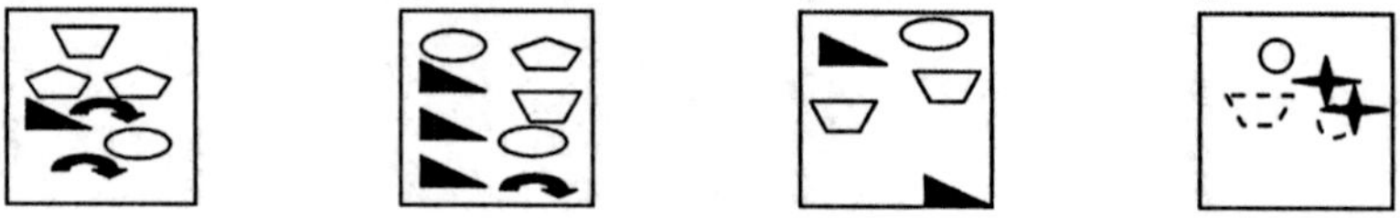

2. Which of the following belong to Set A?

A B C D

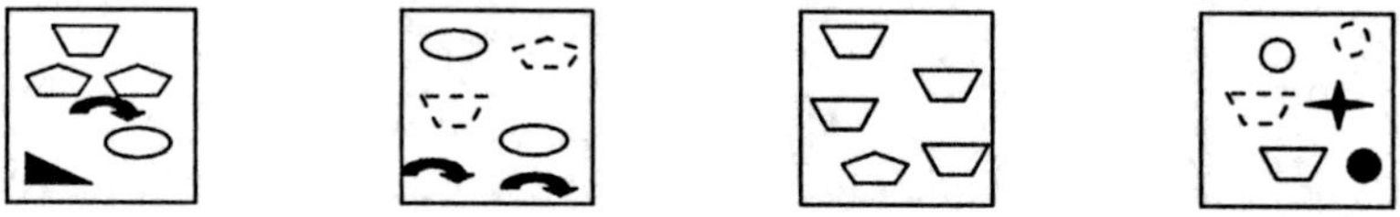

3. Which of the following belong to Set B?

A B C D

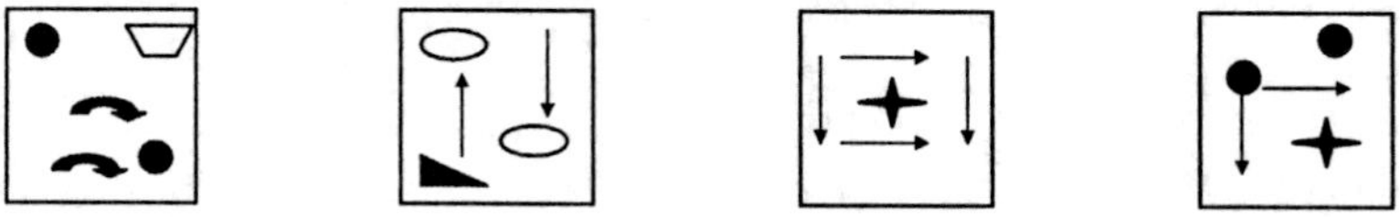

4. Which of the following belong to Set B?

A B C D

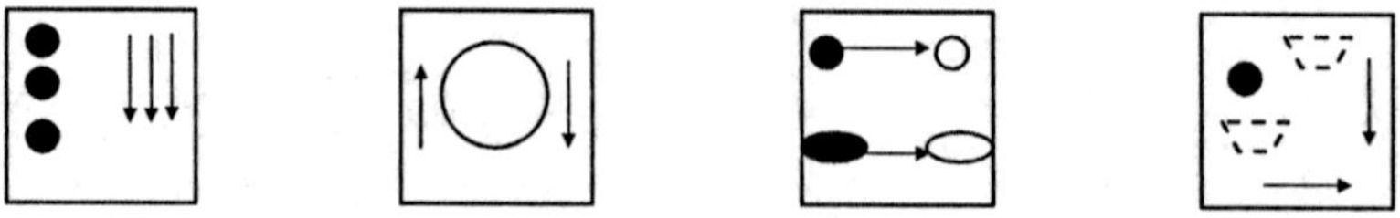

5. Which of the following belong to Set B?

A B C D

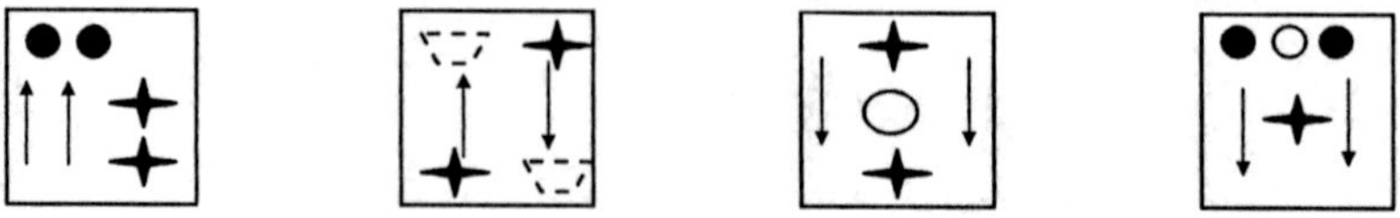

Question 7

Set A

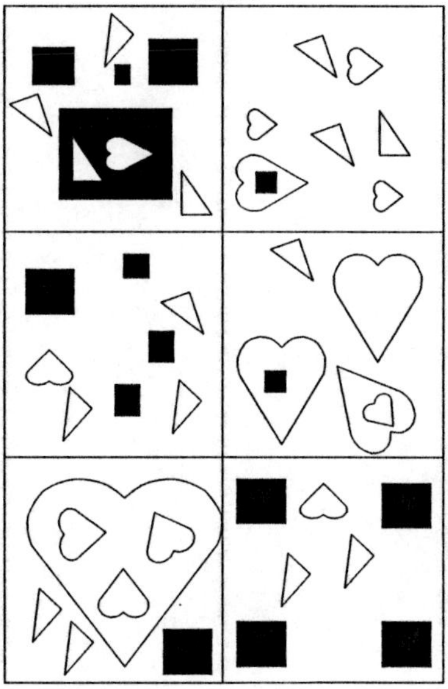

Set B

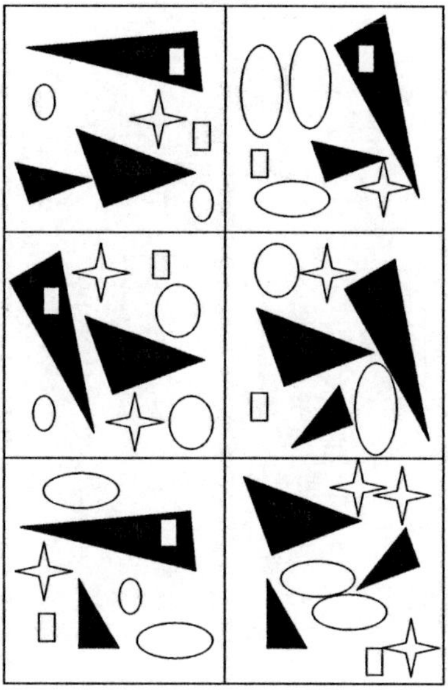

Test Shape 1

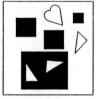

Set A

Set B

Neither

Test Shape 2

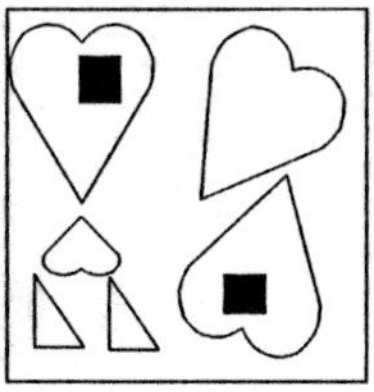

Set A

Set B

Neither

Test Shape 3

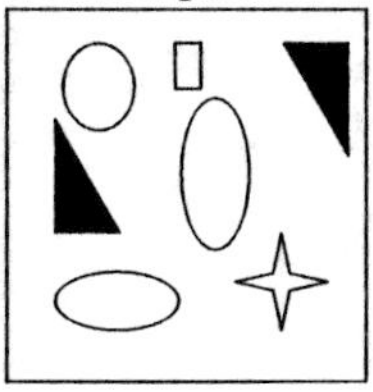

Set A

Set B

Neither

Test Shape 4

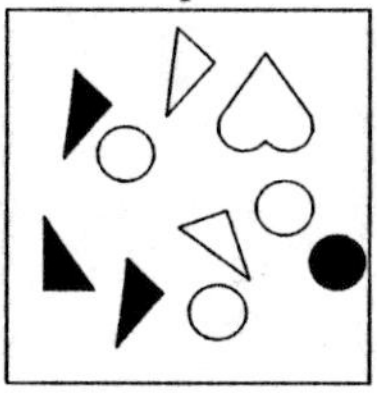

Set A

Set B

Neither

Test Shape 5

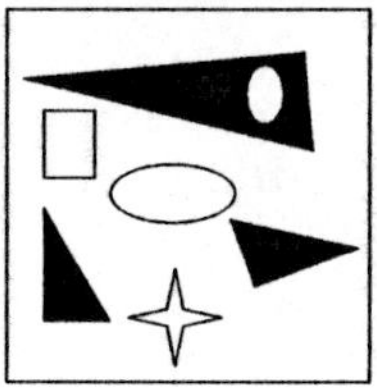

Set A

Set B

Neither

YOU ARE NOW OVER THE HALFWAY STAGE OF THIS SECTION. IDEALLY YOU SHOULD HAVE APPROXIMATELY 7 MINUTES LEFT. (Please note this prompt will not be given in your actual test.)

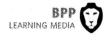

Question 8

Set A

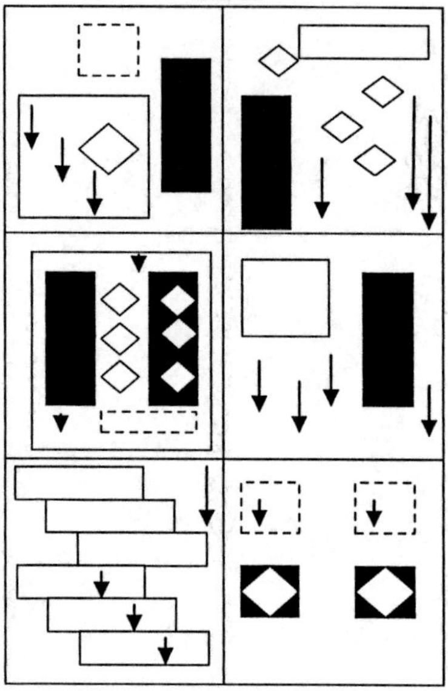

Set B

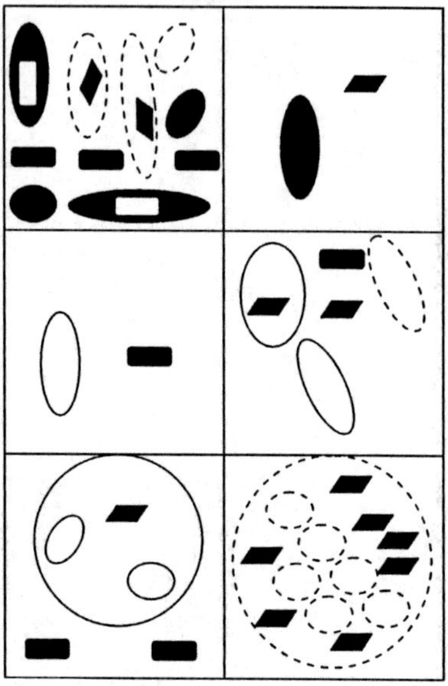

Test Shape 1

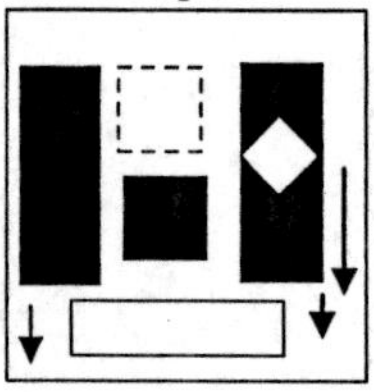

Set A

Set B

Neither

Test Shape 2

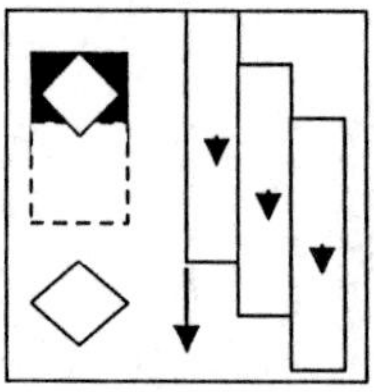

Set A

Set B

Neither

Test Shape 3

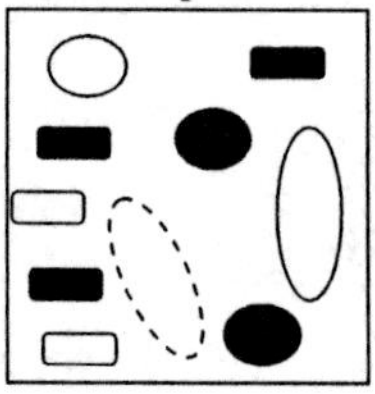

Set A

Set B

Neither

Test Shape 4

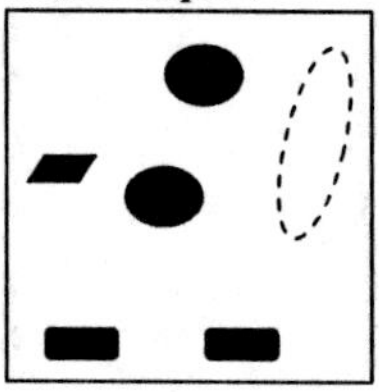

Set A

Set B

Neither

Test Shape 5

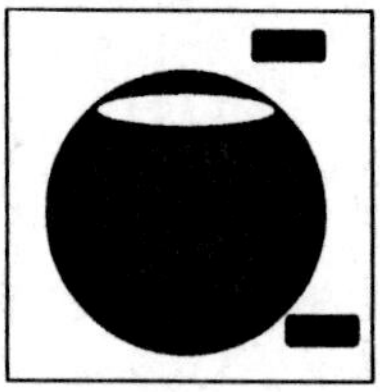

Set A

Set B

Neither

Question 9

Set A

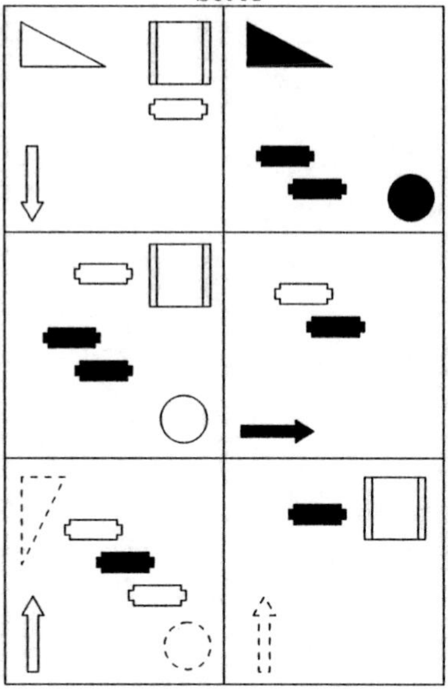

Set B

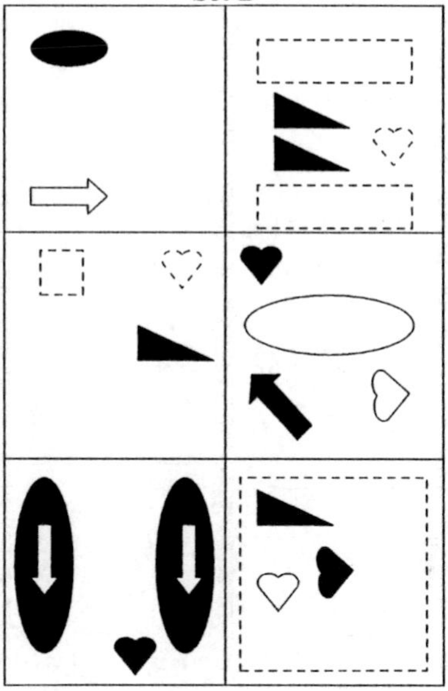

Test Shape 1

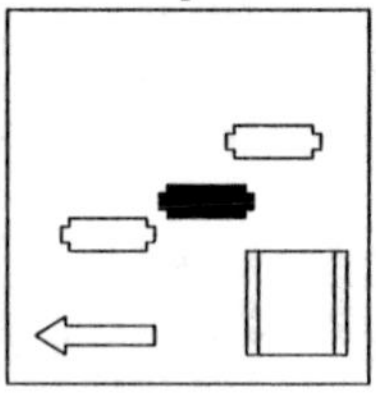

Set A

Set B

Neither

Test Shape 2

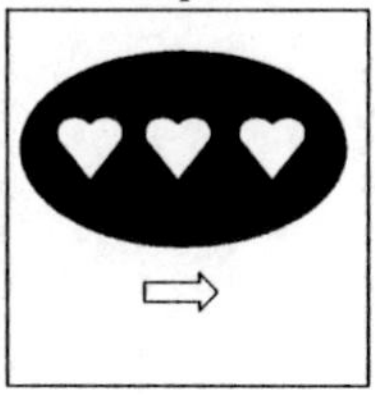

Set A

Set B

Neither

Test Shape 3

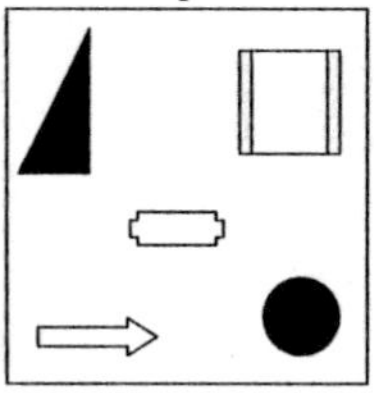

Set A

Set B

Neither

Test Shape 4

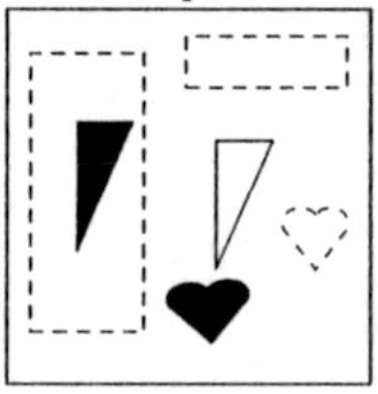

Set A

Set B

Neither

Test Shape 5

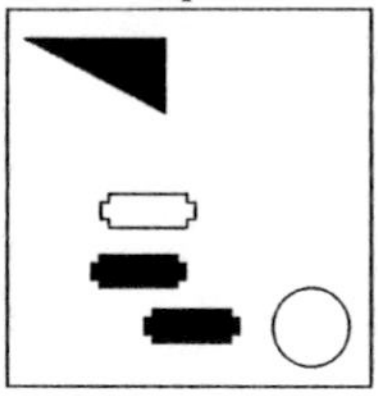

Set A

Set B

Neither

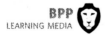

Question 10

Set A

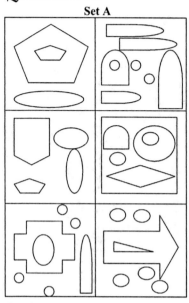

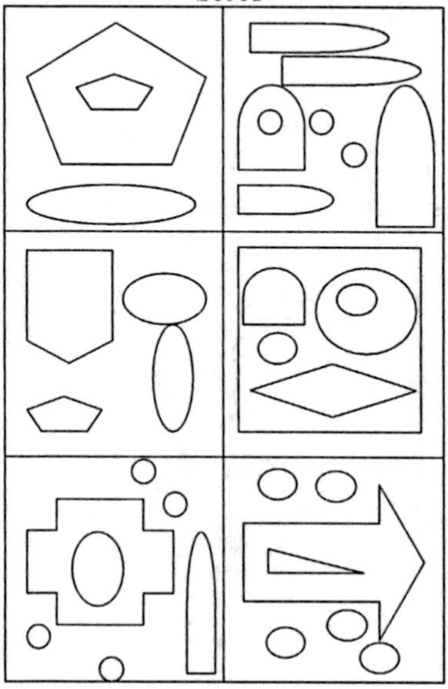

Set B

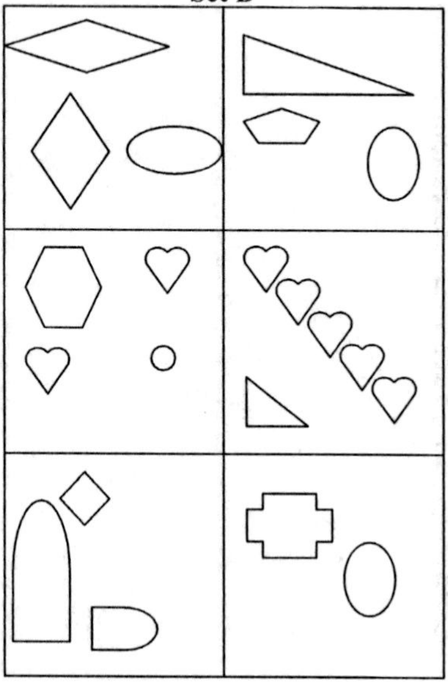

Test Shape 1

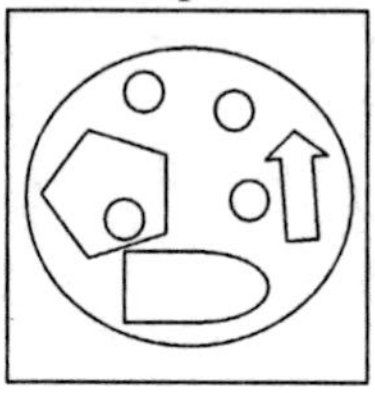

Set A

Set B

Neither

Test Shape 2

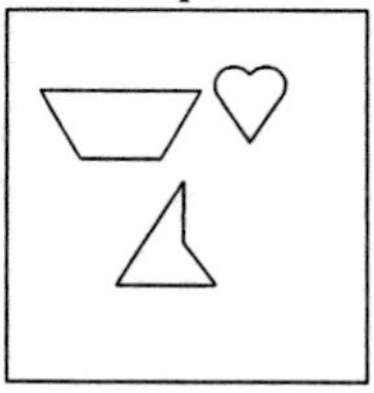

Set A

Set B

Neither

Test Shape 3

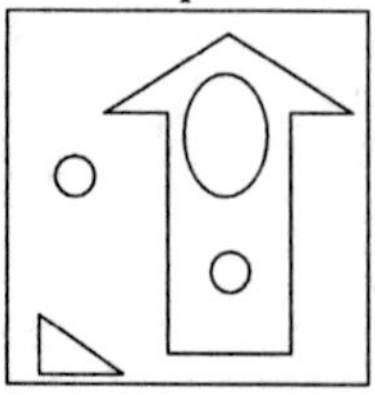

Set A

Set B

Neither

Test Shape 4

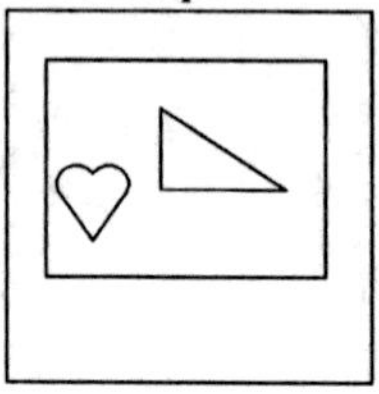

Set A

Set B

Neither

Test Shape 5

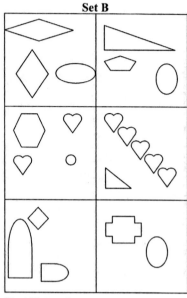

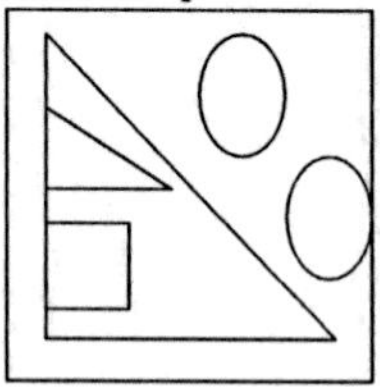

Set A

Set B

Neither

Question 11

Set A

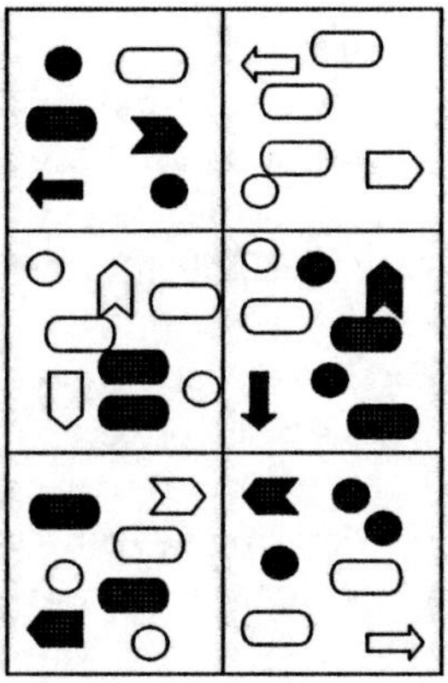

Set B

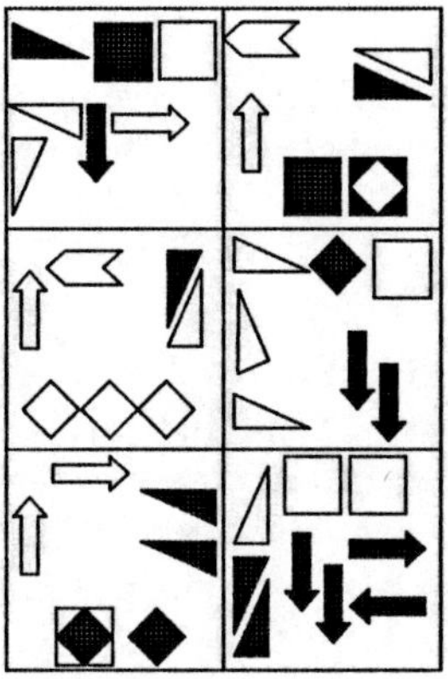

1. Which of the following belong to Set A?

A

B

C

D

2. Which of the following belong to Set A?

A
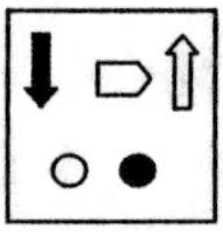
B

C
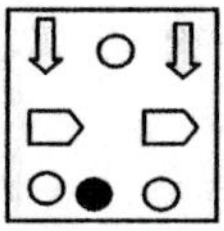
D
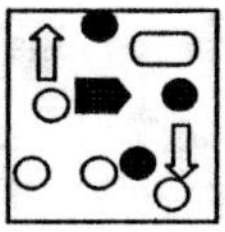

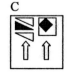

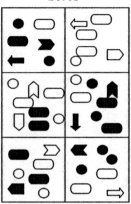

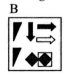

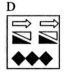

3. Which of the following belong to Set B?

A

B

C

D

4. Which of the following belong to Set B?

A

B

C

D

5. Which of the following belong to Set B?

A

B

C

D

Decision Analysis – 32 minutes

Scenario

A team of scientists have found a vast cave network deep within the Jamaican hills. There are many buildings with strange symbols and codes, some of which have been deciphered by the team and are shown below. Your task is to examine particular codes or sentences and then choose the best interpretation of the code from one of five possible choices.

You will find that, at times, the information you have is either incomplete or does not make complete sense. You will then need to make your best judgement based on the codes rather than what you expect to see or what you think is reasonable. There will always be a best answer which makes the most sense based on all the information presented. It is important that you understand that this test is based on judgements rather than simply applying rules and logic.

Operating codes	Basic codes
1 = opposite	A = warm
2 = increase	B = hazard
3 = merge	C = rain
4 = negative	D = insect
5 = positive	E = sun
6 = past	F = today
7 = present	G = tomorrow
8 = condition	H = danger
9 = similar	I = person
10 = hard	J = he
11 = similar	K = catch
12 = plural	L = building
13 = attribute	M = success
	N = weapon
	O = fly
	P = wind
	Q = winter
	R = fight
	S = fire
	T = word
	U = emotion

Question 1

Examine the following coded message: **J, 10, R, D, (4, 13, D)**

Now examine the following sentences and try to determine the most likely interpretation of the code.

A He fought hard for honey.
B He fought well but lost the battle to cancer.
C Sometimes infections overcome us.
D He caught malaria on holiday.
E He tried hard to fight off the insect bites.

Question 2

Examine the following coded message: **(12, I), K, (12, I, L), 6**

Now examine the following sentences and try to determine the most likely interpretation of the code.

A The people tried to capture the stadium.
B The rounders team will be very good catchers with the crowd in the school cheering.
C If the bouquet is thrown, someone will catch it.
D One of the guests will catch the bouquet in the church.
E The sportsmen tried to pluck the thrown ball out of the air.

Question 3

Examine the following coded message: **(13, S), B, (13, P)**

Now examine the following sentences and try to determine the most likely interpretation of the code.

A Blown hot flames are dangerous.
B Be careful it is hot and windy today.
C Fire and wind are never a good combination.
D Fanning flames with air does not put them out.
E Fire and wind represent a danger.

Question 4

Examine the following code: **(12, I, N), R, (2, M), 6**

Now examine the following sentence and try to determine the **two most likely** interpretations of the code.

A Soldiers fight to win.
B The soldiers battled to enjoy more victory.
C Soldiers must show bravery to enjoy victory.
D The militia battled for increased reward.
E A soldier must fight to success.

Question 5

Examine the following coded message: **I, M, O, (1, H), 13 (E, C), 6**

Now examine the following sentences and try to determine the most likely interpretation of the code.

A I successfully navigated through the storm.
B The pilot navigated through the bad weather.
C I passed safely with flying colours.
D I navigated safely and passed the rainbow.
E I travel better when I see the sun shining.

Question 6

Examine the following coded message: **(4, 13, R), R, M, (H, I, 12)**

Now examine the following sentences and try to determine the most likely interpretation of the code.

A He broke his arm in the battle but defeated the enemy.
B The fight was stopped because the fighter broke his arm.
C My success in the fight overshadows my broken arm.
D He broke his arm fighting the soldiers.
E He broke his leg in the fight and lost to the enemy.

Question 7

Examine the following coded message: **(1, Q), (1, A), (1, 6)**

Now examine the following sentences and try to determine the **two most likely** interpretations of the code.

A Future summers will be freezing.
B Summers will be cold.
C Winters will be cold.
D Future summers will be cold.
E Future winters will be cold.

Question 8

Examine the following coded message: **(1, G), 13(2, E), 10, (I, L)**

Now examine the following sentences and try to determine the most likely interpretation of the code.

A The sun made it difficult for the constructors to work yesterday.
B The heat worsened yesterday, making it difficult to construct.
C Building is difficult in hot conditions.
D Yesterday sunstroke made it impossible for the builders to finish.
E Yesterday the builders did nothing.

Question 9

Examine the following coded message: **(12, I), (12, T), (13, S)**

Now examine the following sentences and try to determine the most likely interpretation of the code.

A Everyone is talking about the heat.
B He is shouting 'fire'.
C The conversation is a hot topic.
D The dialogue is subdued.
E Most people keep conversation cool.

Question 10

Examine the following coded message: **(12, I, R), (12, N), R, (1, 6)**

Now examine the following sentences and try to determine the most likely interpretation of the code.

A The men fought bravely with their hands.
B The crowd used batons during the brawl.
C The army will use arms in the conflict.
D The soldiers fight tomorrow.
E The general proposed to use better weapons in future warfare.

Question 11

Examine the following coded message: **12(I, N), K, (H, I), (4, M), 6**

Now examine the following sentences and try to determine the most likely interpretation of the code.

A Police officers will catch criminals.
B Officers can apprehend thieves with limited success.
C He caught the perpetrator escaping with a dangerous weapon
D Soldiers fought with the suspect but she fled.
E Despite the army officers apprehending the criminal, he got away.

Question 12

Examine the following coded message: **(12, I), 2(4, U), 12(13, D), B, 6**

Now examine the following sentences and try to determine the most likely interpretation of the code.

A The travellers were more afraid of being bitten by a dangerous insect.
B An insect bite can be harmful and cause worry.
C The explorers were very frightened that the bites would cause injury.
D The team was not worried that the bites would be harmful.
E The scientist found that the bites were dangerous and was worried.

Question 13

Examine the following coded message: **(1, G), (1, A), G, 13(2, E), (12, I, U)** Now examine the following sentences and try to determine the most likely interpretation of the code.

A Yesterday it was cold, but tomorrow will be colder and we will be sad.
B Yesterday it was cold, but tomorrow will be warmer and I will be much happier.
C Today it was cold, but tomorrow will be warmer and they will be much happier.
D Yesterday it was warm, but tomorrow will be warmer still.
E Yesterday it was cold, but tomorrow will be warmer and we will be much happier.

Scenario

The team of scientists have stumbled across a new set of codes, which they have called 'specialist codes'.

Operating codes	Basic codes	Specialist codes
1 = opposite	A = warm	♋ = drop
2 = increase	B = hazard	♌ = running
3 = merge	C = rain	♍ = watching
4 = negative	D = insect	♎ = hearing
5 = positive	E = sun	♐ = wisdom
6 = past	F = today	♒ = happy
7 = present	G = tomorrow	♓ = worried
8 = condition	H = danger	☺ = stopping
9 = similar	I = person	♦ = feeling
10 = hard	J = he	
11 = similar	K = catch	
12 = plural	L = building	
13 = attribute	M = success	
	N = weapon	
	O = fly	
	P = wind	
	Q = winter	
	R = fight	
	S = fire	
	T = word	

Question 14

Examine the following coded message: **I, ♦, 8, (C, P)**

Now examine the following sentences and try to determine the most likely interpretation of the code.

A One is sad when the storm arrives.
B I may scream if the storm arrives.
C The gardener is feeling sad about the impending rain.
D Bad weather can make farmers worry.
E A storm causes worry to all.

YOU ARE NOW AT THE HALFWAY STAGE OF THIS SECTION.
IDEALLY YOU SHOULD HAVE AROUND 14.5 MINUTES LEFT.
(Please note that this prompt will not be given in your actual test.)

Question 15

Examine the following coded message: **(4, ♐), O, (13, Q)**

Now examine the following sentences and try to determine the most likely interpretation of the code.

A Flies do not like the cold.
B The humidity makes it ill-advised to travel.
C It is unwise to travel in freezing conditions.
D Pilots do not fly in freezing conditions.
E He unwisely jumped into the ice.

Question 16

Examine the following coded message: **(1, J), ♎, G, 1(2, A), 6**

Now examine the following sentences and try to determine the most likely interpretation of the code.

A She hears that tomorrow is going to be very cold.
B She heard that tomorrow was going to be colder.
C She heard that tomorrow will be colder than today.
D He heard that tomorrow was going to be very cold.
E She heard that tomorrow was going to be cold.

Question 17

Examine the following coded message: **(12, I), ☺, R, (12, I, L), 6**

Now examine the following sentences and try to determine the most likely interpretation of the code.

A The people waited to fight at the stadium.
B The men stopped to fight at the community centre.
C The mob started a fight at the stadium.
D The gladiators' fight was stopped in the ring.
E The fighters will battle in the stadium.

Question 18

Examine the following coded message: **(12, I), ♍, (4, •), (12, I), 7**

Now examine the following sentences and try to determine the most likely interpretation of the code.

A They observe the anxious pupils.
B The group watched an emotional movie with friends.
C People see wonderful things.
D They saw nervous pupils.
E Examiners will oversee the nervous pupils.

Question 19

Examine the following coded message: **(12, I), ♌, L, 12 (H, I), R, 6,**

Now examine the following sentences and try to determine the **two most likely** interpretations of the code.

A People sought shelter during dangerous times.
B The tribe escaped the hut before the militia arrived.
C The fight took place in a village involving many gangsters.
D The inhabitants fled the fighting and sought shelter in the jungle.
E The crowd raced through the stadium to avoid the mob brawl.

Question 20

Examine the following coded message: **(12, I), ♓, (C, P), ♍, (J, ♐), 6**

Now examine the following sentences and try to determine the most likely interpretation of the code.

A The inhabitants kept an eye on the impending bad weather as they were afraid.
B According to the wise man, everyone will see the storm and be frightened.
C The villagers consulted the wise man because seeing the thunder made them afraid.
D The inhabitants were concerned about the storm so saw the wise man.
E The wizard created a storm and made everyone worried.

Question 21

Examine the following coded message: **(12, I), (4, •), 2(13, P), ♌, (12, L), 6**

Now examine the following sentences and try to determine the most likely interpretation of the code.

A People were worried about the cyclone and so prepared by building a shelter.
B You cannot outrun a cyclone.
C The population deserted their homes after the tornado.
D I was afraid of the increasing wind so I ran for shelter.
E The tribespeople were scared about the impending hurricane and so deserted their shelters.

Question 22

Examine the following sentence: **'Forget your problems'**.

Now examine the following codes and try to determine the most likely interpretation of the sentence.

A (♋, ♎)
B (4, ♎)
C ☺, ♓
D ☺, ♓, 6
E H, (4, ♎)

Question 23

Examine the following sentence: **'The couple witnessed the sunset together'**.

Now examine the following codes and try to determine the most likely interpretation of the sentence.

A (12, I), ♍, (E, ♋), 7
B (12, I), ♍, (E, ♋), 6
C (12, I), ♍, (2, E), 6
D (E, ♋), J, (12, I), ♍, 6
E (12, I), (E, ♋), ♍, (4, ♦), 6

Question 24

Examine the following sentence: **'People are falling like flies from the increasing heat'**.

Now examine the following codes and try to determine the most likely interpretation of the sentence.

A I, ♋, (12, O), 13(2, E), 7
B (12, I), ♋, (12, O), (2, H), 7
C (12, I), ♋, O, 13(2, E), 7
D (12, I), ♋, (12, O), 13(2, E), 7
E 12, (I, ♋,) 12, O, 13, 2, (E, 7)

Question 25

Examine the following sentence: **'The journalists were jubilant in writing about the victory'**.

Now examine the following codes and try to determine the most likely interpretation of the sentence.

A 12(I, T), (5, ♦), 13(12, T), M,
B 12(J, I), (5, ♦), 13(12, T), M,
C 8, 12(T, I), (5, ♦), 13(12, T), M,
D 12(T, I), ♦, 13(12, T), M,
E 12(T, I), (5, ♦), 13(12, T), M, (1, G)

Question 26

Examine the following sentence: **'If the storm arrives the tribespeople will be petrified and will leave their shelter'.**

Now examine the following codes and try to determine the most likely interpretation of the sentence.

A 8, (C, E), (12, I), (4, •), L, (1, 6)
B 8, (C, P), (12, I), (4, •), L, 6
C (1, 6), (C, P), (12, I), L, (4, •)
D 8, (C, P), (12, I), (4, •), L, (1, 6)
E 8, (C, P), (12, I), (4, •), (12, L), (1, 6)

Question 27

Examine the following coded message: J, 6, (13,f), T

Now examine the following sentences and try to determine the most likely interpretations of the code.

A Today a wise man will learn about words
B A lady who is good with words is very wise
C The written word is mightier than a man's sword
D The women was an expert in singing
E The man was an expert with words

Question 28

Examine the following coded message: (1,J) (6,s), i, (1, M),

Now examine the following sentences and try to determine the most likely interpretations of the code.

A The man was feeling worried as he had failed
B Failure is not an option
C The woman felt worried after failing
D The man felt worried after failing
E The man was not worried after failing

Situational Judgement Test 2 – 27 Minutes

Scenario 1

Derek is a clinical psychologist working in a mental health service at a NHS trust. A colleague, Ellen, is a qualified nurse and works part-time at the same NHS hospital in a High Dependency / Intensive Care unit. Ellen was involved in a road traffic accident some six months previously whilst travelling back from a late shift. Ellen's health has deteriorated in the months following the accident and Derek is aware that she has not been eating properly and has lost a significant amount of weight. She is often visibly distressed and has been leaving work early to avoid driving through the intersection where the accident took place because it makes her feel panicky.

How **appropriate** is each of the following responses by <u>**Derek**</u> in this situation:

1. **To report Ellen to HR for leaving work early.**
   A. A very appropriate thing to do
   B. Appropriate but not ideal
   C. Inappropriate but not awful
   D. A very inappropriate thing to do

2. **To ignore the situation as he is not Ellen's line manager.**
   A. A very appropriate thing to do
   B. Appropriate but not ideal
   C. Inappropriate but not awful
   D. A very inappropriate thing to do

3. **To gossip with other colleagues openly in the staff room about how awful it is she is not pulling her weight.**
   A. A very appropriate thing to do
   B. Appropriate but not ideal
   C. Inappropriate but not awful
   D. A very inappropriate thing to do

4. **Seek to speak to her in private to express concerns about her wellbeing and encourage her to seek help.**
   A. A very appropriate thing to do
   B. Appropriate but not ideal
   C. Inappropriate but not awful
   D. A very inappropriate thing to do

Scenario 2

Sanjay is a third year medical student who has just begun his clinical training on the Vascular surgery outpatients clinic. He has been asked together with his fellow student and friend Sarah to take a patient history whilst the Consultant finishes with another patient. The clinic is very busy and is running very behind schedule. The patient is an elderly lady who has attended the appointment alone and is obviously quite uncomfortable and uneasy. She expresses her concern about having to have an operation as she has nobody to care for her afterwards.

How **appropriate** is each of the following responses by **Sanjay** in this situation:

1. **Listen to the concerns of the patient and acknowledge their concerns.**
   A. A very appropriate thing to do
   B. Appropriate but not ideal
   C. Inappropriate but not awful
   D. A very inappropriate thing to do

2. **Take the history of the patient and do not engage in any conversation.**
   A. A very appropriate thing to do
   B. Appropriate but not ideal
   C. Inappropriate but not awful
   D. A very inappropriate thing to do

3. **Tell the patient that the operation is going to be a success and they have nothing to worry about.**
   A. A very appropriate thing to do
   B. Appropriate but not ideal
   C. Inappropriate but not awful
   D. A very inappropriate thing to do

4. **Tell the patient the Consultant will be with her shortly who will be able to address her concerns.**
   A. A very appropriate thing to do
   B. Appropriate but not ideal
   C. Inappropriate but not awful
   D. A very inappropriate thing to do

Scenario 3

Michael, a registrar, has just completed a nightshift and is waiting to handover to a day colleague before he can go home to rest. He has to come back later that evening to do another nightshift and is keen to get some sleep. His day colleague however is already 45 minutes late and he has no idea what has happened to him.

How **appropriate** is each of the following responses by <u>**Michael**</u> in this situation:

1. **To ring the medical staffing team to see if his colleague has called in sick.**
   A. A very appropriate thing to do
   B. Appropriate but not ideal
   C. Inappropriate but not awful
   D. A very inappropriate thing to do

2. **To inform the day shift manager and seek guidance on what to do given he needs to get some sleep before his shift later on that evening.**
   A. A very appropriate thing to do
   B. Appropriate but not ideal
   C. Inappropriate but not awful
   D. A very inappropriate thing to do

3. **Leave the ward and go home without waiting for cover.**
   A. A very appropriate thing to do
   B. Appropriate but not ideal
   C. Inappropriate but not awful
   D. A very inappropriate thing to do

4. **Ring his colleague's mobile as he has their number and knows them well.**
   A. A very appropriate thing to do
   B. Appropriate but not ideal
   C. Inappropriate but not awful
   D. A very inappropriate thing to do

Scenario 4

Eleanor has just finished her shift and left the hospital some 30 minutes ago. She is rushing as she is late for an important family dinner. While driving she remembers that she has forgotten to write up in the patient notes some routine eight hourly maintenance IV fluids for a patient. She tries to call the on-call doctor directly but they are not answering.

How **appropriate** is each of the following responses by <u>Eleanor</u> in this situation:

1. **Ring the hospital switch board and ask to be transferred to the ward and to bleep the on-call doctor.**
   A. A very appropriate thing to do
   B. Appropriate but not ideal
   C. Inappropriate but not awful
   D. A very inappropriate thing to do

2. **Do nothing the nursing team will pick up on the error and correct it.**
   A. A very appropriate thing to do
   B. Appropriate but not ideal
   C. Inappropriate but not awful
   D. A very inappropriate thing to do

3. **Turn round and drive back to the hospital immediately and correct the mistake herself.**
   A. A very appropriate thing to do
   B. Appropriate but not ideal
   C. Inappropriate but not awful
   D. A very inappropriate thing to do

4. **Keep trying to call the on-call doctor whilst proceeding to attend to the family matter.**
   A. A very appropriate thing to do
   B. Appropriate but not ideal
   C. Inappropriate but not awful
   D. A very inappropriate thing to do

Scenario 5

Siobhan is a third year dental student who has been nominated as the *team leader for a piece of assessed project work. There are 5 other dental* students who comprise the team and the project involves a piece of research over the period of 2 months culminating in a presentation to academic faculty.

How **appropriate** is each of the following responses by **Siobhan** in this situation:

1. **Arrange a meeting as soon as possible to agree roles and responsibilities for the project team.**
   A. A very appropriate thing to do
   B. Appropriate but not ideal
   C. Inappropriate but not awful
   D. A very inappropriate thing to do

2. **Arrange to see each team member separately to agree their role.**
   A. A very appropriate thing to do
   B. Appropriate but not ideal
   C. Inappropriate but not awful
   D. A very inappropriate thing to do

3. **When meeting the team for the first time agree a code of behaviour for the team to adhere to for the duration of the project.**
   A. A very appropriate thing to do
   B. Appropriate but not ideal
   C. Inappropriate but not awful
   D. A very inappropriate thing to do

4. **Email the team to assign each individual their role and request they provide her with a weekly update.**
   A. A very appropriate thing to do
   B. Appropriate but not ideal
   C. Inappropriate but not awful
   D. A very inappropriate thing to do

Scenario 6

James is a foundation doctor on a general practice rotation. One of his fellow medical students, Rupal, who is attached to James' practice confides in him that she is very upset about her teaching on this rotation. Rupal has exams approaching and she is very anxious as she has not seen many patients with clinical signs. She has a clinical OSCE coming up and therefore needs this experience to pass her exam.

How **appropriate** is each of the following responses by **James** in this situation:

1. **Tell Rupal not to worry she is likely to pass anyway.**
   A. A very appropriate thing to do
   B. Appropriate but not ideal
   C. Inappropriate but not awful
   D. A very inappropriate thing to do

2. **Advise Rupal to contact her medical school straight away as it is unacceptable that she is not receiving adequate teaching from the practice.**
   A. A very appropriate thing to do
   B. Appropriate but not ideal
   C. Inappropriate but not awful
   D. A very inappropriate thing to do

3. **Suggest to Rupal that she should discuss her concerns with the GP responsible for her training so that they can arrange for her to see more patients.**
   A. A very appropriate thing to do
   B. Appropriate but not ideal
   C. Inappropriate but not awful
   D. A very inappropriate thing to do

4. **Offer to help Rupal with her exam revision having recently sat his finals himself.**
   A. A very appropriate thing to do
   B. Appropriate but not ideal
   C. Inappropriate but not awful
   D. A very inappropriate thing to do

5. **Have a word with her trainer telling him that Rupal is not happy at all. She is not getting adequate teaching and he feels something needs to be done about this immediately.**
   A. A very appropriate thing to do
   B. Appropriate but not ideal
   C. Inappropriate but not awful
   D. A very inappropriate thing to do

Scenario 7

There are five minutes to go until Laura finishes her day shift. She has made plans with friends that evening and is keen to leave on time having finished late most days this week. Her bleep suddenly goes off just as she has left the ward. Laura checks her bleep and it is her ward that is bleeping her.

How **appropriate** is each of the following responses by **Laura** in this situation:

1. **Ignore the bleep, she only has 5 minutes left of her shift and doesn't want to be late home.**
   A. A very appropriate thing to do
   B. Appropriate but not ideal
   C. Inappropriate but not awful
   D. A very inappropriate thing to do

2. **Go back to the ward and see what the problem is.**
   A. A very appropriate thing to do
   B. Appropriate but not ideal
   C. Inappropriate but not awful
   D. A very inappropriate thing to do

3. **Ask one of the nurses to answer the bleep for her and explain that she has already left for the day.**
   A. A very appropriate thing to do
   B. Appropriate but not ideal
   C. Inappropriate but not awful
   D. A very inappropriate thing to do

4. **Answer the bleep, and if it is not urgent, explain that she is finishing her shift and kindly ask if they could please bleep the on-call doctor.**
   A. A very appropriate thing to do
   B. Appropriate but not ideal
   C. Inappropriate but not awful
   D. A very inappropriate thing to do

Scenario 8

Penny is an FY2 doctor on a general practice rotation. A competent 88-year-old lady has recently been diagnosed with iron deficiency anaemia. When Penny explains to the patient the possible causes she informs her that she does not want any investigations to find out the cause.

How **appropriate** is each of the following responses by **Penny** in this situation:

1. **Explain to her that it is in her best interests to have it investigated and refer her for a colonoscopy and gastroscopy regardless of how she feels.**
   A. A very appropriate thing to do
   B. Appropriate but not ideal
   C. Inappropriate but not awful
   D. A very inappropriate thing to do

2. **Explore her reasons for not wanting to have any further investigations and allay any concerns if possible.**
   A. A very appropriate thing to do
   B. Appropriate but not ideal
   C. Inappropriate but not awful
   D. A very inappropriate thing to do

3. **Agree that as she is 88 there is no point in investigating her anyway as they are unlikely to do anything about it should anything sinister be found.**
   A. A very appropriate thing to do
   B. Appropriate but not ideal
   C. Inappropriate but not awful
   D. A very inappropriate thing to do

4. **Ask the patient for permission to discuss her options with her daughter who is also a patient at the surgery.**
   A. A very appropriate thing to do
   B. Appropriate but not ideal
   C. Inappropriate but not awful
   D. A very inappropriate thing to do

Scenario 9

Tamsin, a dental nurse, receives a complaint from a patient who informs her that they saw one of her colleagues reading adult pornography in the waiting room. On further investigation she finds out that the pornography she was referring to was Page 3 of 'The Sun' newspaper.

How **appropriate** is each of the following responses by **Tamsin** in this situation:

1. **Tell the patient that Page 3 does not really count as adult pornography and that she should not be concerned.**
   A. A very appropriate thing to do
   B. Appropriate but not ideal
   C. Inappropriate but not awful
   D. A very inappropriate thing to do

2. **Go to a senior immediately. This constitutes adult pornography and is a serious matter.**
   A. A very appropriate thing to do
   B. Appropriate but not ideal
   C. Inappropriate but not awful
   D. A very inappropriate thing to do

3. **Have a private conversation with your colleague regarding the complaint the patient has made and suggest that although this situation may be entirely innocent, perhaps he should apologise to the patient to ensure the matter does not escalate.**
   A. A very appropriate thing to do
   B. Appropriate but not ideal
   C. Inappropriate but not awful
   D. A very inappropriate thing to do

Scenario 10

Ahmed is a foundation doctor on a busy medical firm. It is the night after the mess party and one of his junior colleagues arrives on the ward looking very hung over and still smelling of alcohol.

How **appropriate** is each of the following responses by **Ahmed** in this situation:

1. **Immediately inform the consultant on shift as he is concerned about his junior colleague's ability to work.**
   A. A very appropriate thing to do
   B. Appropriate but not ideal
   C. Inappropriate but not awful
   D. A very inappropriate thing to do

2. **Take his colleague aside and explain to him that as he is hung over and smells of alcohol, as it is best for him to go home for a while and that he should inform medical staffing that he is not able to work.**
   A. A very appropriate thing to do
   B. Appropriate but not ideal
   C. Inappropriate but not awful
   D. A very inappropriate thing to do

3. **Advise his colleague sensitively that perhaps next time he should stop drinking a little earlier in the evening in order to still be fit for his shift the next day.**
   A. A very appropriate thing to do
   B. Appropriate but not ideal
   C. Inappropriate but not awful
   D. A very inappropriate thing to do

Scenario 11

A mother brings her eight-year-old son into A&E. He is having a severe asthma attack and is extremely unwell. His mother tells Jayne, a foundation Doctor, that she ran out of inhalers last month and she has not had a chance to get any more from the GP. She also tells you that his lips went blue last night and he stopped breathing but she did not call an ambulance.

How **important** to take into account are the following considerations for Jayne when deciding how to respond to the situation?

1. **That she is a single mother.**
   A. Very important
   B. Important
   C. Of minor importance
   D. Not important at all

2. **That she ran out of medication a month ago.**
   A. Very important
   B. Important
   C. Of minor importance
   D. Not important at all

3. **That the social services had recently visited the family as concerns of neglect had been raised by the sons' school.**
   A. Very important
   B. Important
   C. Of minor importance
   D. Not important at all

Scenario 12

A medical student is due to meet with her supervisor. Just before her meeting she is asked if she would like to attend a clinical session. The student appreciates the value of this session but is worried about missing her meeting with her supervisor as it is too late to contact them to ask to rearrange.

How **important** to take into account are the following considerations for **the student** when deciding how to respond to the situation?

1. **That she had to rearrange her previous meeting due to personal reasons.**
   A. Very important
   B. Important
   C. Of minor importance
   D. Not important at all

2. **That she cannot contact her supervisor to let them know she won't be attending.**
   A. Very important
   B. Important
   C. Of minor importance
   D. Not important at all

3. **That there will be other clinical sessions that will be valuable to her learning and development.**
   A. Very important
   B. Important
   C. Of minor importance
   D. Not important at all

4. **That her supervisor will agree that the clinical session is more valuable than their meeting.**
   A. Very important
   B. Important
   C. Of minor importance
   D. Not important at all

Scenario 13

A nurse on a ward was approached by an elderly patient concerned that she has frequently overheard the consultant using bad language when speaking to her colleagues. She explains that it is making her uncomfortable and wishes to be moved to a different ward.

How **important** to take into account are the following considerations for **the nurse** when deciding how to respond to the situation?

1. **She has never heard the consultant use bad language.**
   A. Very important
   B. Important
   C. Of minor importance
   D. Not important at all

2. **That the patient feels uncomfortable and wishes to be moved to a different ward.**
   A. Very important
   B. Important
   C. Of minor importance
   D. Not important at all

3. **That other patient's may too have overheard the consultant use bad language.**
   A. Very important
   B. Important
   C. Of minor importance
   D. Not important at all

4. **That the patient has dementia and is easily confused.**
   A. Very important
   B. Important
   C. Of minor importance
   D. Not important at all

Scenario 14

A midwifery student is present during an examination of a pregnant lady. Whilst the patient is undressing for her examination the student notices the midwife appears to be texting on her mobile phone.

How **important** to take into account are the following considerations for **the student** when deciding how to respond to the situation?

1. **That the patient has not noticed that the midwife is on her phone.**
   A. Very important
   B. Important
   C. Of minor importance
   D. Not important at all

2. **That the midwife is having difficulties with her eldest son at school.**
   A. Very important
   B. Important
   C. Of minor importance
   D. Not important at all

3. **That the midwife is responding to comments on facebook.**
   A. Very important
   B. Important
   C. Of minor importance
   D. Not important at all

4. **The midwife is marking one of the students' assessments.**
   A. Very important
   B. Important
   C. Of minor importance
   D. Not important at all

Scenario 15

A nurse approaches a senior doctor regarding a junior doctors' appearance. She is concerned that other members of staff are commenting that the junior doctor is wearing an inappropriate amount of make up.

How **important** to take into account are the following considerations for the **senior doctor** when deciding how to respond to the situation?

1. **A number of patients have complained about the junior doctors' appearance.**
   A. Very important
   B. Important
   C. Of minor importance
   D. Not important at all

2. **The nurse dislikes the junior doctor.**
   A. Very important
   B. Important
   C. Of minor importance
   D. Not important at all

3. **The senior doctor has not seen the junior doctor that day so cannot comment on her appearance.**
   A. Very important
   B. Important
   C. Of minor importance
   D. Not important at all

Scenario 16

Ellie, a third year medical student and her friend Bella are on placement in the Vasuclar clinic at the university hospital. Whilst discussing a case with the consultant Bella's phone rings, she picks it up and looks at the screen before rejecting the call and placing the phone down. The consultant is furious and sends Bella out of the room.

How **important** to take into account are the following considerations for Ellie when deciding how to respond to the situation?

1. **She is aware that Bella's mother is very ill and that Bella has been waiting for a call with an update from her father.**
   A. Very important
   B. Important
   C. Of minor importance
   D. Not important at all

2. **Bella has tried on numerous occasions to explain the situation to the consultant.**
   A. Very important
   B. Important
   C. Of minor importance
   D. Not important at all

3. **Bella is Ellie's best friend and they are housemates.**
   A. Very important
   B. Important
   C. Of minor importance
   D. Not important at all

Scenario 17

Sarah an auxiliary nurse is waiting with a patient for an x-ray on a suspected broken leg. They have been waiting for over an hour and the waiting room is still full.

How **important** to take into account are the following considerations for <u>Sarah</u> when deciding how to respond to the situation?

1. **That the patient is obviously in a lot of pain and discomfort.**
   A. Very important
   B. Important
   C. Of minor importance
   D. Not important at all

2. **That nobody has explained the delay or apologised.**
   A. Very important
   B. Important
   C. Of minor importance
   D. Not important at all

3. **That people who have not been waiting as long are being seen before them.**
   A. Very important
   B. Important
   C. Of minor importance
   D. Not important at all

Scenario 18

James is a medical student on rotation on the paediatric ward. He has been on the ward for over an hour when, taking a patients history, a nurse points out to him that he is not wearing his identification badge, which James explains he left at home by mistake.

How **important** to take into account are the following considerations for <u>James</u> when deciding how to respond to the situation?

1. **That an identification badge should always be worn during clinical sessions.**
   A. Very important
   B. Important
   C. Of minor importance
   D. Not important at all

2. **That patients are aware that he is not yet qualified.**
   A. Very important
   B. Important
   C. Of minor importance
   D. Not important at all

Scenario 19

Laura, a medical student is on a quiet train to visit family for the weekend. She hears a message over the tannoy asking if there are any medically trained passengers on board. The message is repeated four times. Laura suspects that there is a medical emergency and that there are no medically trained people on board. Laura must decide whether to make herself known.

How **important** to take into account are the following considerations for Laura when deciding how to respond to the situation?

1. **That there have been a number of announcements.**
   A. Very important
   B. Important
   C. Of minor importance
   D. Not important at all

2. **That people are beginning to become concerned due to the repeated announcements.**
   A. Very important
   B. Important
   C. Of minor importance
   D. Not important at all

3. **That she is only a medical student and may not be able to assist.**
   A. Very important
   B. Important
   C. Of minor importance
   D. Not important at all

Chapter 11

Entire mock UKCAT exam 2 answers

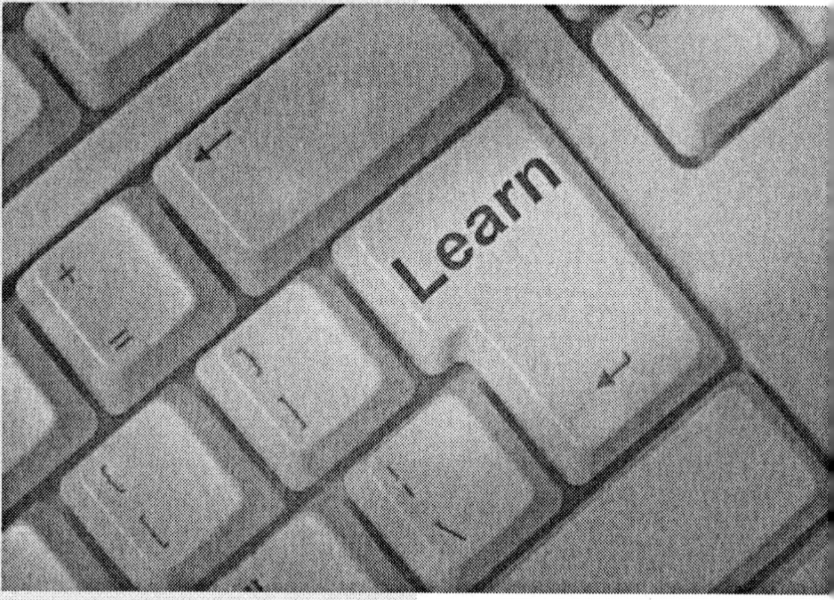

Entire mock UKCAT exam 2 answers

Verbal Reasoning answers and justifications

Question 1

1 **True.** This statement is confirmed by the following: *'In November 2001 the NHS reform bill was published. This followed the recommendations of the July 2001 public inquiry into children's heart surgery at Bristol Royal Infirmary.'*

2 **Can't tell.** Although the passage refers to the CHI gaining the powers of assessment following the implementation of the NHS Reform Act it does not state what NHS organisations are actually assessed against: *'Subsequently the NHS Reform Act 2002 expanded the powers of CHI to include performance assessment of the NHS. This indicated that CHI would publish NHS star ratings in future'.*

3 **False.** This statement is false based on the following in the passage: *'The bill proposed new powers for an NHS inspectorate, including the ability to suspend services at failing trusts, to inspect private health facilities where NHS work was carried out and to publish an annual state-of-the-NHS report'.*

4 **False.** The passage refers to two white papers, *The New NHS* and *A First Class Service – Quality in the NHS.*

Question 2

1. **The correct answer is D.** Broadly, the objective of macroeconomic policies is to maximise the level of national income, providing economic growth to raise the utility and standard of living of participants in the economy.
2. **The correct answer is A.** Price stability - when prices remain largely stable, and there is not rapid inflation or deflation
3. **The correct answer is A.** Where those who are able and willing to have a job can get one
4. **The correct answer is B.** External Balance - equilibrium in the Balance of payments without the use of artificial constraints. That is, the value of exports being roughly equal to the value of imports over the long run.

Question 3

1 **True.** This statement is confirmed by the following in the passage: '*As an alternative, by taking a random sample of patients, one could also hope to achieve a representative result. Such random sampling may be carried out with the help of most statistical textbooks and a random numbers table, or alternatively using mathematical computer software*'.

2 **True.** This statement is confirmed by the following in the passage: '*However, it may be a more practical and feasible option to audit the management of hypertension in a specific ward over a three-month period*'.

3 **Can't tell.** Although the passage states that opinion polls can be used to gauge the opinion of the population as a whole it does not state whether it can or cannot be used to determine opinion of a particular community: '*A common example of sampling in use is at the time of an election. Here opinion polls are commonly constructed in an effort to select samples that are indicative of the population as a whole*'.

4 **False.** The passage states that most but not all statistical textbooks will be able to assist in random sampling: '*Such random sampling may be carried out with the help of most statistical textbooks and a random numbers table, or alternatively using mathematical computer software*'.

Question 4

1. **The correct answer is D.** Three hypotheses have been put forward to explain why stuttering occurs
2. **The correct answer is B.** In contrast, neurogenic speech disorders (resulting from head injuries, strokes, etc.) result in disordered speech under all conditions.
3. **The correct answer is A.** A third hypothesis suggests that stutterers' auditory processing underactivity reduces the left-brain communication of sensory information processed in the rear brain to frontal speech and language areas.
4. **The correct answer is A.** It can be inferred from the passage that although nothing is clinically proven that stuttering is in some way linked to defects in the brain.

Question 5

1 **False.** This statement is contradicted by the following in the passage: '*Perhaps the most significant part of Unfinished Business, however, was its advice regarding the Consultant grade*'.

2 **True.** This statement is confirmed by the following in the passage: '*And so, the following year, MMC was launched. The first stage of the new career path, the Foundation Programme, launched in 2005*'.

3 **Can't tell.** Although the passage refers to the fact that the SHO position was reviewed as part of the report *Unfinished Business*, the passage does not confirm either way that the position actually became obsolete by September 2003: '*His report, Unfinished Business, published in September 2002, signalled the beginning of the end of the SHO grade*'. Also the passage does not confirm that SHO stands for 'Senior House Officer'.

4 **Can't tell.** Although the title 'Sir' in the passage suggests Sir Liam has been knighted, the passage does not indicate the exact date his investiture occurred.

Question 6

1. **The correct answer is C.** According to the authors, Piaget contends that normal children will reach the final stage of development, which is the stage of formal operations, between the age of twelve and fifteen.
2. **The correct answer is D.** Though Arlin's proposed fifth stage produced more questions than answers, it opens the door to understanding the learning needs of adults; to be approached as thinkers.
3. **The correct answer is D.** Jean Piaget states that there are "four invariant stages of cognitive development that are age related"
4. **The correct answer is C.** Arlin's hypothesised fifth stage was the problem-finding stage. This stage focuses on problem discovery.

Question 7

1 **False.** The passage explicitly states that for an individual to become a psychiatrist they must attend medical school; '*In the UK, to become a psychiatrist you must have been to medical school and completed your foundation year training*'.

2 **Can't tell.** Although this is indeed the case the passage neither confirms nor contradicts this statement and therefore it is not possible to confirm whether it is true or false.

3 **True.** This is confirmed by the following in the passage: '*Its reputation, after all, is laden with cultural myths. With its long heritage of colourful characters such as Freud, and coverage in the media and other cultural domains, preconceptions can fuel attitudes to it as a potential career path. While such views are still evident in society as a whole, they also continue in mainstream medicine. This can skew what advice or perspective you gain of psychiatry during medical school. Limited experience of dealing with mental illness and psychological distress means that many doctors are not skilled in dealing with the nuances of mental health problems*'.

4 **Can't tell.** Although it is indeed the case that a psychologist can practice psychotherapy in some instances the passage does not confirm this.

Question 8

1 **The correct answer is A.** Another one called calcium tungstate, CaWO4, has been widely used in X-ray cassettes although this substance has been replaced by other scintillators such as lanthanum oxybromide in many modern cassettes.

2. **The correct answer is C.** For example if a radioactive sample happened to be in liquid form we could mix it with a liquid scintillator so as to optimise the chances of detection of the emitted radiation and hence have a very sensitive detector.

3. **The correct answer is B.** A final example is p-terphenyl in polystyrene which is a scintillator in the form of a plastic. This form can be easily made into different shapes like most plastics and is therefore useful when detectors of particular shapes are required.

4. **The correct answer is A.** This activating element is used to influence the wavelength (colour) of the light produced by the scintillator.

Question 9

1 **True.** This is confirmed by the following in the passage: *'Complaints were subsequently made to the GMC concerning the conduct of two cardiac surgeons and of the Chief Executive of the Trust. They were found guilty in 1998 of serious professional misconduct by the GMC'.*

2 **True.** This statement is confirmed by the following in the passage: *'To make recommendations which could help to secure high quality care across the NHS'.*

3 **True.** This statement is confirmed by the following in the passage: *'A group of parents of children who had undergone cardiac surgery at the BRI organised themselves to provide mutual support. In June 1996 the group first called for a Public Inquiry into the Paediatric Cardiothoracic services at the BRI'.*

4 **True.** This statement is confirmed by the following in the passage: *'To inquire into the management of the care of children receiving complex cardiac surgical services at the Bristol Royal Infirmary between 1984 and 1995 and relevant related issues'.*

Question 10

1 **True.** This is confirmed by the following in the passage: *'A **mini-CEX** is a mini-Clinical Evaluation Exercise. It assesses doctor-patient interactions. Examples include taking a history or giving some bad news to a patient. Again, this is done on the ward with one of your seniors. **CBDs**, or Case Based Discussions, involve presenting a case and answering questions about the diagnosis and management. A **mini-ePAT**, or 360 degree assessment, looks at how well those who work with you think you're doing. They rate your ability across a range of skills including communication, timekeeping and attitude'.*

2 **Can't tell.** Although this is the case the passage does not confirm this and therefore it is not possible to say whether this is true or false: *'The aim of the Foundation Programme is to form a stepping stone between medical school and specialty training – it's a big step up, so that can only be a good thing! It's much more structured than the old pre-registration house officer (PRHO) position. For instance, you must complete various assessments and you have a supervisor who sets objectives with you and monitors your progress'.*

3 **True.** This is confirmed by the following in the passage: *'A **mini-CEX** is a mini-Clinical Evaluation Exercise. It assesses doctor-patient interactions. Examples include taking a history or giving some bad news to a patient'.*

4 **True.** This is confirmed by the following in the passage: *'Each foundation year (FY1 and FY2) is divided into three or four blocks, known as 'firms'. 'FY1 jobs range from general medicine or surgery to ENT or renal medicine. FY2 jobs can also include A&E and general practice'.*

Question 11

1 **False.** This statement is contradicted when the passage refers to the advantages of the new system over the old: *'Importantly, this system would ensure a fair and consistent basis for hospital funding rather than being reliant principally on historic budgets and the negotiating skills of individual managers. Competition between providers would also be encouraged by this system'.*

2 **True.** This statement is supported by the following in the passage: *'Subsequently the government, through the NHS Plan, signalled its intention to link the allocation of funds to hospitals to the activity they undertook'.*

3 **Can't tell.** Although the passage details that 25% of the NHS budget is awarded through SLAs it does not clarify the proportion of this that is awarded on a PbR basis.

4 **True.** This statement is confirmed by the following in the passage: *'It would reward efficiency, support patient choice and diversity and encourage activity for sustainable waiting time reductions'.*

Quantitative Reasoning answers and justifications

1. **The correct answer is C.**
   First identify how much chocolate you would need for one person. This can be calculated by dividing the amount of chocolate need for 4 people by 4:

   256 ÷ 4 = 64 g per person.

   Then multiply the individual sum by 11 to find out the total amount of chocolate needed for 11 people:

   64 × 11 = 704 g of chocolate.

   Chocolate is sold in 200 g bars.

   3 blocks = 3 × 200 = 600 g.

   4 blocks = 4 × 200 = 800 g.

   704 g of chocolate are required, so we would need to purchase **4 bars.**

2. **The correct answer is E.**
   Similarly to the previous question, we need to find out how much margarine is needed per person:

   124 ÷ 4 = 31 g per person

   We then divide the amount of margarine in the recipe by 31 to determine how many people the recipe is based on:

   1,705 ÷ 31 = **55 people**

3. **The correct answer is A.**
   We first need to find out the total amount of ingredients:

   689 (grams of flour) + 100 (grams of sugar) + 124 (grams of margarine) + 256 (grams of chocolate) = 1,169 grams of ingredients

   100 grams of sugar, expressed as a percentage of 1,169 grams of total ingredients is:

   (100 ÷ 1169) × 100 = **8.55%** to 2 decimal places.

4. **The correct answer is D.**
   There are 124 grams of margarine to 256 grams of chocolate present in the recipe. This can be written as 124:256.
   However, this can be reduced further by dividing both numbers by 4:

124 ÷ 4 = 31

256 ÷ 4 = 64

The ratio of margarine to chocolate is therefore **31:64**

5. **The correct answer is D.**
   The ratio of fat:protein = 9.66:29.27
   To express the ratio is its lowest form divide the amount of protein by the amount of fat:

   29.27 ÷ 9.66 = 3.03

   This gives a ratio of fat to protein of approximately **1:3**

6. **The correct answer is A.**
   To answer this question you do not actually have to work out the ratio, just divide the number of calories by the amount of protein. The meat with the smallest number has the best ratio.
   For **Bison:** 143 ÷ 28.44 = 5.02
   For Chicken (skinless): 190 ÷ 28.93 = 6.57

7. **The correct answer is C.**
   First find 1/5 of 2,000 to determine how may calories should come from meat:

   2,000 ÷ 5 = 400 kcal

   Next determine how much chicken this equates to:

   100 g chicken = 190 kcal

   1 kcal = 100 ÷ 190

   400 kcal = (100 ÷ 190) × 400 = **211 g**

8. **The correct answer is A.**
   The correct answer **Bison** can simply be read from the table.

9. **The correct answer is A.**
   To find the fraction, add up the sales from Asia and Australia, and then divide that by the total sales:

   ($17,000 + $21,000)/$133,000 = **2/7**

10. **The correct answer is D.**
    Find the sum of the sales from Asia and Australia. Divide that by the total sales:
    ($17,000 + $21,000) ÷ $133,000 = 0.291

Then multiply by 100 to get the percentage

0.291 × 100 = 29.1%

This is closest to **29%**

11. **The correct answer is A.**
Find the sum of the sales for all the regions then divide by the number of regions:

($12,000 + $23,000 + $21,000 + $30,000 + $17,000 + $30,000) = $133,000 ÷ 6 = $22,333

This is closest to **$22,000**

12. **The correct answer is E.**
Multiply the sales value in South America by 1.75:

$30,000 × 1.75 = **$52,500**

13. **The correct answer is B.**
To determine this, add up all the totals from each group for each year and compare them.

Year 1 = 60 + 55 + 65 + 80 + 85 + 90 = 435 staff

Year 2 = 70 + 60 + 85 + 100 + 95 + 100 = 510 staff

Year 3 = 65 + 45 + 65 + 35 +65 + 25 = 300 Sales staff

14. **The correct answer is B.**
To determine this, add all the staff totals in each group for Year 3:

Year 3 = 65 + 45 + 65 + 35 + 65 + 25 = **300**

15. **The correct answer is E.**
First find out how many staff members there were in Years 1 and 3 in Product group 4:

Year 1 = 80

Year 2 = 35

This means that there were 45 more staff members in Year 1 than in Year 3 (80 – 35 = 45)

Then take the above difference, divide it by the number of staff in Year 1 and multiply it by 100 (to calculate percentage decrease).
(45 ÷ 80) × 100 = **56.25%** (to 2 decimal places).

16. **The correct answer is C.**
Find the total number of staff members in Year 1:

Year 1 = 60 + 55 + 65 + 80 + 85 + 90 = 435

To find the mean, divide the above total by the number of Product groups, which is 6:

435 ÷ 6 = 72.5

17. **The correct answer is D.**
First find out the individual prices of the machines at wholesale. We do this by dividing the total price of 13 Brand G machines by the number of machines (13) therefore the calculation is:

£9,843 ÷ 13 = £757.15 per machine.

Then find the total of 11 Brand G machines at wholesale price, which is:

11 × £757.15 = £8,328.65

Then find the total of the machines sold at RRP, which is:

£923.40 × 11 = £10,157.40

Finally find the difference between the total sold at the RRP and the total paid for the machines at the wholesale price, which is:
£10,157.40 – £8,328.65 = **£1,828.75** (profit made).

18. **The correct answer is D.**
As above, first find out the price of the machines individually at wholesale price for 7 Brand D machines. For 13 Brand D machines the wholesale price is £8,790.00, therefore for 7 Brand D machines the calculation is:

£8,790 ÷ 13 = 676.15 (per washing machine).

676.15 × 7 = £4,733.05 (for 7 Brand D washing machines at wholesale price).

Then find the new selling price with 25% off:

£723.12 × 0.75 = £542.34 (new selling price per washing machine).

£542.34 × 7 = £3,796.38 (retail price for 7 washing machines).

Finally calculate the profit loss. In order to carry out this calculation, we take the above total and subtract it from the cost of the machines bought at the wholesale price:

£4,733.05 – £3,796.38 = **£936.67** (Total profit loss).

19. The correct answer is B.

First find the total of 1 Brand B machine at wholesale price which is:

£7,685.00 ÷ 13 = £591.15

The RRP of 1 Brand B washing machine is £699.29

Then find the profit (difference between the two totals):

£699.29 – £591.15 = £108.14

Finally find the percentage difference from the original wholesale price:

(£108.14 ÷ £591.15) × 100 = **18.3%** (to the nearest decimal point).

20. The correct answer is E.

The washing machine is sold at 5/8 of the price. This is equivalent to a saving of 3/8. This can be converted into a percentage by the following calculation:

(3 ÷ 8) × 100 = **37.5%**

21. The correct answer is D.

From the table, 30 ml is two tablespoons, so 60 ml would be **4 tablespoons**.

22. The correct answer is A.

From the table you can see that you need 1 fluid ounce of Tabasco and 2 fluid ounces of Worchester. This gives the ratio of Worchester to Tabasco as **2:1.**

23. The correct answer is D.

From the table find out how many fluid ounces 4 cups and 1 gallon are respectively, then divide the 1 gallon by the 4 cups.

1 gallon = 128 fluid ounces

4 cups = 32 fluid ounces

128 ÷ 32 = **4** times that Lloyd could perform the recipe

24. The correct answer is C.

Convert all ingredients into cups using the table then add them all together:

4 cups tomato juice = 4 cups of tomato juice

5 fluid ounces of lemon juice = 5/8 of a cup (since 1 cup = 8 fluid ounces)

60 ml Worchester sauce = 1/4 cup Worchester sauce
2 tablespoons Tabasco = 1/8 cup Tabasco
4 cups + 5/8 cup + 1/4 cup + 1/8 cup = **5 cups**

25. The correct answer is E.
In the graph we are given information about the total chain production, and standard chains on their own. However there is no information for the number of substandard chains alone. This is for us to work out.

In September the total chain production was 85 and the total standard production was 65. To find the substandard total, subtract the total standard chains from the total chain production:

Substandard chain production = Total chain production – Standard chain production

85 – 65 = 20 substandard chains produced

We then need to calculate this as a percentage of the total chain production:

(Total number of substandard chains ÷ total number of chain production) × 100

ie (20 ÷ 85) × 100 = 23.5%

26. The correct answer is D.
First calculate how many standard and substandard chains there were in both October's and November's total sales value:

October	Standard	–	80
	Substandard	–	20
November	Standard	–	85
	Substandard	–	10

We then find out the cost of one standard chain and one substandard chain:

Standard chains cost £5.70 per 100.

For one chain it is £5.70 ÷ 100 = £0.057 per standard chain.

Substandard chains cost £2.85 per 100.

For one chain it is £2.85 ÷ 100 = £0.0285 per sub standard chain.

We then find the sales value of the standard and substandard chains for each month:

October	Standard	–	80 × 0.057 = £4.56
	Substandard	–	20 × 0.0285 = £0.57
November	Standard	–	85 × 0.057 = £4.845
	Substandard	–	10 × 0.0285 = £0.285

We then add the total sales values of both months:

October £4.56 + £0.57= £5.13

November £4.845 + £0.285 = £5.13 therefore **no change**

27. **The correct answer is E.**
In October, 20 substandard chains and 80 standard chains were produced. Therefore we can write this as 20:80.

Dividing each side by 20 shows the ratio in its simplified form: **1:4.** Hence for every substandard chain produced there are 4 standard chains.

28. **The correct answer is E.**
Take the substandard chains and divide them by the total chain production and multiply this figure by 100:

(10 ÷ 70) × 100 = **14.29%**

29. **The correct answer is E.**
It tells you **c** is the **y** intercept, read from the graph where the line touches the y axis. Giving you **c = 10**

30. **The correct answer is C.**
Take a segment from the graph and divide the change in **y** by the change in **x**. For example, take from x = 0 to x = 2.

Change in **y** = 20 – 10 = 10

Change in x = 2 – 0 = 2

Gradient (m) = 10 ÷ 2 = **5**

31. **The correct answer is B.**
Substitute in the values given then solve.

y = mx + c

3 = 2x + 0

3 ÷ 2 = x

x = **1.5**

32. The correct answer is A.
The correct answer is A. Substitute in the values given then solve.

$y = mx + c$

$9 = 12m + 3$

$6 = 12\ m$

$6 \div 12 = m$

m = **0.5**

33. The correct answer is B.
To calculate the number of Bulgarian Levs you can exchange for £45.00, you need to calculate the following:

£45.00 × 21 (BGL Exchange rate) **= 945 Levs**

34. The correct answer is D.
To calculate how much 677 Bangladesh Takas are worth in Pounds Sterling you need to perform the opposite of the calculation in the above question:

677 ÷ 2.4 = **£282.10** (to 2 decimal places).

35. The correct answer is E.
First find a 10% increase in the exchange rate for the Cuban Peso:

(10 ÷ 100) × 213 CUPs = 21.3

Then add the 10% increase to the original exchange rate:

21.3 + 213 = 234.3 (new exchange rate for Cuban Peso)

Now find out how many Cuban Pesos are needed to make £45.00:

£45.00 × 234.3 = **10,543.5 CUPs**

36. The correct answer is C.
This question requires you to identify the actual exchange rate. We can work this out by the following calculation:

6,790 ÷ 1,900 = **3.6** (to 1 decimal place).

Abstract Reasoning answers and justifications

Question 1

Set A

The set contains large circles and squares consisting of dashed, or solid lines, which may be shaded or unshaded. There are also chevrons and quadrilateral shapes.

- The rule in this set is that when two large circles are present there must be one square, while when there are two squares only one circle is present.
- All the other shapes are distracters.

Set B

The set contains shaded triangles, circles and arrows.

- The rule in this set is that when there is one triangle present there must be three circles, while when there are two triangles present there must be two circles.
- All the other shapes are distracters.

Test Shape 1 Answer: Set B
This test shape contains two triangles and two circles. Therefore it belongs to Set B.

Test Shape 2 Answer: Set A
This test shape contains one square and two circles. Therefore it belongs to Set A.

Test Shape 3 Answer: Set A
The test shape contains a square and two circles, features of Set A.

Test Shape 4 Answer: Set A
This test shape contains a square and two circles. Therefore the shape belongs to Set A.

Test Shape 5 Answer: Set B
This test shape contains two triangles and two circles. Therefore the shape belongs to Set B.

Question 2

Set A

This set contains circles and crescents with no straight edges.

- The rule in this set is that all shapes must have curved lines only.

Set B

The various shapes may be shaded or unshaded with solid or dashed lines.

- The rule in this set is that each box contains two different shapes which must be drawn from straight lines only.

Test Shape 1 Answer: Neither
The test shape contains shapes composed of straight and curved lines and therefore belongs to neither set.

Test Shape 2 Answer: Set A
The test shape contains circles, and therefore belongs in Set A.

Test Shape 3 Answer: Neither
This test shape contains both curved and straight lines, features of neither set.

Test Shape 4 Answer: Neither
This test shape contains three squares, but as there are more than two shapes, the test shape cannot belong to Set B.

Test Shape 5 Answer: Set B
As both shapes are drawn from solid lines and are different, the test shape belongs to Set B.

Question 3

Set A

The set contains shaded and unshaded shapes drawn from solid, or dashed lines.

- The rule in this set is that shapes must not contain any right angles.

Set B

This set contains shaded and unshaded shapes drawn from solid lines.

- In contrast to Set A, the rule in this set is that each shape must have at least one right angle.

- Also, there must be at least one downwardly facing arrow.

1. **Correct answer A:** The shapes have solid or dashed lines and do not contain any right angles, therefore it belongs to Set A.

2. **Correct answer B:** The shapes have solid or dashed lines and do not contain any right angles, therefore it belongs to Set A.

3. **Correct answer C:** There are both shaded and unshaded shapes, at least one contains a right angle and there is at least one downward facing arrow present, therefore it belongs to Set B.

4. **Correct answer D:** There are both shaded and unshaded shapes, at least one contains a right angle and there is at least one downward facing arrow present, therefore it belongs to Set B.

5. **Correct answer C:** There are both shaded and unshaded shapes, at least one contains a right angle and there is at least one downward facing arrow present, therefore it belongs to Set B.

Question 4

Set A

The set contains a large centrally placed shape and some smaller shaded shapes.

- The rule in this set is that there are always four small shaded shapes which each contain at least one curved line.
- Also, the large shape is composed of straight lines which may be solid or dashed.

Set B

The set contains various shapes drawn from straight and curved lines which may be shaded or unshaded. However, all shapes must have solid lines.

- The rule in this set is that there is always at least one arrow facing downwards outside of the shapes, and no arrows facing upwards.
- Also, there are always four identical large shapes and at least two edges of each large shape must be in contact with another large shape.

Test Shape 1 Answer: Neither
The large shape does not possess straight lines only, and so does not comply with Set A. The test shape cannot belong to Set B because there are not four large shapes.

Test Shape 2 Answer: Set B
The test shape contains four repeated large unshaded shapes that touch at two points and are drawn of solid lines as well as a downward pointing arrow. Therefore, the test shape belongs to Set B.

Test Shape 3 Answer: Set A
The large centrally placed quadrilateral is drawn of straight lines and divided into two compartments, a feature of Set A. The smaller shaded shapes also correspond to Set A and repeated number sequence of four is also present. The set therefore belongs to Set A.

Test Shape 4 Answer: Neither
The test shape contains four unshaded circles with overlapping borders drawn of solid lines, which are all common features to Set B. Three arrows face downwards and correspond with Set B. However, one arrow faces upwards. Therefore, the test shape does not belong to Set B.

Test Shape 5 Answer: Set A
The large arrow is composed of dashed lines and divided into two by a solid line and corresponds with Set A. The four small shaded test shapes are repeated from Set A and complete the rule.

Question 5

Set A

The set contains a large centrally placed shape with solid straight lines and two smaller shapes that are identical with each other.

- The rule in this set is that the large shape must possess at least one line of symmetry.
- Also, one of the small shapes must be shaded and the other shape unshaded. The small shaded shape must be within the large shape, while the smaller unshaded shape must be positioned at the bottom left of the box.

Set B

The set contains curved shapes and arrows facing right. All shapes may be drawn of solid or dashed lines and may be shaded or unshaded.

- The rule in this set is that large shapes are always placed on the left hand side of each cell.
- Also, the number of arrows corresponds to the number of large curved shapes.
- Also, the arrows correspond to the large shapes with respect to the type of line used and whether they are shaded or unshaded.

1. **Correct answer A:** The largest shape has at least one line of symmetry, the two smaller shapes are identical, the shaded one is within the large shape, the unshaded positioned at the bottom left of the box, therefore it belongs to Set A.

2. **Correct answer B:** The largest shape has at least one line of symmetry, the two smaller shapes are identical, the shaded one is within the large shape, the unshaded positioned at the bottom left of the box, therefore it belongs to Set A.

3. **Correct answer D:** The largest shape has at least one line of symmetry, the two smaller shapes are identical, the shaded one is within the large shape, the unshaded positioned at the bottom left of the box, therefore it belongs to Set A.

4. **Correct answer C:** The largest shape is located on the left of the box, the number of arrows corresponds to the number of large curved shapes and have the same type of line (ie solid or dashed), therefore it belongs to Set B.

5. **Correct answer D:** The largest shape is located on the left of the box, the number of arrows corresponds to the number of large curved shapes and have the same type of line (ie solid or dashed), therefore it belongs to Set B.

Question 6

Set A

The set contains shaded curved arrows, triangles and stars; and unshaded quadrilateral shapes, ovals and pentagons. There are no number patterns between shapes.

- The rule in this set is that there must be only one pentagon in each cell.

Set B

Set B contains right and downward facing arrows, shaded stars and circles; and unshaded, dashed circles and quadrilateral shapes.

- The rule in this set is that there must be two circles and two arrows in each cell.
- The stars and quadrilateral shapes are distracters.

1. **Correct answer B:** The shapes have solid lines, and these is only one pentagon present, therefore it belongs to Set A.

2. **Correct answer C:** The shapes have solid lines, and these is only one pentagon present, therefore it belongs to Set A.

3. **Correct answer D:** There are at least two circles and two arrows present, therefore it belongs to Set B.

4. **Correct answer C:** There are at least two circles and two arrows present, therefore it belongs to Set B.

5. **Correct answer A:** There are at least two circles and two arrows present, therefore it belongs to Set B.

Question 7

Set A

Set A contains shaded squares and unshaded triangles and hearts with solid lines. There are no patterns in the total numbers of shapes.

- The rule in this set is that when there are four shaded squares there must be one unshaded heart. Alternatively, when there is one shaded square, there must be four unshaded hearts.
- The triangles are distracters.

Set B

Set B contains shaded triangles, unshaded ovals, squares and stars.

- The rule in this set is that when there are three shaded triangles there must be two unshaded ovals. Alternatively, when there are three ovals there must only be two triangles.
- The remaining shapes are distracters and follow no pattern.

Test Shape 1 Answer: Set A
The test shape contains four shaded squares and one unshaded heart. This satisfies the rules for Set A.

Test Shape 2 Answer: Neither
The test shape contains four unshaded hearts and two shaded squares. Although these are the correct shapes to belong to Set A, there is an incorrect ratio of hearts to squares. Therefore, the test shape does not belong to either group.

Test Shape 3 Answer: Set B
The test shape includes two shaded triangles and three unshaded ovals. Therefore the test shape includes both the correct type of shapes and the correct ratio of shapes to belong to Set B.

Test Shape 4 Answer: Neither
The test shape contains shapes corresponding to Set A. While there is one unshaded heart, which is a prerequisite to belonging to Set A, there are no shaded squares. Therefore the test shape cannot belong to Set A. Also, while there are three shaded triangles, there are no ovals and so the test shape does not belong to Set B.

Test Shape 5 Answer: Set B
As there are three shaded triangles and two unshaded ovals, the test shape belongs to Set B.

Question 8

Set A

Set A contains squares and rectangles which may be shaded or unshaded, with solid or dashed lines. Arrows may be present in odd or even numbers.

- The rule in this set is that the number of quadrilateral shapes must add up to an even number.
- Also, one or more downward facing arrows must be present.

Set B

Set B contains a mixture of curved and straight lined shapes which may be shaded or unshaded, with solid or dashed lines.

- The rule in this set is that elliptical shapes (that is, circles and ovals) are present in odd numbers.
- Also, there must be an equal number of elliptical as quadrilateral shapes.

Test Shape 1 Answer: Set A
The test shape contains a total of six combined rectangles and squares. Also, there are three downward facing arrows present. Therefore the test shape belongs to Set A.

Test Shape 2 Answer: Neither
The combined number of rectangles and squares is seven, which is an odd number. Therefore the test shape cannot belong to Set A. There are no circular shapes, which rules out Set B.

Test Shape 3 Answer: Set B
Test Shape 3 contains shapes corresponding to Set B. There are five ovals and five corresponding non elliptical shapes, satisfying the rules of Set B.

Test Shape 4 Answer: Set B
There are three ovals with three corresponding smaller shaded shapes, satisfying the rules of Set B.

Test Shape 5 Answer: Neither
The test shape contains two elliptical shapes and two straight lined shapes. The rules of Set B require an odd number of elliptical shapes, thus ruling out Set B.

Question 9

Set A

The set contains triangles, squares, circles and straight arrows. Shapes may be shaded, or unshaded, and drawn from dashed or solid lines. Shapes may be placed in any combination and there is no number pattern or obvious rules of symmetry.

- The rule in this set is that triangles must be in the top left, squares in the top right, straight arrows in the bottom left and circles in the bottom right.
- All other shapes are distracters.

Set B

Set B contains dashed quadrilaterals, shaded triangles and straight arrows and ovals which may be shaded, or unshaded.

- The rule in this set is that shaded ovals must always accompany unshaded arrows in equal numbers.

- Also, dashed quadrilaterals must always accompany shaded triangles in equal numbers.

Test Shape 1 Answer: Neither
Although the arrow is positioned correctly for the test shape to belong to Set A, the square is placed in the bottom right and not the top right, which is a requirement of Set A. Therefore the test shape belongs to neither set.

Test Shape 2 Answer: Set B
The test shape contains one straight arrow and one shaded oval therefore it belongs to Set B.

Test Shape 3 Answer: Set A
The test shape contains a triangle, a square, a straight arrow and a circle, all located in the correct positions for the test shape to belong to Set A.

Test Shape 4 Answer: Neither
Although the ratio of quadrilaterals to triangles is correct, the test shape cannot belong to Set B because only one of the triangles is shaded. Therefore the test shape does not belong to either group.

Test Shape 5 Answer: Set A
The test shape contains a shaded triangle in the top left corner and an unshaded circle in the bottom right corner. Therefore the test shape belong to Set A.

Question 10

Set A

Set A contains various unshaded shapes with solid lines which have curved or straight lines. There are no repeated or positional patterns or rules of symmetry.

- The rule in this set is that each box must contain shapes with a combined total of ten angles.
- The circles act as distracters.

Set B

As in Set A there are various unshaded shapes with solid lines which have curved or straight lines. Again, there are no repeated or positional patterns or rules of symmetry.

- The rule in Set B is that each box must contain shapes with a combined total of eight angles.

Test Shape 1 Answer: Neither
The test shape contains one hexagon with five angles, one irregular shape with two angles, and one arrow with seven angles, making a total of 14 angles. As the total number of angles equals neither eight nor ten, the test shape belongs to neither set.

Test Shape 2 Answer: Neither
The test shape includes two quadrilateral shapes with four angles, and one heart with one angle, giving a total of nine angles. As the total number of angles equals neither eight, nor ten, the test shape belongs to neither set.

Test Shape 3 Answer: Set A
The arrow contains seven angles and the triangle contains three angles, giving a total of ten angles. Therefore the test shape belongs to Set A.

Test Shape 4 Answer: Set B
The test shape contains one heart, one triangle and one rectangle. As the total number of angles is eight the test shape therefore belongs to Set B.

Test Shape 5 Answer: Set A
The test shape contains two triangles, one square and two ovals. As the total number of angles is ten the test shape belongs to Set A.

Question 11

Set A

Set A contains shaded and unshaded arrows that face in all directions. There are no number or positional patterns.

- The rule in this set is that up and down arrows or chevrons must appear together, while left and right arrows or chevrons must also appear together.
- The shaded and unshaded circles and ovals are distracters.

Set B

The set contains circles, triangles, squares and arrows, which may be shaded or unshaded.

- The rule in this set is that when there are three squares positioned along the bottom there must be two triangles positioned on the right.
- However, when there are three triangles positioned along the left there must be two squares positioned along the top.
- The arrows are distracters.

1. **Correct answer C:** There are opposite arrows (or chevrons) present, therefore it belongs to Set A.

2. **Correct answer B:** There are opposite arrows (or chevrons) present, therefore it belongs to Set A.

3. **Correct answer A:** There are three squares along the bottom of the box and two triangles on the right, therefore it belongs to Set B.

4. **Correct answer D:** There are three squares along the bottom of the box and two triangles on the right, therefore it belongs to Set B.

5. **Correct answer C:** There are three triangles on the left and two squares at the top of the box, therefore it belongs to Set B.

Decision Analysis answers and justifications

Question 1

Answer: E

J, 10, R, D, (4, 13, D)

The code combines the words: he, hard, fight, insect, (negative, attribute, insect).

A Is incorrect as the statement introduces 'honey'.
B Is incorrect as the statement does not use all the codes and introduces 'cancer'.
C Is incorrect as the statement does not use all the codes and introduces 'infections'.
D Is incorrect as the statement does not use all the codes and introduces 'holiday'.
E **Is the correct answer as it uses all the codes and the rules within the brackets. 'Negative' is combined with 'attribute' and 'insect' to give 'bites'.**

Question 2

Answer: A

(12, I), K, (12, I, L), 6

The code combines the words: (plural, person), catch, (plural, person, building), past.

A **Is the correct answer as it uses all the codes and the rules within the brackets. 'Plural' and 'person' are combined to imply 'people'. 'Catch' is replaced with 'capture.' Also, 'plural, person, building' are combined to give 'stadium'.**

B Is incorrect as the statement is not set in the past tense. Also, 'rounders' and 'school' are introduced.

C Is incorrect as 'bouquet' and 'thrown' have been introduced.

D Is incorrect as 'bouquet' has been introduced.

E Is incorrect as 'ball' has been introduced.

Question 3

Answer: A

(13, S), B, (13, P)

The code combines the words: (attribute, fire), hazard, (attribute, wind).

A **Is the correct answer as it uses all the codes and the rules within the brackets. 'Attribute' and 'fire' are combined to imply 'hot flames'. 'Attribute' and 'wind' are combined to imply 'blown', and 'hazard' is replaced with 'dangerous'.**

B Is incorrect as it introduces 'today'.

C Is incorrect as it refers to fire and wind rather than attributes of fire and wind.

D Is incorrect as it does not use 'hazard'.

E Is incorrect as it refers to fire and wind rather than attributes of fire and wind.

Question 4

Answers: B & D

(12, I, N), R, (2, M), 6

The code combines the words: (plural, person, weapon), fight, (increase, success), past.

A Is inaccurate as the present tense is used.

B Is the most accurate interpretation. 'Plural', 'person' and 'weapon' are combined to imply 'soldiers'. 'Fight' is replaced with 'battled'. 'Increase' and 'success' are combined to imply 'more victory'.

C Is inaccurate as the code ignores 'fight' and introduces 'bravery'.

D Is also correct. 'Person', 'plural' and 'weapon' are combined to imply 'militia', 'fight' is replaced with 'battled', and 'increase' and 'success' are combined to imply 'increased reward'.

E Is incorrect as 'plural', 'person' and 'weapon' are not combined correctly. Also, the sentence is not set in the past tense.

Question 5

Answer: D

I, O, M, (1, H), 13 (E, C), 6

The code combines the words: person, fly, success, (opposite, danger), attribute (sun, rain), past.

A Is incorrect as 'opposite' and 'danger' are not combined. Also 'attribute' is incorrectly combined with 'sun' and 'rain' to give 'storm'.

B Is incorrect as 'opposite' and 'danger' are not combined. Also, success is not referred to.

C Is incorrect as 'attribute' is not combined with 'sun' and 'rain'.

D Is the correct answer as 'person' is interpreted as 'I', 'success' with 'passed', 'fly' with 'navigate'. 'Opposite' and 'danger' are combined to imply 'safely' and 'attribute' is combined with 'sun' and 'rain' to imply 'rainbow'. The statement is also set in the past.

E Is incorrect as 'attribute' is not combined with 'sun' and 'rain'. '(Opposite, danger)' is also ignored.

Question 6

Answer: A

(4, 13, R), R, M, (H, I, 12)

The code combines the words: (negative, attribute, fight), fight, success, (danger, person, plural).

- A **Is the correct answer as it uses all the codes and the rules within the brackets. 'Negative', 'attribute' and 'fight' are combined to imply 'broke his arm', while 'danger', 'person' and 'plural' are combined to imply 'enemy'. 'Fight' is replaced with 'battle' and 'success' is implied by 'defeated the enemy'.**
- B Is incorrect as it does not mention success.
- C Is incorrect as it does not combine '(danger, person, plural)'.
- D No reference is made to success.
- E Is incorrect as it does not refer to success and introduces 'lost'.

Question 7

Answers: B & D

(1, Q), (1, A), (1, 6)

The code combines the words: (opposite, winter), (opposite, warm), (opposite, past).

- A Is incorrect, as 'freezing' is not the opposite of 'warm'.
- B **Is correct as it uses all the codes and rules. Although 'future' is not explicitly stated as in D, 'opposite' and 'past' are combined to derive the future tense, 'will'.**
- C Is incorrect as it does not combine 'opposite' and 'winter'.
- D **Is correct, as it uses all the codes and rules within the brackets. 'Opposite' and 'winter' are combined to imply 'summer', opposite and past are specifically combined to imply 'future', and 'opposite' and 'warm' are combined to imply cold.**
- E Is incorrect as it does not combine 'opposite' and 'winter'.

Question 8

Answer: D

(1, G), 13(2, E), 10, (I, L)

The code combines the words: (opposite, tomorrow), attribute (increase, sun), hard, (building, person).

- A Is incorrect as an attribute of increasing sun, ie in this case sunstroke, is not identified.

B Is incorrect as 'person' is not used with 'building' to make 'builders'.

C Is incorrect as 'opposite' and 'tomorrow' are not combined to make 'yesterday'; also 'building' and 'person' are not combined.

D Is the best answer as it uses all the codes and the rules within the brackets even though 'finish' is added. 'Opposite' and 'tomorrow' are combined to imply 'yesterday'. 'Attribute', 'increase' and 'sun' are combined to imply 'sunstroke', and 'building' and 'person' are combined to imply 'builders'. 'Hard' is replaced with 'impossible'.

E Is incorrect as 'attribute' is not combined with 'increase' and 'sun'. Also, 'hard' is not referred to.

Question 9

Answer: A

(12, I), (12, T), (13, S)

The code combines the words: (plural, person), (plural, word), (attribute, fire).

A Is the correct answer as it uses all the codes and the rules within the brackets. 'Attribute' and 'fire' are combined to imply 'heat', 'plural' and 'word' are combined to imply 'talking', and 'plural' and 'person' are combined to imply 'everyone'.

B Is incorrect as only one person is mentioned and 'fire' is used rather than an attribute of fire.

C Is incorrect as persons are not mentioned. Also, 'topic' is introduced.

D Is incorrect as 'attribute' and 'fire' are not combined and 'subdued' is introduced. Also persons are not mentioned.

E Is incorrect as 'attribute' and 'fire' are not combined and 'cool' is introduced.

Question 10

Answer: C

(12, I, R), (12, N), R, (1, 6)

The code combines the words: (plural, person, fight), (plural, weapon), fight, (opposite, past).

A Is incorrect as 'opposite' and 'past' are not combined to imply the future tense.

B Is incorrect as the statement does not combine 'opposite' and 'past' to infer the future.

C Is the correct answer as it uses all the codes and the rules within

the brackets. 'Plural', 'person' and 'fight' are combined to imply 'army'; 'plural' and 'weapon' are combined to imply 'arms'; 'opposite' and 'past' are combined to imply future tense; and 'fight' is replaced with 'conflict'.

D Is incorrect as the statement does not refer to weapons.

E Is incorrect as 'plural' and 'person' are ignored, and 'general' is introduced.

Question 11

Answer: E

12(I, N), K, (H, I), (4, M), 6

The code combines the words: plural (person, weapon), catch, (danger, person), (negative, success), past.

A Is incorrect as the statement is set in the future and does not use all of the code.

B Is incorrect as the sentence is not set in the past tense.

C Is incorrect as 'plural' is not combined with 'person' and 'weapon'. Also, 'negative' and 'success' are not combined.

D Is incorrect as 'catch' is ignored. The statement also introduces 'fought'.

E **Is the correct answer as it uses all the codes and the rules within the brackets despite 'he' being introduced. 'Plural' is combined with 'person' and 'weapon' to imply 'army officers', while 'danger' is combined with 'person' to imply 'criminal'. 'Catch' is replaced with 'apprehending', and 'negative' and 'success' are combined to imply 'got away'. The statement is also set in the past.**

Question 12

Answer: C

(12, I), 2(4, U), 12(13, D), B, 6

The code combines the words: (plural, person), increase (negative, emotion), plural (attribute, insect), hazard, past.

A Is incorrect as 'plural (attribute, insect)' are not combined. Also the sentence introduces 'more'.

B Is incorrect as 'plural' is not combined with '(attribute, insect)'. Also, '(plural, person)' are not combined.

C **Is the correct answer as it uses all the codes and the rules within the brackets. 'Plural' is combined with '(attribute, insect)' to give 'bites', '(plural, person)' are combined to give 'explorers', and 'increase' is combined with '(negative, emotion)' to give 'very**

frightened'. 'Hazard' is interpreted as 'injury'.

D Is incorrect as it does not combine 'increase (negative, emotion)'.

E Is incorrect as it does not combine '(plural, person)'.

Question 13

Answer: E

(1, G), (1, A), G, 13(2, E), (12, I, U)

The code combines the words: (opposite, tomorrow), (opposite, warm), tomorrow, attribute (increase, sun), (plural, person, emotion)

A Is incorrect as it does not combine 'attribute (increase, sun)' to imply 'warmer'.

B Is incorrect as it introduces 'I' and does not combine '(plural, person, emotion)'.

C Is incorrect as it does not combine '(opposite, tomorrow)' to make 'yesterday'.

D Is incorrect as it does not combine '(opposite, warm)' and ignores '(plural, person, emotion)'.

E **Is the correct answer as it uses all the codes and the rules within the brackets. '(Opposite, tomorrow)' are combined to imply 'yesterday', '(opposite, warm)' are combined to imply 'cold'. 'Tomorrow' is used directly, '(attribute, increase, sun)' are combined to infer 'warmer', and '(plural, person, emotion)' are combined to imply 'we will be much happier'.**

Question 14

Answer: B

I, ♦, 8, (C, P)

The code combines the words: person, feeling, condition, (rain, wind).

A Is incorrect as the condition is not used.

B Is the correct answer as it uses all the codes and the rules within the brackets. 'Person' is replaced with 'I', 'feeling' is replaced with 'scream', and 'rain' and 'wind' are combined to imply 'storm'.

C Is incorrect as 'rain' and 'wind' are not combined. Also no condition is used.

D Is incorrect as no condition is used and 'farmers' is introduced.

E Is incorrect as no condition is used and 'person' is replaced with 'all'.

Question 15

Answer: C

(4, ♐), O, (13, Q)

The code combines the words: (negative, wisdom), fly, (attribute, winter).

A Is incorrect as 'flies' is introduced and ('negative', 'wisdom') are not combined.

B Is incorrect as 'attribute' and 'winter' are not combined.

C **Is the correct answer as it uses all the codes and the rules within the brackets. 'Negative' and 'wisdom' are combined to give 'unwise', 'fly' is replaced with 'travel' and 'attribute' and 'winter' are combined to give 'freezing'.**

D Is incorrect as 'pilots' is introduced and 'negative' and 'wisdom' are not combined.

E Is incorrect as 'fly' is not referred to. Also 'jumped' is introduced.

Question 16

Answer B

(1, J), ♎, G, 1(2, A), 6

The code combines the words: (opposite, he), hearing, tomorrow, opposite (increase, warm), past.

A Is incorrect as it is not set in the past tense.

B Is the correct answer as it uses all the codes and the rules within the brackets. It correctly combines 'opposite' and 'he' to imply 'she'. 'Hearing' is replaced with 'heard'. 'Tomorrow' is used directly. 'Opposite' is applied to 'increase, warm' to imply 'colder'.

C Is incorrect as it introduces the word 'today'.

D Incorrect as it does not combine 'opposite' and 'he'.

E Incorrect as it does not correctly combine 'opposite' with 'warm' and 'increase' to make 'colder'.

Question 17

Answer: A

(12, I), ☺, R, (12, I, L), 6

The code combines the words: (plural, person), stopping, fight, (plural, person, building), past.

A **Is the best answer as it uses all the codes and the rules within the brackets. 'Plural' and 'person' are combined to give 'people'. 'Stopping' is replaced with 'waited'. 'Fight' is used directly. 'Plural, person, building' are combined to give 'stadium'.**

B Is incorrect as it incorrectly combines 'plural' and 'people' to mean 'men'.

C Is incorrect as it does not refer to stopping, and introduces 'started'.

D Is incorrect as it introduces 'ring' and 'gladiator', and does not combine 'plural, person, building'.

E Is incorrect as it does not use 'stopping' and is set in the future.

Question 18

Answer: A

(12, I), ♍, (4, •), (12, I), 7

The code combines the words: (plural, person), watching, (negative, feeling), (plural, person), present.

A **Is the best answer. 'Plural' and 'person' are combined to imply 'they'. 'Watching' is replaced with 'observe'. 'Negative' and 'feeling' are combined to imply 'anxious', and 'plural' and 'person' are again combined, this time to imply 'pupils'.**

B Is incorrect as 'negative' and 'feeling' are not combined. Also the statement is set in the past.

C Is incorrect as '(plural, person)' is only used once.

D Is incorrect as the statement is set in the past.

E Is incorrect as the statement is set in the future.

Question 19

Answers: B & E

(12, I), ♌, L, 12 (H, I), R, 6

The code combines the words: (plural, person), running, building, plural (danger, person), fight, past.

A Is incorrect as 'dangerous' is introduced. Also, 'plural' is not combined with 'danger' and 'person'. Also, running is not referred to.

B Is the correct answer: '(plural, person)' is combined to give 'the tribe', while 'running' is substituted for 'escaped'. 'Building' is substituted for 'hut'. 'Plural (danger person)' is combined to imply 'the militia'. The sentence is set in the past tense.

C Is incorrect as 'village' is introduced. 'Plural' and 'person' are not referred to, while 'building' and 'running' are not used.

D Is incorrect as 'jungle' is introduced. 'Plural' is not combined with 'danger' and 'person'.

E **Is also the correct answer as it uses all the codes and the rules within the brackets. 'Plural' and 'person' are combined to imply 'crowd', 'running' is replaced with 'raced', 'building' is replaced with 'stadium'. 'Plural' is combined with 'danger' and 'person' to imply 'mob', and fight is replaced with 'brawl'.**

Question 20

Answer: D

(12, I), ♓, (C, P), ♍, (J, ♐), 6

The code combines the words: (plural, person), worried, (rain, wind), watching, (he, wisdom), past.

A Is incorrect as the statement ignores combining 'he' and 'wisdom' to give 'wise man'.

B Is incorrect as the statement is set in the future.

C Is incorrect as 'attribute (rain, wind)' is incorrectly combined to give 'thunder'. Also, 'consulted' is introduced.

D **Is the correct answer as it uses all the codes and the rules within the brackets. 'Plural' and 'person' are combined to imply 'inhabitants'. 'Worried' is replaced with 'concerned', and 'rain' and 'wind' are combined to imply 'storm'. 'Watching' is replaced with 'saw', and finally 'he' is combined with 'wisdom' to imply 'wise man'.**

E Is incorrect as watching is not referred to.

Question 21

Answer: E

(12, I), (4, ♦), 2(13, P), ♌, (12, L), 6

The code combines the words: (plural, person), (negative, feeling), increase (attribute, wind), running, (plural, building), past.

A Is incorrect as 'plural' and 'building' are not combined and 'running' is also ignored.

B Is incorrect as 'negative' and 'emotion' are not used. Also, '(plural, building)' is not included.

C Is incorrect as 'negative' and 'emotion' are not combined.

D Is incorrect as it ignores combining '(plural, person)' and '(plural, building)'.

E **Is the correct answer as it uses all the codes and the rules within the brackets. 'Plural' and 'person' are combined to imply 'tribespeople', while 'negative' and 'emotion' are combined to imply 'scared'. 'Increase' is applied to 'attribute' and 'wind' to imply 'hurricane'. 'Running' is replaced with 'deserted', and 'plural' and 'building' are combined to give 'shelters'.**

Question 22

Answer: C

☺, ♓

The code combines the words: stopping, worried.

A Is incorrect as the code introduces a reference to hearing.
B Is incorrect as there is no reference to 'forget'.
C **Is the most accurate interpretation as 'stopping' is used to mean 'forget' and 'problems' is indicated by 'worried'.**
D Is incorrect as the code uses the past tense.
E Is incorrect as 'danger' is introduced.

Question 23

Answer: B

(12, I), ♍, (E, ♋), 6

The code combines the words: (plural, person), watching, (sun, drop), past.

A Is incorrect as the code implies that the statement is set in the present and not the past.
B **Is the most accurate interpretation. 'Plural' is combined with 'person' to imply 'couple'. 'Sun' is combined with 'drop' to imply 'sunset', 'watching' is replaced with 'witnessed', and the statement is set in the past.**
C Is incorrect as the statement combined 'increasing' and 'sun' which would imply 'hotter'.
D Is incorrect as the code ignores 'couple' and introduces 'he'.
E Is incorrect as the code introduces 'negative' and 'feeling', which the statement does not suggest.

Question 24

Answer: D

(12, I), ♋, (12, O), 13(2, E), 7

The code combines the words: (plural, person), drop, (plural, fly), attribute (increase, sun), present.

A Is incorrect as the code suggests an individual person rather than many people.

B Is incorrect as the code suggests an increase in danger.

C Is incorrect as the code does not suggest 'flies', rather it suggests 'fly'.

D **Is the most accurate interpretation as 'attribute' is combined with 'increase' and 'sun' to imply 'increasing heat', 'plural' is combined with 'fly' to imply 'flies' and '(plural, person)' is combined to imply 'people'. 'Drop' is replaced with 'falling' and the statement is set in the present tense.**

E Is incorrect as the code incorrectly combines the brackets.

Question 25

Answer: A

12(I, T), (5, ♦), 13(12, T), M

The code combines the words: plural (person, word), (positive, feeling), attribute (plural, word), success.

A **Is the most accurate interpretation as 'plural' is combined with 'person' and 'word' to imply 'journalists'. 'Positive' is combined with 'feeling' to imply 'jubilant', 'attribute' is combined with 'plural' and 'word' to imply 'writing', and 'victory' is denoted by 'success'.**

B Is incorrect as the code introduces the word 'he'.

C Is incorrect as the code introduces a condition.

D Is incorrect because the code does not specify the type of feeling.

E Is incorrect as the code implies the event took place yesterday.

Question 26

Answer: D

8, (C, P), (12, I), (4, •), L, (1, 6)

The code combines the words: condition, (rain, wind), (plural, person), (negative, feeling), building, (opposite, past).

A Is inaccurate as rain and sun combined does not imply a storm.

B Is inaccurate as the code implies that the statement is set in the past.

C Is inaccurate as the code ignores the condition 'if'.

D Is the most accurate interpretation even though 'leaving' is not present in the code. 'Rain' and 'wind' are combined to imply 'storm', 'plural' and 'person' are combined to imply 'tribespeople', and 'negative' and 'feeling' are combined to imply 'afraid'. Also, 'building' is replaced with 'shelter' and 'opposite' and 'past' are combined to imply future.

E Is incorrect as the plural of 'building' is used, which implies more than one shelter.

Question 27

Answer E

J, 6, (13,f), T

The code combines the words He, was, (attribute, wise), words

A This is incorrect as it introduces the words today and learn

B This is incorrect as it introduces the word lady

C This is incorrect as it introduces the words sword and mightier

D This is incorrect as it introduces the words women and singing

E This is the correct answer as it uses all of the words with expert replacing wise

Question 28

Answer D

(1,J) (6,s), i, (1, M),

The code combines the words (Opposite, He), (Past, Feeling), Worried, (Opposite, Success),

A This is incorrect as it is written in the present tense

B This is incorrect as it does not use many of the words in the code

C This is incorrect as it uses the word woman

D This is the correct answer as uses all the words and he becomes man

E This is incorrect as it stipulates the man is not worried

Situational Judgement answers and justifications

Scenario 1

1. **Appropriate but not ideal** – Ellen leaving work early will be putting the quality of healthcare provision at risk. She clearly has problems that need addressing but the more ideal route would be to encourage Ellen to seek assistance from her employer.
2. **A very inappropriate thing to do** – good teamwork and supporting colleagues especially when they are facing challenging situations is very important within healthcare and ignoring the situation would be a very inappropriate thing to do.
3. **A very inappropriate thing to do** – gossiping is not the professional behaviour expected of a healthcare professional and is not acceptable.
4. **A very appropriate thing to do** – seeking to speak to Ellen privately, showing empathy for her situation and encouraging her to seek support and assistance would be a very appropriate thing to do.

Scenario 2

1. **Appropriate but not ideal** – listening and demonstrating empathy is a key skill that healthcare professionals must possess although more could be done to address her concerns.
2. **Inappropriate but not awful** – although not awful ignoring the patient would be very negative and add to the patients worry. Demonstrating a compassionate approach towards the patient and acknowledging their concerns, even as a medical student is very important.
3. A **very inappropriate thing to do** – all surgical procedures carry varying degrees of risk. Providing the impression that this is not the case, especially as a medical student, is not acceptable.
4. **A very appropriate thing to do** – the Consultant will be in a position to address the concerns of the patient and to request the intervention of the Social Care team to ex[lore post surgery support.

Scenario 3

1. **A very appropriate thing to do** – for all Michael knows something serious may have happened to his colleague so seeking to establish whether any messages have been received would be an appropriate thing to do.
2. **A very appropriate thing to do** – again taking to steps to seek assistance as to what to do in this matter and to raise the fact that he is back on

the ward later that evening would be a very appropriate thing to do.

3. **A very inappropriate thing to do** – leaving the ward and the care of the patients exposed would be a very inappropriate thing to do.
4. **A very appropriate thing to do** – seeking to contact his colleague would be an appropriate thing to do to establish his whereabouts and whether he is coming in.

Scenario 4

1. **A very appropriate thing to do** – attempting to speak to the on-call doctor as soon as possible to inform them of the error is a very appropriate thing to do.
2. **A very inappropriate thing to do** – taking no action to correct the mistake would be a very inappropriate thing to do.
3. **Appropriate but not ideal** – although this would be an appropriate course of action it would not be ideal as the mistake could be rectified by the telephone.
4. **Inappropriate but not awful** – although continuing to call the on-call doctor would not be awful there are more appropriate actions that can be taken to correct the situation.

Scenario 5

1. **A very appropriate thing to do** – effective team working and communication is a key component to delivering high quality care. Establishing roles and responsibilities at the earliest opportunity would be a very appropriate thing to do.
2. **Appropriate but not ideal** – although appropriate, it is not ideal as effective team working requires clear communication within the whole group which would not be achieved through individual meetings despite team members being clear on their role.
3. **A very appropriate thing to do** – this would be a very appropriate thing to do to ensure the smooth working of the team.
4. **A very inappropriate thing to do** – again effective team working should involve clear communication and give the members the opportunity to interact and feed in ideas and suggestions.

Scenario 6

1. **Inappropriate but not awful** – it may simply be that Rupal is panicking and just needs some reassurance, however it would not be appropriate to just ignore her concerns. Although she may very well pass with her current knowledge James cannot say that for sure and he should at least try and address her concerns.

2. **Inappropriate but not awful** – although this may address this matter immediately, it seems slightly drastic and there are other ways to address the problem in the first instance. If despite trying to alleviate Rupals' concerns no action is taken then this may need to be the next step.
3. **A very appropriate thing to do** – this is a very appropriate thing to do. It may be that her trainer is unaware of how she feels and can do something to remedy the situation. By advising her to explain her concerns to her trainer James is trying to do something about the situation but is also being fair to his colleague. At least then Rupals' trainer has a chance to address the matter without the medical school becoming involved.
4. **Appropriate but not ideal** – it would be perfectly appropriate for James to offer to help Rupal with her studies, having been through the exams himself he would understand her concerns, however this is not addressing the issue of Rupal feeling she has seen a lack of patients with clinical signs.
5. **A very inappropriate thing to do** – James would be overreacting and making the assumption that his colleague has not been teaching the medical student. This action would demonstrate poor team working and communication skills.

Scenario 7

1. **A very inappropriate thing to do** – by not answering the bleep, Laura may be compromising patient safety and putting a patient at risk. Also, she is technically still working.
2. **A very appropriate thing to do** – Laura can return to the ward and handover the duty to the on-call doctor, if it is appropriate to do so. Realistically, her shift hasn't ended so she still has responsibilities on the ward. As Laura has literally just left the ward it is probably quicker for her to go back to the ward rather than trying to find a phone to call them back. If there was an emergency she would be acting in the patient's best interest by dealing with it herself especially as she is likely to know the patient better than the on-call doctor. Also, if it is something that could be handled quickly she would be able to complete the task and still be able to leave on time.
3. **A very inappropriate thing to do** – by asking a nurse to say she is not there is putting patient safety at risk as the nurse will not be able to deal with the situation if it is a medical emergency, Laura cannot guarantee they will get be able to get through to someone else. It is also putting the nurse in an awkward position by asking her to lie.

4. **Appropriate but not ideal** – by answering the bleep but asking the nurse to phone the on-call doctor themselves if it is not urgent will allow Laura to leave on time without compromising patient safety. As Laura is still on duty, it is preferable for her to handover to the on-call doctor herself, rather than putting the responsibility back onto the nurse, who is still well within her rights to bleep her at this time. However, these approaches allow her to possibly leave on time if it is a matter that can be deferred to the on-call doctor.

Scenario 8

1. **A very inappropriate thing to do** – a competent patient's decision cannot be overridden, hence they cannot be referred for investigations that they have declined.
2. **A very appropriate thing to do** – the patient needs clear and complete information in order to make an informed decision and therefore Penny should present them with the risks and benefits of undergoing any further investigations. Penny should also try to understand the reasons behind the patient's decision. Their decisions may be based on fear or false health beliefs which may be able to be addressed. This does not mean that the patient should be persuaded to change their mind; but it is imperative their decision is based on fact.
3. **A very inappropriate thing to do** – this option is ageist, although the patient is 88 years old they may be completely fit and healthy and have an excellent quality of life. To inform them not to bother to have any investigations and that they will be denied treatment is false and unethical.
4. **Inappropriate but not awful** – the next of kin cannot consent for the patient or override their decision and the patients consent must be sought before breaking her confidentiality. However, by speaking to the patients' daughter it may encourage her to discuss her decisions with her family.

Scenario 9

1. **Inappropriate but not awful** – it could be debated endlessly on whether reading Page 3 of The Sun can be seen as adult pornography. However, regardless of personal opinion the patient was obviously upset and so she should be reassured that her concerns will be addressed.
2. **Inappropriate but not awful** – although the patient is upset there is no legal or patient safety issue here. There is no conclusive evidence that the colleague has done anything wrong. The issue needs to be addressed in view of a patient making a complaint, however a simple apology may prevent the escalation of a somewhat minor issue.

3. **A very appropriate thing to do** – although this incident may have been completely innocent, a patient is upset and may make a complaint. It is common courtesy both to the patient and to the colleague to inform them of what has happened. By suggesting the colleague apologise, it does not mean that he is being accused of any wrong doing. However, it may prevent the matter from escalating and indeed it shows professional courtesy to apologise to an upset patient even if the complaint is unwarranted.

Scenario 10

1. **Appropriate but not ideal** – although a little over the top, if Ahmed is concerned about patient safety his intentions are good. There are more appropriate actions that could be taken as this shows little sensitivity to his junior colleague.
2. **A very appropriate thing to do** – this is the sensitive and tactful option. By taking the colleague aside and gently telling them that perhaps it is not best for them to be on the wards and why, it avoids any patient safety issue and protects the colleague from getting into serious trouble. Obviously, someone will need to cover, and so by suggesting they inform medical staffing that they are not able to cover their shift the patients are being protected, by ensuring there is adequate cover for the day if needed.
3. **Inappropriate but not awful** – It does not deal with the situation immediately at hand, however, Ahmed's colleague should have been more responsible and ensured that they were fit to work their shift the following day. Although at this stage there is no need for Ahmed to reprimand his colleague, it would be sensible to just delicately inform them that perhaps next time they should stop drinking a little earlier.

Scenario 11

1. **Not important at all** – this is irrelevant to the child's treatment and although it may be a reason for why the mother did not call an ambulance it has no bearing on how the child will be treated.
2. **Very important** – although not immediately important to the treatment of the child, this is a serious issue and raises concerns about safeguarding and child protection. This cannot be ignored as the child may be at risk.
3. **Important** – again, this has no bearing on the immediate treatment of the child, however this will need to be explored further as the child is possibly not receiving the correct medication at home.

Scenario 12

1. **Important** – the fact that the meeting has already been rearranged once already is important to consider, especially if the meeting itself is for something of high importance.
2. **Very important** – it is professional courtesy for the student to communicate effectively with her supervisor, especially given that she has already re-arranged the meeting once already.
3. **Very important** – if the opportunity is likely to arise again their may be no need to re-arrange or miss her meeting with her supervisor. This demonstrates skills such as time management and forward planning.
4. **Important** – although her supervisor will agree the importance of attending clinical sessions, the student needs to take responsibility of their own learning and development as it is not the sole responsibility of her supervisor.

Scenario 13

1. **Of minor importance** – this may be the case however this does not factor into how the nurse should respond to the patients' complaint, which should be followed up properly.
2. **Very important** – the patients' health, wellbeing and safety should be the main concern at all times.
3. **Important** – this may well be the case, and although the nurse has no evidence of this – it still needs to be addressed, however it doesn't directly address the immediate issue with the patient.
4. **Not important at all** – to assume that she is confused about what she heard is unfair. The complaint should be followed up regardless as patient safety and wellbeing should be the main focus.

Scenario 14

1. **Not important at all** – the fact that the patient has not noticed the midwife on the phone is irrelevant and should have no influence on the students' actions. The question is about whether the patient is receiving the best level of care.
2. **Important** – although not best practice there may be a genuine reason why the midwife needs to be on her phone. The patient is not in danger and their care is not necessarily being affected. Sometimes a little compassion needs to be displayed
3. **Very important** – the fact that the midwife is using her phone in an inappropriate manner is very important.
4. **Not important at all** – although there may be apparent consequences for the student if she decides to follow up what she has witnessed – assessments should be marked professionally and objectively so should not be a major concern to the student in deciding what to do.

Scenario 15

1. **Very important** – the views of patients about the appearance and behaviour of staff is very important and so must be the considered.
2. **Of minor importance** – this has no influence on the situation, however if the nurse dislikes the junior doctor they may not be truthfully and objectively presenting the facts of the situation.
3. **Very important** – in any situation it is important that the facts are established before a course of action can be decided.

Scenario 16

1. **Very important** – there was a perfectly reasonable explanation why Bella would have her phone on. The consultant was obviously not aware, if they were it would be highly unlikely that they would respond in that manner.
2. **Very important** – the fact that Bella has tried to make the consultant aware of her personal problems is very important.
3. **Important** – the fact that they are friends and housemates possibly means that Ellie knows what Bella is going through and if appropriate can explain the situation to the consultant so that they can make time to speak with Bella.

Scenario 17

1. **Very important** – the patients' health and wellbeing should always be a priority.
2. **Of minor importance** – although obviously frustrating this should have no impact on the course of action Sarah should take. There may be factors influencing waiting times of which Sarah is unaware.
3. **Of minor importance** – patients will be seen in order of level of seriousness hence it is often the case that some people get seen sooner. However if the wait is inappropriate Sarah should raise her concerns with someone as they may have been mistakenly overlooked

Scenario 18

1. **Very important** – clinical guidelines state that an identification badge be worn when in contact with patients. Clinical guidelines are in place to protect patients and the public and so must always be adhered to.
2. **Very important** – medical students should always introduce themselves as so and ask permission from the patient to be present, otherwise the patient may believe they are being treated by a fully qualified practitioner, which is not the case.

Scenario 19

1. **Very important** – the fact that there have been a number of announcements implies that there are no medically trained people on board and the situation may be urgent. Laura should respond quickly and offer as much assistance as she can.
2. **Of minor importance** – Laura should respond calmly and decide what is the best course of action, irrespective of how others around her are behaving.
3. **Of minor importance** – although not yet qualified it may be the case that she has enough knowledge to assist in an emergency. Without knowing the details she is not in a position to say one way or the other.

Chapter 12

Closing thoughts

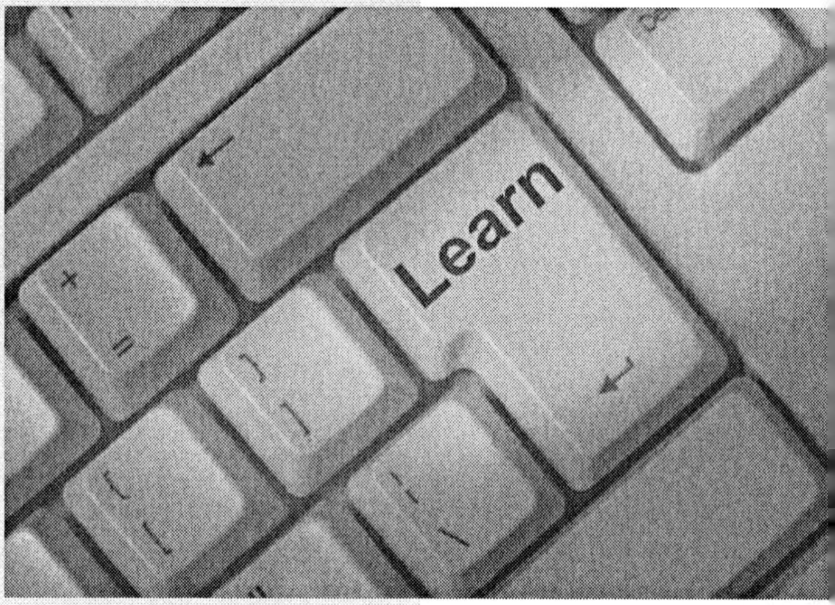

Chapter 12

Closing thoughts

The aim of this guide has been to provide you with an insight into the UKCAT and give you the opportunity to practise the various questions you will come up against. Our hope is that, by following the principles and steps contained in this guide, you will be able to complete your UKCAT confidently and with excellent results.

We strongly recommend that you do seek more information from the medical or dental schools to which you are applying, and also from the official UKCAT website, to ensure that you are fully prepared for your UKCAT.

From all at BPP Learning Media we would like to wish you every success in securing your place at medical or dental school.

Good luck!

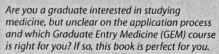

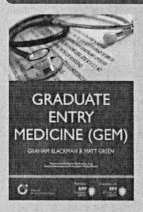

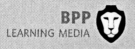

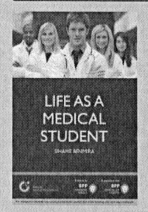

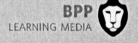